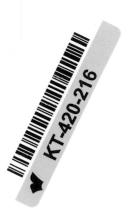

Equine Geriatric
Medicine
and Surgery

Equine Geriatric Medicine and Surgery

JOSEPH J. BERTONE, DVM, MS, DACVIM

Professor, Equine Medicine
College of Veterinary Medicine
Western University of Health Sciences
Pomona, California

Special thanks to Keith Chandler for his extensive review of the manuscript.

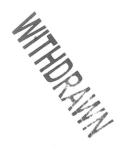

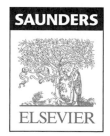

SAUNDERS

ELSEVIER

SAUNDERS
ELSEVIER

W.B. Saunders Company
An Imprint of Elsevier Inc.
11830 Westline Industrial Drive
St. Louis, Missouri 63146

EQUINE GERIATRIC MEDICINE AND SURGERY
© 2006 Elsevier Inc. All rights reserved.
Back cover photos © 2006 Katie Barrett

ISBN-10: 0-7216-0163-4
ISBN-13: 978-0-7216-0163-2

Notice

Veterinary Medicine is an ever-changing field. Standard safety precautions must be followed but as new research and clinical experience broaden our knowledge, changes in treatment and drug therapy may become necessary or appropriate. Readers are advised to check the most current product information provided by the manufacturer of each drug to be administered to verify the recommended dose, the method and duration of administration, and contraindications. It is the responsibility of the treating veterinarian, relying on experience and knowledge of the patient, to determine dosages and the best treatment for each individual patient. Neither the Publisher nor the author assumes any liability for any injury and/or damage to persons or property arising from this publication.

The Publisher

ISBN-10: 0-7216-0163-4
ISBN-13: 978-0-7216-0163-2

Publishing Director: Linda Duncan
Senior Editor: Liz Fathman
Managing Editor: Jolynn Gower
Editorial Assistant: Stacy Beane
Publishing Services Manager: Melissa Lastarria
Project Manager: Andrea Campbell
Designer: Julia Dummitt

Printed in the United States of America

Last digit is the print number: 9 8 7 6 5 4 3 2 1

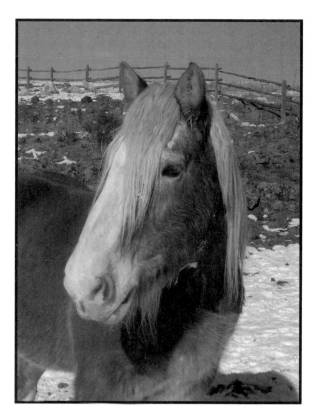

I would like to dedicate this work to Tina
and John Bertone, Mel, Tina, Peter, Linda
and Carmine, Jennifer, John, Jeb
and Olivia.

I would also like to dedicate this
to all the great old horses.

Contributors

Gordon J. Baker, BVSc, PhD, MRCVS, DACVS
Professor and Head (Retired)
Equine Medicine and Surgery
College of Veterinary Medicine
University of Illinois,
Urbana, Illinois
Dentistry in the Geriatric Horse

Joseph J. Bertone, DVM, MS, DACVIM
Professor, Equine Medicine
College of Veterinary Medicine
Western University of Health Sciences
Pomona, California
What Is an "Old Horse" and Its Recent Impact?
Neurologic Disease in Geriatric Horses

Mark Bowen, BVetMed
Department of Veterinary Clinical Sciences
Royal Veterinary College
University of London
Hatfield
Hertfordshire, United Kingdom
Cardiac Disease in the Geriatric Horse

Carolyn L. Butler, MS
Lincoln, Nebraska
Euthanasia and Grief Support Techniques in an Equine
Bond-Centered Practice

Elaine M. Carnevale, DVM, PhD
Equine Reproduction Lab
Colorado State University
Fort Collins, Colorado
Reproductive Disorders

Julie A. Cary, DVM, MS, DACVS
New River, Arizona
Geriatric Musculoskeletal Disorders of the Horse

Keith J. Chandler BVMS, CertEP, MRCVS
Lecturer in Equine Medicine
Veterinary Clinical Studies
University of Edinburgh
Roslin
Midlothian, Scotland
Dentistry in the Geriatric Horse
Eye Disease in Geriatric Horses

Noah D. Cohen, VMD, MPH, PhD,
  DACVIM
Associate Professor
Large Animal Medicine & Surgery
College of Veterinary Medicine
Texas A&M University
College Station, Texas
Gastrointestinal Medicine

Elizabeth G. Davis, DVM, DACVIM
Clinical Instructor
Clinical Sciences
Kansas State University
Manhattan, Kansas
Respiratory Disease in the Geriatric Equine Patient

Thomas J. Divers, DVM, DACVIM,
  DACVECC
Professor of Medicine
Clinical Science
Cornell University
Ithaca, New York
Urinary Tract Disorders in Geriatric Horses

Lydia L. Donaldson, VMD, PhD, DACVA
Assistant Professor
Marion duPont Scott Equine Medical Center
Virginia–Maryland Regional College of Veterinary
  Medicine
Leesburg, Virginia
Anesthetic Considerations for the Geriatric Equine

Daniel Q. Estep, PhD, CAAB
Vice President
Animal Behavior Associates, Inc.
Littleton, Colorado
Interactions with Horses and the Human-Animal Bond

A. T. Fischer, DVM, DACVS
Chino Valley Equine Hospital
Chino, California
Abdominal Surgery in the Geriatric Equine

Robert E. Holland Jr.,
Holland Management Services, Inc.
Lexington, Kentucky
Conditions, Diseases and Injuries of the Older Horses
  for Horse Owners

James D. Kenney DVM
Clarksburg, New Jersey
Manual Therapy, Acupuncture, and Chinese Herbal Medicine in the Geriatric Equine

Laurel Lagoni, MS
Director and Co-Owner
Emotional Support Resource Center
Fort Collins, Colorado
Euthanasia and Grief Support Techniques in an Equine Bond-Centered Practice

Katharina L. Lohmann, Med Vet, DACVIM
Graduate Assistant
Department of Large Animal Medicine
College of Veterinary Medicine
University of Georgia
Athens, Georgia
Gastrointestinal Medicine

Maureen T. Long, DVM, PhD, DACVIM
Assistant Professor
Large Animal Medicine
College of Veterinary Medicine
University of Florida
Gainesville, Florida
West Nile Virus and the Geriatric Horse

Rachel E. Long, BS
Equine Medicine Research Associate
Department of Clinical Sciences
Colorado State University
Fort Collins, Colorado
What Is an "Old Horse" and Its Recent Impact?

Nancy S. Loving, DVM
Loving Equine Clinic
Boulder, Colorado
Field Approach and Wellness Management of Geriatric Horses

Celia M. Marr, BVMS, MVM, PhD, DEIM, MRCVS
Senior Lecturer and Head of Equine Medicine and Surgery Group
Veterinary Clinical Sciences
Royal Veterinary College
North Mymms
Hertfordshire, United Kingdom
Cardiac Disease in the Geriatric Horse

Andrew G. Matthews, BVM & S (Distinction), PhD, FRCVS
Honorary Fellow
Department of Veterinary Clinical Sciences
University of Edinburgh
Honorary Lecturer
Weipers Centre for Equine Welfare
University of Glasgow
Kilmarnock
Ayrshire, Scotland
Eye Disease in Geriatric Horses

William H. McCormick, VMD
President, CEO
Middleburg Equine Clinic, Inc.
Middleburg, Virginia
Manual Therapy, Acupuncture, and Chinese Herbal Medicine in the Geriatric Equine

Kenneth Harrington McKeever, PhD, FACSM
Department of Animal Science
Rutgers, the State University of New Jersey
New Brunswick, New Jersey
Aging and How It Affects the Response to Exercise in the Horse

Nicola J. Menzies-Gow, MA, VetMB, PhD, DECEIM, MRCVS
Lecturer in Equine Medicine
Department of Veterinary Clinical Sciences
Royal Veterinary College
North Mymms
Hertfordshire, United Kingdom
Liver Disease in the Geriatric Horse

Nat T. Messer IV, DVM, DABVP
Associate Professor
Veterinary Medicine and Surgery
University of Missouri
Columbia, Missouri
Endocrine Dysfunction in the Aged Horse

Gillian A. Perkins, DVM, DACVIM
Lecturer
Department of Clinical Sciences
College of Veterinary Medicine
Cornell University
Ithaca, New York
Urinary Tract Disorders in Geriatric Horses

Sarah L. Ralston, VMD, PhD, DACVN
Associate Professor
Animal Science
Cook College
Rutgers, The State University of New Jersey
New Brunswick, New Jersey
Nutrition of the Geriatric Horse

Bonnie R. Rush, DVM, MS, DACVIM
Professor
Clinical Sciences
Kansas State University
Manhattan, Kansas
Respiratory Disease in the Geriatric Equine Patient

Donna L. Shettko, DVM
Assistant Professor
College of Veterinary Medicine
Western University of Health Sciences
Pomona, California
The Equine Geriatric Foot

Josie L. Traub-Dargatz, DVM, MS
Professor of Equine Medicine
Clinical Science
Colorado State University
Fort Collins, Colorado
What Is an "Old Horse" and Its Recent Impact?

Tracy A. Turner, DVM, MS, DACVS
Anoka Equine Veterinary Services
Elk River, Minnesota
Geriatric Musculoskeletal Disorders of the Horse

Beth A. Valentine, DVM, PhD, DACVP
Associate Professor
Department of Biomedical Sciences
College of Veterinary Medicine
Oregon State Universitiy
Corvallis, Oregon
Neoplasia

Preface

There was a time, not too long ago, that it seemed that a 16-year-old horse was past its prime and horses over 20 years old were "old horses" rarely being treated with anything more than deworming medications and vaccinations. Almost all were on a short list to euthanasia, or relegated to renderers, pet food, or the human food supply abroad. Well clearly that has changed. In polling audiences, this author and editor has found that the majority of veterinarians (with a few years experience) are convinced they manage many more old horses now than they did in the 1980s or before. Society seems far less comfortable with euthanasia of healthy horses, even if they happen to have some years on them. This trend is clearly evident in the publication of the American Association of Equine Practitioners', Care Guidelines for Equine Rescue and Retirement Facilities, 2004. Search the web and in excess of 30 retirement homes for horses are available. That is supply trying to meet demand.

Horse owners and trainers have discovered, many of them a long time ago, that the older horses get, the greater value these individuals can have outside the show ring, or as active campaigners, or as child care givers. They bring comfort to many owners that just like to know that the pasture isn't empty and that an old friend is putting the space to good use.

Geriatric medicine and surgery is not glamorous work. The Geritol Derby and the Barren Mare's Cup are having trouble finding sponsorship. However, many veterinarians know that working with older horses and the clients who care for them can be very satisfying. These horses may not be campaigners or trophy winners, but often they are part of a family. They may be a tradition in the barn like old boots or a comfortable old saddle. They may be a child's (or an adult's) best friend, a challenged individual's best chance for therapy, or a troubled youth's best shot at rehabilitation. Let's continue to service these horses and owners in the best way we can. Both are a little different from what we normally do. Both need some special care.

Table of Contents

CHAPTER 1

What Is an "Old Horse" and Its Recent Impact?

Josie L. Traub-Dargatz,

Rachel E. Long,

Joseph J. Bertone

W e do not know for sure if the population of older horses is growing relative to all horses, or not at all, due to lack of trend data for the equine population. However, it seems that society is more inclined to avoid euthanasia of older horses when the horses are physically comfortable. We can also be safe to assume that older horses are receiving more medical and surgical attention than they may have received 15 or more years in the past. Therefore, it seems logical to try to identify the special needs and management considerations in these horses.

WHAT IS AGING AND THE DISPOSABLE SOMA THEORY?

Horses, like humans, are not programmed to die. Aging occurs because in the evolutionary past, when life expectancy was much shorter, natural selection placed a limited priority on long-term maintenance of the body. Aging is caused by an accumulation of cell and tissue damage that occur secondary to normal biochemical responses and actions.

The disposable soma theory explains aging by organ selection and choice processes. In other words, how best should an organism allocate its metabolic resources, primarily energy, between keeping alive and progeny production? One way to think of this theory is that the conservation of energy dictates how long an organism lives. No species is immune to the hazards of life. To be successful procreators, all an individual needs to do is acquire the tools to stay alive and in good condition until most of

the individuals of that generation of a species have died from accident or disease. Hence, the optimum course is to invest fewer resources in the maintenance of somatic tissues than are necessary for indefinite survival. The result is that aging occurs through the gradual accumulation of unrepaired somatic defects, but the level of maintenance will be set so that the deleterious effects are not apparent until an age when survivorship in the wild environment would be extremely unlikely.[1]

WHAT IS AN OLD HORSE?

The most common question from the authors asked to participate in the writing of this textbook was "How do you define an old horse?" This is a very good question with almost no definitive answer. And the answer may not be simply an identified chronological age.

Age can be defined in horses in 3 ways, largely by what is used to define age in humans. The usual age characterizations include: the chronological age, or how many years has the horse been alive; the physiologic age, or how well the animal is functioning versus a younger animal; and the demographic age, or how the animal compares chronologically with other animals of the same species. However, all three of these fall short in terms of equine health compared with human and other companion animal health. The reason for the short fall is the reality of horse use, or *functional age*.

Functional age, as defined herein, always takes into account the horse's use. So a horse is not simply an older horse. Broodmares may be defined in terms of reproductive capability, which, from data presented in this text, may be any horse over 16 years old. However, 16 years old is prime of life in what is often their second career as hunters, barrel racers, stock, and polo horses. The horse's actual, chronological age must be modified by the horse's use. It is an older racehorse, broodmare, or barrel horse. One should become even more specific in determining functional age by adding if the horse is an older Thoroughbred or Standardbred racehorse, knowing that Standardbreds may have more longevity in the profession. And then, let us look at the older Thoroughbred race horse that then becomes the young hunter. Therefore, not only does functional age take into account what the horse does, but it also can be a fountain of youth as the horse changes profession. Clearly, as the horse becomes chronologically older, functional age begins to lose relevance. This concept is not new because horseowners, trainers, and veterinary practitioners have recognized the importance of the functional age of the horse for some time.

Functionality is far more relevant to a horse's age than mortality. Hence, the demographic age, as defined in human gerontology, has almost no relevance to the population of horses. In human gerontology, demographic age is related to survivorship relative to the rest of the population. As defined, the age at which one becomes demographically old is when there is only 25 percent survivorship at or above that specific age.[2] In real terms, the demographic age has almost no relevance to the life of a horse, unless one looks at the demographic age of broodmares, for example, and defines age by functionality. Therefore, an old broodmare may be defined as a mare that surpasses the point at which only 25 percent —or some other number—of mares are expected to be fertile. As yet, we have little data to identify this or other specific age characterizations.

PHYSIOLOGIC AGE

Some physiologic and functional characteristics are different between older and younger horses.

We know that the older horse population does have some differences from younger animals. Arterial blood gases of horses more than 20 years of age had a reduced partial pressure of arterial oxygen (PaO_2) and partial pressure of arterial carbon dioxide ($PaCO_2$) compared with horses 3 to 8 years of age. While on the other hand, the alveolar-to-arterial pressure gradient of oxygen and pH were increased in the older horses. This indicated that there was a reduction in transfer of oxygen from alveoli to capillaries in the older horse. The lower $PaCO_2$ and increased pH seem to represent

hyperventilation by the animal to maintain arterial PaO_2.[3]

There are hematologic differences between younger and older horses. Hemoglobin is increased[4,5] and total lymphocytes are decreased in older horses.[4] Specifically, B and T cell and CD4 and CD8 counts were decreased. However, an increase of the CD4:CD8 ratio, which is interpreted as a nonspecific indicator of inflammation or immunodeficiency, was also noted.[6] Immunoglobulin levels, total and specific levels of IgG, IgG (T), IgM, or IgA do not seem different.[5] However, there was a decreased gross response to vaccination with equine influenza.[5] Exercise, physiological, musculoskeletal, and other system deficiencies are presented throughout the text.

HOW OLD DO HORSES GET?

What is the age of the oldest horse? What is the background of this horse? Using the key words "oldest" and "horse" on Internet search systems or in library databases, we found some interesting citations. Most revolve around one of the oldest horse trainers (Charlie Whittingham) or one of the oldest jockeys (Pincay or Shoemaker) rather than information on the oldest horse. Another citation that comes up is about an ancient clay horse found in Syria by Dr. Thomas Holland. This clay statue, estimated to be 4300 years old, is a likeness of the modern horse, evidence that the type of horse we have today dates back much longer than originally thought.[7]

A short news item in the Journal of Equine Veterinary Practice from 1994 entitled "America's Oldest Horses" describes a nationwide search conducted by Purina Mills as part of the company's 100th anniversary.[8] In the search, more than 2000 equine owners submitted information about their beloved senior horses. The winner was Theodore Edward (Teddy) Bear a Shetland pony that was 52 years old in 1994. According to Dr. Scott King of Purina Mills Senior Feed Division, "Teddy" just received a birthday card at his home in Virgina Beach, Virginia from Purina Mills to celebrate his 60th birthday. Runners-up in the Purina Mills survey were two standard-sized horses that were both 46 years of age in 1994. One was a Florida Cracker horse and the other a Morgan. In addition to the three oldest equids, 6 other horses were honored for their interesting stories of activity and companionship. These equids ranged in age from the late 20s to early 30s.

According the Guinness Book of World Records, the oldest horse on record was "Old Billy," an English draft horse who lived to the grand old age of 62 years. Perhaps more remarkable is that Old Billy did not retire from pulling barges until the age of 59.[9]

Based on a response to our request for information on the oldest reproductively sound Thoroughbred mare and stallion, the Jockey Club's public relations department responded that, according to their records, the oldest Thoroughbred mare to have a foal was "Betsy Ross," who was 30 years old in 1937 when she had her last foal; and the oldest Thoroughbred stallion to sire a foal was McGee, who was 31 years old when he sired his last foal crop in 1931.

The National Animal Health Monitoring Systems (NAHMS) Equine '98 Study estimated that approximately 8 percent of the equine population is 20 years of age or older.[10] Based on data from the initial phase of the NAHMS Equine '98 study, the leading cause of death among equids 30 years of age or older was "old age." Old age accounted for approximately 30 percent of the equine deaths in 1997, followed by colic (17.5% of deaths) and injury/wounds/trauma (10.5% of deaths). The overall death rate for all ages of equids in 1997 was 2.5 percent. The death rate (death due to natural causes or euthanasia) in equids 20 years of age or more was 11 percent, and that death rate in equids between 30 days and 20 years of age was approximately 1.3 percent.

The following information is based on data from the final phase of the NAHMS Equine '98 Study collected in the spring of 1999 for horses residing on operations with 3 or more horses on January 1, 1998. The percent of resident horses that died or were euthanized in the previous 12 months was 2 percent, close to the estimate for 1997 from the NAHMS Equine '98 Study. The death rate in horses 20 years and older was approximately 8 percent, somewhat lower than the estimate for 1997. However, the populations in the 1997 estimate included all kinds of equids and those on small and large operations. The data from 1998 included only horses on operations with 3 or more horses or horse foals on January 1, 1998. The leading causes of death in 1997 and 1998 were the same, lending more credibility to these observations.[9] More detailed data were collected in the spring of 1999 regarding the "old age" death category during 1998. Approximately 64 percent of the horses that were reported dead due to old age had been euthanized. The common specific causes of death in the 20 years of age or older were weight loss and inability to ambulate.

There are only limited data on the ages of the equine population over time. The NAHMS study mentioned previously was only conducted throughout a 1-year period, therefore trends over time cannot be compared unless the study is repeated. The American Veterinary Medical Association (AVMA) Center for Information Management published a U.S. Pet Ownership and Demographics Sourcebook in which information about population of pets, breeds of pets, demographics of pet ownership, and use of and expenditure for veterinary medicine services were reported. Horse ownership is one of the categories included by the AVMA in this report. They published reports in 1987, 1991, and 1996. Their estimates are separated by age with the oldest category including horses of 11 years and older. The percentage of horses in their report that are in this oldest age category (11 years of age or older) was 27.5 percent, 34.7 percent, and 31.0 percent, respectively, for 1987, 1991, and 1996. The methods used to estimate the number of horses in the United States and the percentage by age group were similar across the three periods reported. The data do not include estimates for horses on farms, at racetracks, or at boarding facilities (e.g., horses not at households.) It would appear from these data that the percent of older horses in 1991 and 1996 was slightly higher than in 1987, perhaps indicating that horses residing at households are living longer in the 1990s.[5,11]

Certainly from a clinician's point of view there appear to be more equine owners committed to care of their older horses. The care of older horses has been the focus of many recent articles for both horse owners and veterinarians. Realizing that geriatric horses, like geriatric humans, have unique health and nutritional needs has resulted in an ever-growing market for products that address these needs. For example there are nutritional products designed specifically for the older horse, advancement in equine dental equipment has improved the dental health in older horses, and diagnostic testing and drugs to treat Cushing's syndrome have been developed.

The first commercially available specialty feed for older horses was introduced in the late 1980s in response to requests from the equine industry for a feed that would better meet the needs of the older horse than those already on the market. The feed was Golden Times, which was distributed in a local market area in Colorado (personal communication from Ginger Rich, Memphis, TN). Following a favorable reception of this feed, a national distributor introduced a geriatric horse feed in 1991 called Equine Senior (personal communication, Les Brewer, St. Louis, MO). Since that time most of the major equine feed companies now market an equine geriatric feed to meet the needs of the equine industry (Ginger Rich, Memphis, TN).

TABLE 1-1

Percent of Older Equids Compared to All Equids Seen at the Veterinary Teaching Hospital

1973-1976	210/6584 or 3.19%
1977-1980	371/7008 or 5.29%
1981-1984	549/8416 or 6.52%
1985-1988	543/7598 or 7.15%
1989-1992	686/7492 or 9.16%
1993-1996	851/7907 or 10.76%
1997-2000	1005/8431 or 11.92%

In a review of the medical records database at Colorado State University Veterinary Teaching Hospital to determine the percentages of patients 15 years of age or older that were examined, we found a steady increase in the percentage of older equine patients over time from 1973 to 2000 (Table 1-1 and Fig. 1-1). It is clear from this information that geriatric horses make up an ever-increasing percentage of the equine population. Subsequent chapters will deal with specific conditions of these geriatric horses.

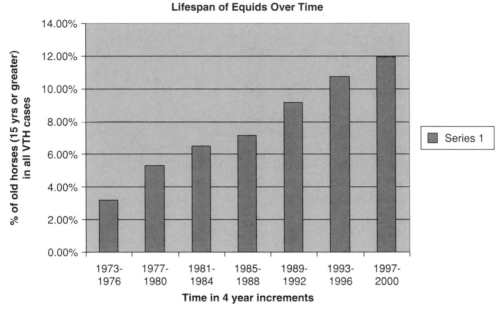

Figure 1-1 Percent of older equids compared with all equids seen at the veterinary teaching hospital.

REFERENCES

1. Kirkwood TBL: Evolution theory and the mechanisms of aging. In Tallis RC, Fillit HM, eds. Geriatric Medicine and Gerontology, ed 6. London, Churchill Livingstone, p 31-35.
2. Grundy EMD: The epidemiology of aging. In Tallis RC, Fillit HM, eds. Geriatric Medicine and Gerontology, ed 6. London, Churchill Livingstone, p 3-20.
3. Aguilera-Tejero E, Estepa JC, Lopez R, et al: Arterial blood gases and acid-base balance in healthy young and aged horses. Equine Vet J 30:352-4, 1998.
4. McFarlane D, Sellon DC, Gaffney D, et al: Hematologic and serum biochemical variables and plasma corticotropin concentration in healthy aged horses. Am J Vet Res 59:1247-51, 1998.
5. Ralston SL, Nockels CF, Squires EL: Differences in diagnostic test results and hematologic data between aged and young horses. Am J Vet Res 49:1387-92, 1988.
6. McFarlane D, Sellon DC, Gibbs SA: Age-related quantitative alterations in lymphocyte subsets and immunoglobulin isotypes in healthy horses. Am J Vet Res 62:1413-7, 2001.
7. Wilford JN: Ancient clay horse is found in Syria, New York Times, January 3, 1993.
8. America's oldest horses. J Equine Vet Pract, 1994.
9. Mary Scott Book of Horses: A complete medical reference guide for horses and foals, Siegal M, Barlough J, Blankenship V, eds, Harper-Collins Publishers, 1996, p 350.
10. Part I: Baseline Reference of 1998 Equine Health and Management, USDA: APHIS:VS, Centers for Epidemiology and Animal Health, N280.898.
11. U.S. Pet Ownership and Demographics Sourcebook, American Veterinary Medical Association (AVMA) Center for Information Management, 1987, 1991, 1996.

CHAPTER 2

Interactions with Horses and the Human–Animal Bond

Daniel Q. Estep

This chapter describes the ways that people interact with horses and the attachments that form between horses and humans. These patterns of attachment and interaction can affect the ways that horses behave around their owners and the veterinary staff. They can also affect the kinds of services that owners request of veterinarians for their horses. All of this ultimately affects the ways that veterinarians and their staff deal with horses and their owners and the kinds and nature of services offered to horse owners. As you will see in the following chapters, older horses sometimes require special care and services. Whether you choose to offer these services and whether owners choose to accept them will depend in part on the kinds of relationships horses and owners have had in the past and the kind of relationships they have currently.

INTERACTIONS AND RELATIONSHIPS

There is considerable diversity in the ways that people use the terms *relationship* and *interaction*. To avoid confusion, these terms and their relationships to each other need explanation. One view of social relationships is that of Hinde.[1] In this theory, social structures are made up of social relationships, and social relationships are composed of social interactions. Although this system was developed to describe relationships within species, it can also be applied to interspecific relationships such as those between people and horses.

Interactions are the building blocks of relationships. They consist of the individual behaviors directed toward others, such as a horse that kicks a person or a veterinarian that examines a horse's teeth. Relationships are made up of a series of interactions over time. The series of interactions between a mare and her foal would define the mare-foal relationship. The interactions that a veterinarian has with a horse define the horse-veterinarian relationship. Social structure emerges from the nature, quality, and patterning of all the relationships among all of the individuals in the system. All of the relationships that horses have with other horses describe the social structure of horses. All of the relationships that horses have with people describe the social structure of humans and horses.

Although the system is hierarchical (social structures are built on relationships, relationships are built on interactions), it is dynamic and there is interaction across levels. Relationships can change over time as interactions change. For example, the relationship between a mare and her foal changes as the foal matures and the interactions change between them. Past relationships can influence current interactions. A horse that has had painful and frightening relationships with veterinarians in the past will likely have a fearful and troublesome interaction with a veterinarian trying to treat her. Being aware of past relationships can help to predict future behavior, whether it is interactions with other horses or with people.

HUMAN–ANIMAL BONDS AND ATTACHMENT

Interest in the relationships between people and companion animals was greatly stimulated in the late 1960s and early 1970s by the work of two psychologists, Samuel Corson and Boris Levinson. Both found that animals could be beneficial in the psychological therapy of children and adults. This work stimulated others to investigate the relationship between people and pets that became known as the "human–companion animal bond." Since it was coined, this term has rarely been defined. It seems to mean different things at different times, and there are a number of assumptions associated with it.[2] It is generally assumed that the bond is a type of mutual relationship that has the same meaning for both participants. Its existence seems to preclude the existence of other kinds of interactions or relationships that may exist between people and their pets. That is, it seems to oversimplify the complexity of most human-animal interactions and relationships. The bond is also assumed to be a good thing, meaning that it results in positive consequences for both people and animals. Finally, there seems to be an assumption that there is only one kind of bond that can form between animal and human, as reflected in the commonly seen phrase "The Bond." These assumptions are not always true.

In the human and animal behavior literature, the terms *bond* and *attachment* are often used interchangeably and often have different meanings, depending on the author. *Attachment* can refer to an emotional feeling, a process, or a specific behavior.[3,4] As it is used here, the term *attachment* or *bond* refers to an internal process that motivates behaviors to keep an individual in close proximity to the object of attachment and behaviors that reflect emotional distress when there is involuntary separation from the object of attachment.

Attachments are not always mutual. A young owner may be very attached to her horse, but the horse may not be similarly attached to the owner. Similarly, an old mare may be very attached to her owner, but the owner may no longer be attached to her and thus sells her to another person.

A bond or attachment implies a relationship or group of relationships between an animal and a person. The interactions upon which the relationship and attachment are based may not always be positive or friendly. Even in the closest and most positive of human relationships, there are occasional negative interactions, such as conflicts involving threats and punishment between parents and children. Similarly, conflicts, threats, aggression, and fear can occur in human-animal relationships characterized by strong attachments. Owners who are very attached to their horses may still use fear-provoking and painful techniques to train them. Having strong attachments to an animal does not always seem to deter neglect, harsh treatment, or even cruelty.

It has often been assumed that the human–companion animal bond was a good thing. Certainly there is evidence that owning or interacting with an animal can improve the quality of life for people under some conditions.[2,5] What has been assumed but rarely examined is that the relationship is also good for the animal. Despite the rosy claims about the value of the bond to people, we know that relationships with animals are not always beneficial. Animals can injure or kill people, destroy property, or create legal problems for people. It is also likely that having relationships with people can produce negative consequences for animals as well. Injuries, fears, stress-related problems, and even death can result from relationships with people, even when the intentions of the people are to do no harm to the animal.

It has never been clear whether there are different kinds of attachments that can form between animals and people (and vice-versa) or whether there are only different degrees of attachment that form between different people and animals. Does the groom who looks after a racehorse have a different kind of attachment to this horse than the little girl who rides her pleasure horse on weekends, or is it only a matter of degree?

HOW ANIMALS AND PEOPLE PERCEIVE EACH OTHER

The kinds of interactions and relationships that can develop between animals and people are highly diverse. When two animals or a person and an animal interact, there is almost always communication between them; that is, the actions of one confer information that causes a change in the behavior of the other. When both partners are members of the same species and share the same communication system, communication is likely to be effective because both partners share the same perception of the signals sent. If the communication partners are of different species, such as people and horses, the communication systems will not be shared, and miscommunication and misinterpretation can occur. Each partner may perceive an interaction differently. Thus, a young rider may perceive her hug of the neck of her horse as being friendly while the horse may perceive it as threatening.

The Swiss zoologist Heini Hediger has pointed out that animals and people have a tendency to perceive and treat other animals as if they were members of their own species, if they sense a familiarity in the others.[6] In humans, this leads to anthropomorphism, the attribution of human characteristics to animals, and in animals it leads to zoomorphism, an analogous attribution of animal characteristics to animals of different species or to humans. In both animals and people, it leads individuals to direct species-typical behavior toward other species and to the expectation that the others will behave appropriately. This is not always the case and can lead to serious problems. For example, it can result in people who lecture their horses on why they should not kick their stalls and in horses that lay back their ears as a threat to people who threaten them.

Anthropomorphism can lead to other problems as well. People who do not know much about the biology or species-typical behavior of other animals and how they learn may assume that animals are motivated to behave for the same reasons as people. The attribution of the human motives of stubbornness, guilt, spite, and revenge to animals is quite common and can lead to inappropriate and cruel treatment of the animals. Beating a stubborn horse is unlikely to motivate him to do what the person wants him to do.

To understand the interactions and relationships that arise between animals and people, it is important to understand how all the participants perceive each other. Hediger has made important contributions to our understanding of the ways that animals can perceive humans and vice versa.[6] He has stated that to humans, animals can take on innumerable roles, "from dead merchandise up to a deity."[6] Humans can be perceived by animals in a variety of ways as well. Hediger describes five major perceptions or roles that humans can take on for animals. These are as predator, prey, a part of the environment without social significance, a symbiont, and a member of the animal's own species. It is unlikely that any mammal or bird perceives humans as belonging exclusively to only one of these categories. These categories probably form a continuum, and an animal probably perceives any given human somewhere along the continuum or as belonging to a combination of categories. These categories are useful as reference points to help describe how animals perceive humans and why they interact with them the way that they do.

How Horses Perceive People

Horses can perceive people in several of the ways described by Hediger. How they perceive any particular person depends on a number of factors influencing the horse, including genetic predispositions, experiences early in life, and later experiences. Some horses may view people as predators and react to them with extreme fear, flight responses, and defensive aggression. This is most likely with horses that have been farther removed from domestication, such as feral horses, those that have not been socialized to people from an early age, and those that have had consistently aversive experiences with people. Anyone who has tried to interact with "wild" mustangs from feral groups knows how difficult and dangerous these animals can be and can appreciate how the animals might perceive them as a predator.

It is unlikely that horses ever perceive people as prey. As large herbivores, horses are not known to stalk, kill,

and consume other animals. Horses may perceive people as socially insignificant parts of the environment. Horses that are well socialized to people, that are around them frequently, and for whom the people have little meaning probably think of people as insignificant and just ignore them. People that pass by horses at work, at pasture, or in stalls and who do not interact with the horses and provide no rewards or punishments are socially insignificant and will likely be ignored.

A caretaker approaching a horse with food or a person stopping to pet a horse will not be socially insignificant and could be considered a symbiont. Symbiosis involves the living together of members of different species to their mutual benefit. There is communication between the two individuals, but in general they do not respond to each other as predator, prey, or conspecific. Communication signals between them may be modifications of species-typical signals or new signals that have specifically arisen between the two. A person approaching with a bucket of grain may lead to a friendly approach by the horse. The person approaching with the grain bucket is a new signal for the horse that had no meaning before it happened the first time. The friendly approach is a species-typical signal by the horse that is easily interpreted by the person. It is likely that most horses that are well socialized to people and have had mostly good experiences with them perceive people as symbionts—foreign creatures that provide some rewards and some punishments. This is also the kind of perception most favored by most people interacting with horses, whether they recognize it or not.

Perhaps the most interesting kind of perception that animals can develop toward people is to view them as conspecifics. Some animals clearly do this, directing species-typical behaviors such as courtship, play, and threats toward people. Why this happens is not thoroughly understood, but it is thought that early socialization of the animal with people may predispose it. If the young animal is reared in the absence of conspecifics but in the presence of people, such perceptions are even more likely.[6,7] Young horses will sometimes direct play toward humans and, rarely, adult horses will threaten people in dominance interactions.[8] Since such behavior by horses can be dangerous to people, it is seldom tolerated and frequently punished. The behavior often declines or disappears, but it is unclear if the perception of the person changes from conspecific to something else.

How People Perceive Horses

As quoted earlier, human perceptions of animals vary dramatically "from dead merchandise up to a deity." The history of human interactions with horses reflects this diversity. Many cultures throughout history have owed much to the horse. As Clutton-Brock puts it, "It may be argued that without the horse human history would have been entirely different . . . There would have been no Crusades and no foreign empires for, without fast transport and fast movement of goods, weapons and food, invaders are powerless."[9] Some societies have honored the horse and even treated them as sacred. Others have abused, neglected, and even eaten them. Such different perceptions exist even within the same societies, such as modern America, where famous racehorses are honored and revered while other horses are slaughtered for food. "In their attitudes to their animals humans have always been as confused as they are in any other relationship, mixing compassion with cruelty and altruism with commercial greed."[9] Despite this confusion, most people in Western societies probably perceive horses as symbionts or even as conspecifics. People provide food, shelter, and medical care to the horse, and the horse provides work, sport, recreation, and/or companionship.

FACTORS INFLUENCING PERCEPTIONS, INTERACTIONS, RELATIONSHIPS, AND BONDS

There are a number of factors that seem to influence how animals and people will perceive each other and that influence the kinds of interactions and relationships that develop between them. This ultimately influences the development of attachments.[4] The first of these is similarities in communication systems. The more similar two species are in their communication, the more likely they are to influence each other, to behave as symbionts or conspecifics, and to form social attachments. The less the overlap in communication, the more likely the individuals are to perceive and respond to each other as predator and prey or not to respond at all. Although horses and people do not have many similarities in their communication systems, both species heavily depend on visual signals for communication and are more likely to attend to the visual cues given by others. This may facilitate communication between them. Horses, like people, have a complex social organization that probably predisposes them to living in complex social groups with people.[10] When left to themselves, horses form stable, long-term groups composed of mares with their foals and a stallion attached to the group. The individuals in the groups form attachments to each other, there are dominance relationships among them, and they cooperate and coordinate their activities with each other. These are all things that would facilitate living with people.

Perhaps the most important factor in developing symbiotic and conspecific relationships and attachments between animals and people is sensory contact or familiarity. The more time a person and animal spend together, the more likely they are to form attachments.

People and animals form attachments to what is familiar, and the more time spent together, the more familiar each becomes to the other. With all other things being equal, the more time that two individuals spend together, the less likely they are to perceive each other as predator and prey or to ignore each other. This factor can influence attachments to inanimate objects and places as well. Horses may become attached to a specific activity ball or even a specific pasture, so that when they are gone, the animal becomes distressed. The longer a person has a given horse, the more likely it is that both horse and owner will form strong attachments to each other. Older horses may be owned longer and both owner and horse may be strongly attached.

For most species of mammals and birds, conspecific perceptions and attachments are most easily established early in life, during a sensitive period for socialization. As a general rule, the younger the individual is when exposed to others, the more likely the individual is to form conspecific perceptions and attachments and the less likely she is to develop perceptions of the other as predator, prey, or socially insignificant. Symbiotic and conspecific perceptions and attachments can be formed at later ages, but it generally requires more time and effort to form these perceptions and attachments. The exact time of the sensitive period for socialization in horses is unknown and is the subject of some debate; however, it appears that exposures to people during the first few days of life can be beneficial in developing more positive perceptions and attachments to people.[11] There is a common belief, but no scientific evidence, that children exposed to horses are more likely to have positive feelings about horses as adults.

Physical contact, feeding, and other positive reinforcers and the absence of punishment seem to facilitate symbiotic and conspecific perceptions and attachments in most species. In general, punishment tends to promote predator–prey perceptions. Punishment is thought to diminish positive social perceptions by increasing the distance between the individual and the punishing object. Punishment can also produce fear that can also inhibit positive perceptions and attachments. Feeding and brushing horses can increase positive perceptions of people by horses and to the extent that it is rewarding to people, it may also increase perceptions and attachments to horses in people as well. Hitting a horse, performing a painful veterinary procedure, or frightening a horse with sudden movements or unusual objects can promote prey-like reactions such as flight, struggle, and defensive aggression. Horses that nuzzle people, follow them around, and approach them probably also elicit symbiotic or conspecifics perceptions from people.

Some experts have suggested that people have selectively bred companion animals for those traits that make the animals better companions and that predispose people to form attachments to them.[12] For example, certain breeds of dogs and cats possess neotenic physical and behavioral traits such as big eyes, a rounded, sloping forehead, large ears, and a short muzzle or nose. Neoteny is the persistence of infantile or juvenile characteristics into adulthood. Many adult companion animals also possess neotenic behavioral traits, such as playfulness and care-soliciting. It is thought that neotenic physical and behavioral characteristics tend to elicit caregiving responses from people and thus increase attachment. It is also thought that animals that show signs of affection, intense greeting behaviors, highly expressive displays, and the appearance of paying attention to people are also more likely to elicit stronger attachments from people.[13] These ideas were developed with dogs and cats in mind, animals that have significant roles as companions to people. Horses have not been bred for the same reasons as dogs and cats, but they probably share some of these characteristics and elicit some of the same perceptions and attachments.

A final factor that influences human perceptions and attachments to animals is what is known as social support.[14] It is not uncommon for pet owners to rely on their companion animals for support. The experience of grief counselors suggests that owners who believe their pets have pulled them through a rough time in their lives, who believe they rescued their pets from death or near death, who spent their childhoods with their pets, who have relied on their pets as their most important source of social support, and who anthropomorphize their pets to a significant degree are more likely to have strong attachments to the animal. Horses, like dogs and cats, can provide social support for people and thus this can be a factor affecting attachment of people to their horses.

RELATIONSHIP-CENTERED VETERINARY PRACTICES

It should be clear at this point that the relationships between animals and people can be quite complex. When veterinarians attempt to care for the medical and behavioral needs of animals, this may affect the relationships that the animal has with her owner, as well as the relationship that the animal and the owner have with the attending veterinary staff. It has been recognized in recent years that when people have strong attachments to their animals and those bonds are threatened by illness, behavior problems, or death of the animal, the person can have a strong emotional reaction. When this happens in the context of veterinary treatment, the emotional needs of the people as well as the medical needs of the animals need to be addressed. To meet these needs, the concept of the Bond-Centered Practice was created.[14] Bond-Centered Practices provide quality medical care for patients while meeting the emotional needs of clients through support services such as animal owner education, pet loss education and support, and referral to veterinary specialists and human psychological specialists. Grief support for owners of geriatric horses is discussed more fully in Chapter 22 of this book.

Recently, Hetts and Estep[2] have suggested a broadening of the concept called "relationship-centered practice." In this view, the totality of the human-animal relationship is assessed for the patient, the client, and their families as well as for the patient and the veterinary staff. It is not enough to simply acknowledge that there is a bond between animal and owner. The nature of the relationship must be assessed and taken into account when medical care recommendations are made. For example, an owner may be strongly bonded to her jumping horse that has a leg injury. The way she is training and competing with her horse may be causing stress to the horse and risks further injury. These aspects of the relationship should be taken into account when making health care recommendations to the owner.

Relationship-centered practices also assess the relationships that the patient has with the veterinary staff and adjusts interactions with the animal to make them as positive and safe as possible for both animal and staff members. Staff members might use positive reinforcers, such as food, when possible, to facilitate certain procedures or they might try to minimize procedures that they know the animal finds aversive.

Relationship-centered practices provide useful services to clients and their animals, and this can translate into stronger attachment or client loyalty to the veterinary practice. Stronger loyalty can result in higher profits. Offering a relationship-centered practice can also result in higher employee satisfaction, whereby staff members feel they are offering valuable, safe, and humane services to both clients and patients. Higher employee satisfaction may translate into higher employee retention and more efficient practice management.

IMPLICATIONS FOR GERIATRIC HORSES AND THEIR OWNERS

The behavior of old horses, their relationships with people, and their attachments to people and animals has received no scientific study. Similarly, the subject of human relationships and attachments to old horses has received no study. What is available is speculation based on the knowledge described above for younger horses and other companion animals. There are several implications of this knowledge that are worthy of mention.

First, we know that, all other things being equal, the more time that an animal and a person spend together, the stronger the attachments are between them. It follows that for most owners of old horses who have had the animals for a long time, there likely is a strong attachment between them. It also follows that if the horse and owner have been in the practice for a long time, the veterinarians and other staff members will develop strong attachments to both horse and owner. Recognizing and acknowledging these bonds will allow the veterinarian to provide the best quality of medical care for the animal, emotional support for the owner, and emotional support for herself and her staff. It is important for the veterinary staff to take care of their own emotional needs when dealing with animals they have attachments to.

Second, because we know that relationships are dynamic and can change over time, veterinarians should not expect the relationships between long-time clients and their old horses to always be the same. Nor should they expect that the relationship of the veterinary staff to the horse to be the same as it was when the horse first came to the practice. Just how these relationships may change is not clear. Horses that are in pain with the diseases of old age, that have deteriorating vision and other senses, or that are unable to interact with their owners as they did when they were younger may show a weakening of their bonds to their owners. It is also possible that the bonds of the owners to the horses may be weakened by changes in the behavior of their aging horse. The horse is no longer able to do the things that gave the owner such pleasure in the past.

Third, since we know that perceptions and attachments between animals and people are not always mutual, veterinarians should not be surprised if the relationship for one of the parties is becoming stronger as the horse ages while for the other it may be becoming weaker. Because the development of perceptions and attachments depend on so many different factors and because each party may experience things differently, it is possible that a horse's attachments grow stronger with age as his owner's attachments grow weaker. The reverse is also possible for a different pair of horses and people.

Finally, we should not underestimate the importance of social support as a factor affecting the strength of the bond between person and horse. Particularly if the person is older herself, she may depend on the older horse companion as a significant source of social support. This may strengthen bonds even if other factors are not favoring the strengthening of bonds. It may be helpful for veterinarians to ask the owners of older horses how they feel about their animals. Asking the owner a series of open-ended questions that allow the owner to talk freely about their relationship with their horse may be helpful in assessing the strength of the bonds between owner and horse. This in turn will help the veterinarian assess the owner's emotional needs with regard to their aging horse.

REFERENCES

1. Hinde RA: Interactions, relationships and social structure. Man 11:1, 1976.
2. Hetts S, Estep DQ: The human-companion animal bond. In Schoen AM, Wynn SG, eds: Complementary and alternative veterinary medicine. St. Louis, Mosby, 1998.
3. Voith VL: Attachment of people to companion animals. Vet Clin North Am Sm Anim Pract 15:289-295, 1985.
4. Estep DQ, Hetts S: Interactions, relationships and bonds: The conceptual basis for scientist-animal relations. In Davis H, Balfour D, eds: The inevitable bond: examining scientist-animal interactions. New York, Cambridge University Press, 1992.
5. Robinson I, editor: The Waltham book of human-animal interaction: benefits and responsibilities of pet ownership. Tarrytown, Elsevier Science, 1995.
6. Hediger H: Man as a social partner of animals and vice-versa. Symp Zool Soc London 14:291, 1965.
7. Roy MA: An introduction to the concept of species identity. In Roy MA, editor: Species identity and attachment. New York, Garland STPM Press, 1980.
8. Crowell-Davis SL: The effects of the researcher on the behavior of horses. In Davis H, Balfour D, editors: The inevitable bond: examining scientist-animal interactions. New York, Cambridge University Press, 1992.
9. Clutton-Brock J: Horse power: A history of the horse and the donkey in human societies. Cambridge, MA, Harvard University Press, 1992.
10. Fraser AF: The behaviour of the horse. Wallingford, CAB International, 1992.
11. Waring GH: Horse behavior: The behavioral traits and adaptations of domestic and wild horses, including ponies Park Ridge, Noyes Publisher, 1983.
12. Messent PR, Serpell JA: An historical and biological view of the pet-owner bond. In Fogle B, editor: Interrelations between people and pets. Springfield, IL, CC Thomas, 1981.
13. Serpell JA: In the company of animals. Oxford, Basil Blackwell, 1986.
14. Lagoni L, Butler C, Hetts S: The human-animal bond and grief. Philadelphia, WB Saunders, 1994.

CHAPTER 3

Field Approach and Wellness Management of Geriatric Horses

Nancy S. Loving

In the role as field practice veterinarians, we are often charged with the care of a horse for its lifetime. Technology and advances in medicine have given us tools to keep horses alive longer and, in many cases, to assist them to remain athletically active into old age. Historically, we have considered a horse to be "aged" when it crosses over into its 20s, when it is "long in the tooth." Despite this rule of thumb, just as some humans have aged beyond their years at the relatively young age of 65, some horses are old by their late teens even in the best of circumstances. In the majority of cases, with good nutrition and preventative management, horses are living well into their late 20s and 30s and doing so with a good quality of life. The equine veterinarian is a critical member of a caregiving team. Clients look to us for advice in all matters of management. Ours is an important role: that of devising successful strategies to provide older horses with the greener pastures they deserve. It is our job to educate the horse owner as to their care options based on financial resources, emotional commitment, and available time to manage suggested strategies.

ADVANTAGES OF FIELD PRACTICE

A field practitioner has the privilege of evaluating a horse in its home environment. Attention to the tiniest management details is a luxury afforded to veterinarians who are able to directly visit the farm. Your client can walk you out to the haystack so you can assess the quality and storage conditions of the feed. You can look at the state of the watering systems and assess the quality of the water.

A visual inspection might alert you to a tank heater that is shorting out in the water tank. You can stroll through the barn and gain an immediate impression of the quality of the air or the efficiency of the ventilation. Bedding is available for your review, as are the size and configuration of the stalls and runs. You can see whether feeders are employed to minimize sand ingestion and waste, and whether they are configured to maximize airway health. You are at liberty to make suggestions to modify herd hierarchy as necessary to eliminate competition over food or space. Evaluation of fencing, safety hazards, and appropriation of living arrangements for all horses on the farm is more easily accomplished when you can visibly see conditions firsthand. You can arrange to meet with a barn manager, horse owner, farrier, and other members of a horse's support system for a consult on the horse's home turf. This is an enviable position to be in when tendering care to any horse. Besides the normal plethora of medical issues that need to be addressed in equine wellness management, insights gleaned by viewing a horse's environment are invaluable in addressing specific concerns of the geriatric horse.

PREVENTIVE MEDICAL MANAGEMENT OF THE OLDER HORSE

A veterinarian is routinely called out to the farm at least once or twice a year to render routine vaccinations and deworming, to clean sheaths, to provide dental care, and to discuss nutrition. While there, the field practitioner has an opportunity to discuss other geriatric medical concerns of which an owner may be unaware. Sufficient time should be scheduled to allow for this educational process.

A thorough physical examination is important to check for a heart arrhythmia, chronic lung changes, enlarged lymph nodes, vision problems, blocked tear ducts, low-grade pyrexia, skin growths, or healing problems. Body condition should be appraised with careful hands-on assessment of flesh covering the ribs, the topline, and the rump. Annual or biannual blood profiles may outline problems with kidney or liver function that could be controlled with dietary management strategies. Gait evaluation and hoof assessment are helpful to detect musculoskeletal concerns that may be managed to improve a horse's comfort.

It is important to implement an aggressive deworming and vaccine schedule as basic health management strategies for the aged horse. Old horses tend to lose efficiency in immune function with age. Some disease conditions, like Cushing's syndrome (described below), reduce the effectiveness of an older horse's immune system. Years of exposure to inhaled allergens (dust, pollens, and molds) compromise the efficiency of the respiratory tract to fend off infectious agents.

There are many variable approaches of endoparasite control, as an interval or fast rotational program, an annual or slow rotational strategy, or a seasonal treatment program. Each of these tactics has some reason to recommend it, so it is best to tailor a parasite control program to each owner and each farm in keeping with what will work best for their individual needs. In all cases, the appropriate dose of anthelmintic should be administered at appropriate intervals and periodic fecal examinations should be evaluated to assess efficacy. A hard-keeping horse may benefit from daily deworming with pyrantel tartrate (Strongid-C, Pfizer) whereas other individuals may flourish well with bolus dewormers administered at 2-month intervals, particularly if paddocks are cleaned of manure at least twice a week.

Routine immunizations should be adjusted to accommodate local threat of disease vectors. Eastern and Western encephalitis, West Nile virus, and tetanus toxoid vaccines should be administered at least once a year, and equine influenza boosters should be administered two to four times a year. A strategy for protection against other diseases such as rabies, rhinopneumonitis, Venezuelan encephalitis, Potomac horse fever, and Strangles is determined by geographic location and endemic risk.

LIVING ARRANGEMENTS

Shelter is important for the aged horse. The older horse is not always as efficient at regulating body temperature; hence he is more sensitive to cold or inclement weather. Instead of stall confinement, you could discuss the use of appropriate blankets to keep a horse warm and dry in adverse weather conditions, the use of flysheets in hot and buggy climates. Advise the owner of the dangers of overheating a horse by applying blankets at inappropriate times.

A paddock or pasture with a run-in shed is an ideal living arrangement. This allows an old horse the ability to move around at will to minimize discomfort from arthritis. Ample bedding in the areas where a horse prefers to lie down also improves his comfort. Outdoor living also assists in minimizing challenge of the airways from irritating substances such as molds and spores or the ammonia that builds up in stalls of closed-up barns.

MAINTAINING BODY CONDITION

Nutritional Concerns

A considerable challenge for the older horse is that of maintaining body condition. Typically, diet and dental efficiency are places to look in determining quality of care.

As a horse ages, it assumes nutritional needs more closely aligned with those of a young, growing horse. Both require a relatively high protein (12%–14%) and high fat (7%–10%) diet as well as an excellent source of quality fiber.[1] The calcium-to-phosphorus ratio should be maintained as close to 1:5:1 as possible.[1] For the aged horse, increased nutritional demands are met by various commercial "senior" feed products formulated with the older horse in mind. Such "senior" products are easy to chew, even for a horse with compromised dentition; these feeds are easy to digest, are nutrient-dense, and are quite palatable. Soybean products also provide a good source for higher protein needs[1] and may be a wise alternative to calcium-rich alfalfa products.

Horses that are still capable of chewing hay should be offered high-quality roughage that is free of dust or mold. Respiratory problems, such as chronic obstructive pulmonary disease, can result from irritation to the airways by molds and dust that are inhaled from poor-quality hay. Hay that is too coarse or stemmy can elicit choke, particularly in horses with poor dentition. One alternative is to offer hay cubes, which are more easily chewed than regular hay. Hay cubes can be moistened to facilitate chewing. Straight grass hay cubes are available, and it is possible to find a cubed blend of grass hay and alfalfa. A diet of straight alfalfa with or without beet pulp is overly rich in dietary calcium, leading to an increased likelihood of developing kidney stones.

Feeding the correct amount of food is equally as important as the horse's ability to consume it or derive balanced nutrients from it. It is important to keep the body condition score of an aged horse as close to the ideal of 5 (Fig. 3-1) as possible. Too fat (scores of 7, 8, or 9)

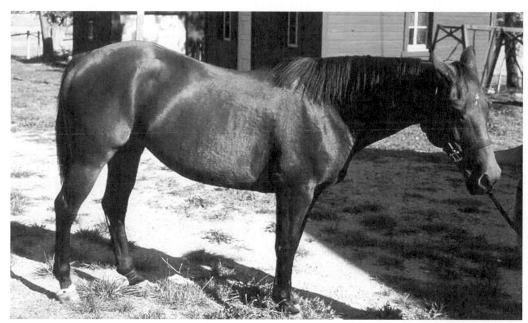

Figure 3-1 This is the same horse as in Figure 3-3, only in this photo she is 16 years old. Her body condition score is close to the ideal.

(Fig. 3-2, A-C) leads to a higher risk of laminitis and additionally adds stress to the joints and limbs of an aged horse. Too thin (scores of 2, 3, or 4) (Fig. 3-3) renders such a horse more susceptible to developing infections or to becoming anemic due to undernutrition. A thin horse has a hard time staying warm in inclement weather. It takes more feed to keep a thin horse warm than a fat one. To add calories without relying on a grain supplement, the horse can be supplemented with 1 to 2 cups of vegetable oil per day or rice bran, both of which are high-fat foods. Soaked beet pulp pellets are an excellent means of presenting the horse with a high-fiber, high-calorie, palatable, and easily digested food. Many old horses that get too thin can be improved in body condition with careful attention to the finer details of feeding.

It has been suggested that older horses have reduced plasma vitamin C relative to levels of younger horses. Supplementation with vitamin C (5-10 g. ascorbic acid twice a day[1]), B-complex vitamins (2-4° of brewer's yeast twice a day[1]), and vitamin E (4000 IU/day) may improve the immune function of an older horse.

Any dietary changes should be started slowly in adding the new components, especially when adding in richer food materials. Allow 2 weeks to gradually increase the volume of the new feedstuffs to the desired amount. This gives time for the intestinal flora to adjust and limits attacks of diarrhea or colic related to feeding changes.

Although sand colic is not a syndrome peculiar solely to old horses, it is a cumulative condition; with age comes the opportunity for accumulated dirt and sand to irritate the large bowel. Attention should be paid to limiting incidental ingestion of sand or dirt. Advise owners of feeding out of appropriate feed containers (tire feeders, on mats or shavings) that will limit ingestion of this material. Sound management practices will limit development of colic, diarrhea, or malabsorption syndrome that develops as a result of "sand" ingestion.

FEEDING PATTERNS

As you observe older horses in the pen or pasture, you will see them dozing more often than the younger horses. An aged horse does not run for his food; he walks serenely, not wasting extra energy or concussion on his ancient legs. After eating for a while, the aged horse often tends to leave the food before it is all finished. In addition to ensuring a balanced ration, it is also important to consider availability of food, particularly if geriatric horses are mixed in with younger ones. Bullying between horses in groups can be a real problem where there is a mix of age groups grazing the same pasture. It can benefit the geriatric horse to be fed separately from grazing cohorts. The old-timer should have forage available at all times so he can snack small meals periodically throughout the day.

DENTAL CONCERNS

The body condition of a geriatric horse often declines in spite of an abundance of feed. Some horses seem to

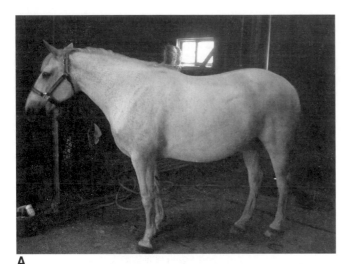

A

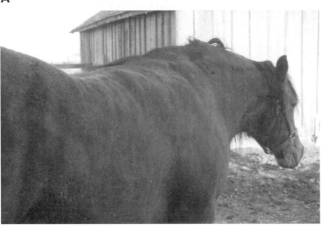

B

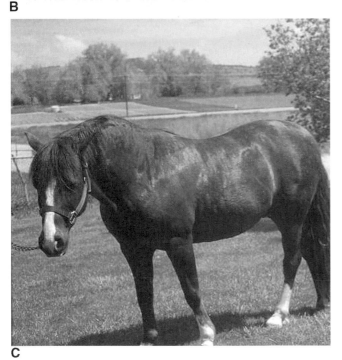

C

Figure 3-2 A-C, Varying degrees of overweight body condition lead to a higher risk of laminitis and add stress to the joints and limbs of an aged horse.

lose weight in the presence of ample food and a good appetite. Not only do many older horses have trouble absorbing their feed as well as they used to, but their teeth are an important variable to consider. Although called "long in the tooth" in reference to lengthy incisors, an elderly horse actually has shortened grinding teeth in the back of its mouth. By the mid-20s, there is no more tooth left to erupt from the sinus cavities of the head; what is left of the cheek teeth is eventually ground down to nubs. Loose cheek teeth fall out of the jaws in many old horses, leaving behind nothing but gaps in the dental arcade. As the opposing tooth has nothing to grind against, it tends to overgrow into the space where the other had been. The resulting wave mouth makes chewing hay or pasture grasses difficult and tedious, and at times painful. Horses with dentition problems tend to "quid" their hay, rolling it into balls of wadded up feed that is then spit out onto the ground.

Many horses have sharp edges on their teeth that need to be filed away (floated) to prevent ulcers on the insides of the mouth and gums. If the incisors have grown overly long with age, then opposing cheek teeth are unable to touch, creating another reason why a horse may have difficulty grinding its feed. Poorly ground hay and forage reduces a horse's ability to obtain sufficient nutrition from its digestion. Further, the coarse, fibrous nature of inadequately ground feed material sets up risks of developing esophageal choke, impaction colic, or diarrhea. Some horses with dental disease or periodontal disease are opposed to drinking cold water, as it can cause discomfort where teeth are loose or missing. Offering warm (room temperature) water may help reduce the risk of impaction colic in horses with sensitive mouths.

Regular dental care is an especially important part of successful management of the older horse. As part of a regular preventative maintenance program, a veterinarian should schedule visits at least twice a year. If an owner notices that a horse is having trouble chewing, is dropping a lot of grain or pellets, or is quidding, it is past time for dental care. Overly long incisors can be reduced with diamond-edged tools; long hooks on the back molars can be ground down with power tools. The remaining teeth can be shaped to be used to their best advantage.

Some old horses do not have sufficient length or number of teeth to help in eating (Fig. 3-4). These horses are candidates for being fed a mash made by soaking complete feed pellets or beet pulp pellets or both in ample water. A mash or gruel is easily gummed by the horse, swallowed, and digested well. Water added to pelleted feed increases fluid intake to avert impaction colic. Moistening the food with sufficient water (half

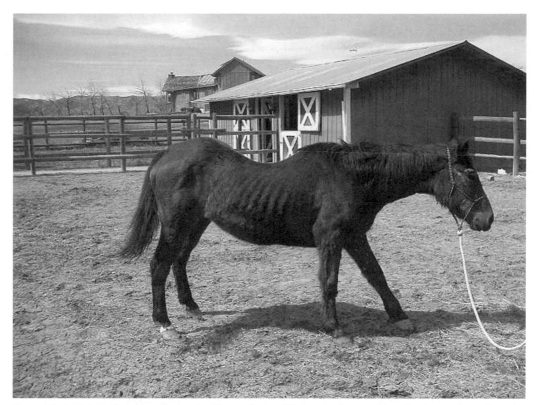

Figure 3-3 This is the same horse in Figure 3-1 at 33 years of age. Here she is weak and too thin.

a gallon of water per pound of pelleted feed) also minimizes the risk of esophageal choke in horses with inadequate dentition. It is also thought that routine washing of the mouth with water may decrease the risk of developing periodontal disease.[2]

ACTIVITY LEVEL OF THE GERIATRIC HORSE

The Active Aged Horse

Not all old horses are retired. Many are still in active work, even into their 30s. In fact, regular exercise is the best thing for those that are sound enough in limb and body to do so. Regular exercise gives the geriatric equine some focus in life and the response from these animals to exercise can be quite dramatic. Good muscle tone keeps an older horse feeling better for longer. Sagging ligaments and muscles result as a consequence of diminished intensity of exercise along with an age-related decline in muscle strength. It is important to check for comfortable saddle fit on the older horse because the saddle that may have fit him well as a teenager will no doubt need some adjustment for an aging body.

An elderly horse that is exercised should be carefully warmed up and cooled down. His musculoskeletal structures may take a little longer to loosen up than when he was a frisky, young horse. It is important to remind the owner to spend a little time to loosen away the creaks and stiffness before asking the aged horse to put in a more strenuous effort. Practical advice on training and conditioning is important as guidance for the horse owner. Too much speed, distance, or rigorous maneuvers may tire an older horse unless he has remained fit to the task.

Many of the older horse set make wonderful riding companions for young humans who do not weigh very much and who demand little of their mount. The bond between a young person and an old horse is satisfying for all. Not only does a child's smile light up when he or she sits proudly astride this horse, but the horse also enjoys the attention, the grooming, and the love that is showered upon him.

Arthritic Conditions and Body Changes

Many older horses have arthritic conditions, not only by virtue of the work they performed as a young and active horse but also due to natural and cumulative "wear and

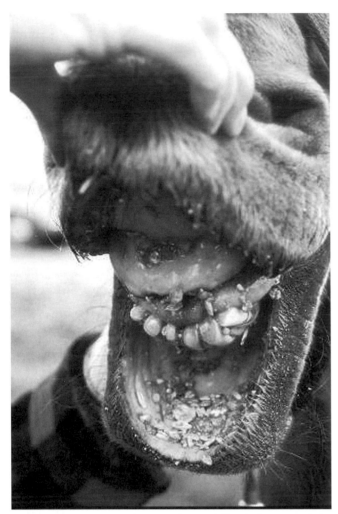

Figure 3-4 Missing incisors makes it difficult for an aged horse to crop pasture grass, whereas other missing teeth have significant adverse effects on optimal utilization of nutrients.

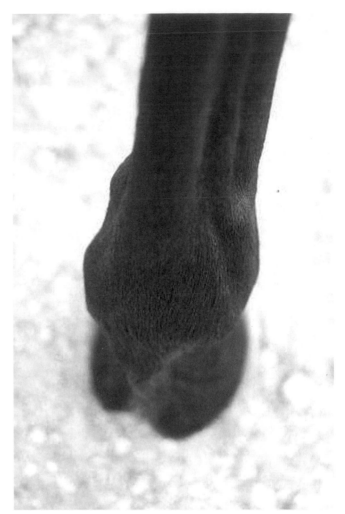

Figure 3-5 Joint distention related to fetlock arthritis.

tear" on the joints with time (Figs. 3-5 and 3-6). Arthritis is evidenced by chronic lameness, stiff gait, and bony enlargements around the joints (Fig. 3-7, A and B). Technology has provided us with effective medications to manage and treat these horses. Previously, the only therapy available was to give the horse "bute" whenever necessary to keep him comfortable. Now we have the option of using products such as intramuscular polysulfated glycosaminoglycans or intravenous hyaluronic acid or to inject ailing joints directly with potent anti-inflammatory medications, such as corticosteroids.

It is not uncommon for old horses to have trouble rising after lying down. This is often due to pain in the hocks making it difficult for the horse to push himself to his feet. Some of these old, creaky horses are reluctant to lie down at all and subsequently spend all their time on their feet. They will sleep standing up, with the occasional episode of suddenly starting to fall. They may have abrasions on the fetlocks where they have drooped yet caught themselves

before fully falling. There are usually telltale signs that a horse has been lying down, such as shavings or dirt on the belly, body, or tail. Whether the horse has trouble getting up or refuses to lie down in the first place, there are solutions to help his plight. Directly injecting the hock joints with anti-inflammatory medications (corticosteroids, hyaluronic acid) has proved to give excellent relief from arthritis pain. However, should the horse be spending long periods of time lying down or repeatedly have difficulty rising from recumbency, then these are signs that euthanasia may be the kindest option. Regularly scheduled hoof trims enable the horse to maintain a solid base of support for good traction. In general, a regular trimming/shoeing schedule provides the best foot care possible to help an aged horse to be comfortable in his exercise or his retirement. Competent farrier care minimizes stress on the joints and hoof structures and should be included as a regular part of routine preventative maintenance. Farriery, in itself, can become an issue when the joints are arthritic; the patient may not want to stand with the limb flexed for any amount of time. In these cases the affected animals benefit

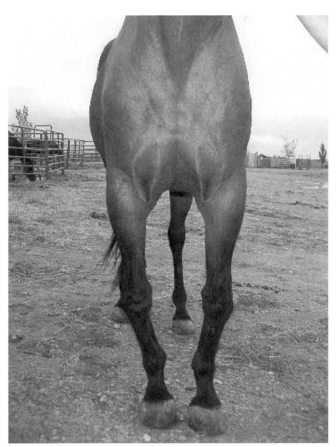

Figure 3-6 Aged horse with advanced carpal osteoarthritis.

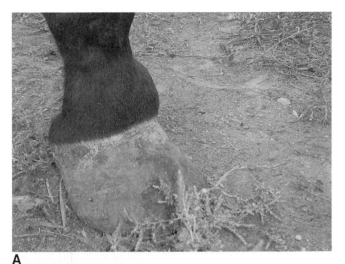

A

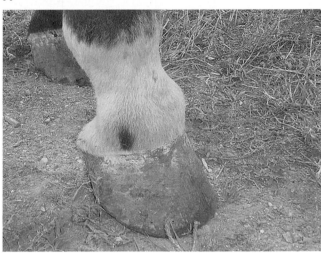

B

Figure 3-7 **A** and **B**, Osteoarthritis of the pastern or coffin joints is called *ringbone*.

from nonsteroidal therapy, such as phenylbutazone, on the morning the farrier is due to attend. Acupuncture is also helpful in providing relief from musculoskeletal pain. Oral "nutraceutical" products such as glucosamines have been reported to give pain relief to ailing joints. Medical and alternative/complementary therapies may keep an older horse feeling younger for longer while improving his quality of life. He may be supported well enough to render him useful for light riding purposes; continued activity further improves his quality of life. Allowing an aged horse to live in a large paddock or pasture is better for the health of his joints than restricting confinement to a stall. Consistent movement keeps the joints "lubricated" and the muscles in tone.

SPECIFIC ORGAN PROBLEMS

An older horse is a high-risk candidate for developing liver disease, kidney disease, or anemia. Unlike the propensity seen in small animals to develop liver or kidney disease, these problems in horses are not that common, but they do occur. As a field practitioner, screening for internal problems is an important aspect of wellness management in an attempt to head off a problem before it becomes overtly serious. Function of the internal

organs can be checked periodically by blood chemistry profiles. Chronic infections may show up as white blood cell abnormalities on a complete blood cell count. Anemia is evidenced by abnormalities in red blood cell counts.

Because dietary strategies differ vastly depending on the organ problem, it is important to carefully screen horses with persistent weight loss and depressed appetites for the specific cause of their poor condition. The syndromes that elicit these problems are varied, and each needs to be addressed specifically.

Renal Disease

Poor kidney function is associated with kidney and bladder stones, weight loss, and decreased appetite. Diet is important in managing failing kidneys. Steer the horse owner away from feeding legume diets, as the high calcium content can worsen kidneys already in trouble, resulting in dangerously high levels of calcium in the bloodstream. Protein levels should be limited to maintenance of 8 to 10 percent. A balanced calcium-to-phosphorus ratio should be achieved as close to 1:2:1 as possible. Beware of feeds such as wheat bran, which is high in phosphorus, or beet pulp or legume hays, which are high in calcium. Ideal feed materials for horses with renal disease are grass hay and a corn-based grain mix.[1]

Liver Disease

Liver failure is associated with weight loss, jaundice, malaise, and decreased appetite. In advanced cases, neurologic signs may appear. Horses with liver disease should be restricted in their protein to maintenance levels and restricted in fat intake. Sufficient calories can be provided using at least 50 percent grass hay supplemented with grains (corn or processed milo) or concentrates, and beet pulp.[1] B complex vitamins and vitamin C should be supplemented in a liver-compromised horse, since the liver is the normal site of production of these vitamins.

Cushing's Disease

Older horses tend to develop their own set of disease conditions. One common disease of the aging horse is pituitary pars intermedia dysfunction, often referred to as equine Cushing's disease (ECD.) This syndrome results from abnormal function of the pituitary gland with the resulting imbalance in hormonal function altering glucose and cortisol metabolism. It has been noted that 70 percent of horses older than 20 years of age showed some obvious or subclinical signs of dysfunction of the pituitary gland.[3] In light of this frequency, a field practitioner cannot ignore this possibility when considering wellness management of older horses. Affected horses often have long, shaggy fur coats that do not fully shed out in the spring (Fig. 3-8, A-C). Many other signs of Cushing's disease may seem to be "normal" indications of old age, but a collection of signs when taken together may hint at an impending problem.

A Cushing's horse often displays external features that are obvious if you stand back at a distance and analyze the suspect horse: You may notice a pot-bellied appearance that results from a loss of muscle mass and tone. On first impression, this may be attributed to sagging muscles of old age. The orbits around the eyes may seem puffy and protrusive due to redistribution of fat deposited there (Fig. 3-9).

An owner may complain that the horse displays a low energy level, whereas others comment that the horse has an increased appetite but with no apparent weight gain. Many owners notice that a horse with ECD seems to drink more than usual, as much as three or four times more. With excess thirst comes excess urination. The stall may seem wetter than usual, more urine spots are evident,

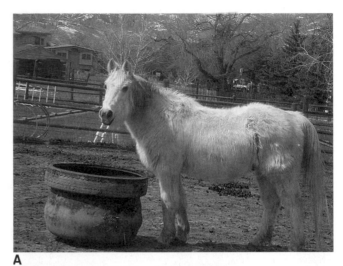

A

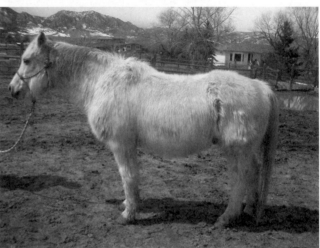

B

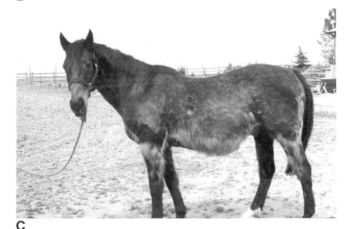

C

Figure 3-8 A-C, Hirsute hair coat typical of equine Cushing's disease.

and water buckets are drained frequently. It is important to rule out boredom or an overzealous attack on the salt blocks as a cause of excess thirst and urination before jumping to conclusions that a horse is affected by ECD.

Because of high circulating levels of corticosteroids created by abnormal feedback from the diseased pituitary

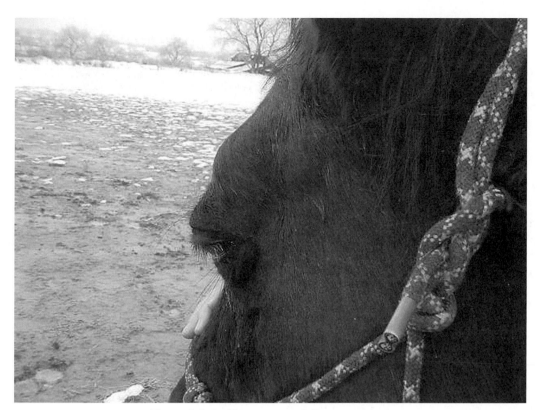

Figure 3-9 Puffiness around the eye orbits.

gland in the brain, these horses have poorly functioning immune systems. Despite regular deworming schedules at frequent intervals, the horse may appear unthrifty due to persistent gastrointestinal parasitism. Some ECD horses are slow to heal wounds. Some experience hyperhidrosis. Frequent viral or bacterial infections occur, with one common development being a chronic sinus infection (Fig. 3-10) that responds poorly to antibiotics. Oral ulcerations and gum disease are also frequent findings in horses affected with ECD. Gastric ulcers also seem to be associated with ECD. It has been the author's observation that some male horses have persistently swollen sheaths that do not respond to cleaning or anti-inflammatory medications.

One of the biggest problems seen with ECD is the eventual development of chronic laminitis as a result of the influence of ever-persistent high levels of corticosteroids and also due to changes in carbohydrate and fat metabolism. It is often the crippling effects of laminitis that necessitate euthanasia of ECD horses. Our goal in prolonging the life of a Cushing's horse is to curtail the development of laminitis. Once laminitis has occurred in these horses, the prognosis is poor for any continued quality of life, since it is difficult to resolve the problems in the feet while the metabolic derangements persist. Feeding a high-fat and high-fiber diet improves glucose and insulin metabolism in ECD horses. Grains or molasses-containing products should

be avoided, as they upset an already altered carbohydrate metabolism.

Medications such as trilostane, cyproheptadine, or pergolide are available to control the effects of ECD in aged horses; these medications have their best effect before laminitis develops, so it is of benefit to recognize the early warning signs of this problem.

A variation on ECD should be considered in the older horse: peripheral Cushing's syndrome. Despite dietary restriction, it is difficult to reduce the weight on affected horses. Fat stores accumulate, especially in the crest of the neck, in the rump areas, and within the prepuce of male horses. Affected horses are often difficult to breed due to infertility issues. This malady resembles classic ECD in many outward signs exhibited by the horse, but instead of being a primary problem within the pituitary gland, the source of the high level of circulating corticosteroids originates from 11, β-hydroxysteroid dehydrogenase enzyme activity in local intestinal sources.[4] These sites include the liver or the adipocytes of the omentum. Adipocytes are responsive to endocrine signals; the more fat cells present as occurs with obesity, the greater the risk is of hormonal perturbations.[4] Many of these horses are erroneously diagnosed as hypothyroid; although there may be some degree of diminished thyroid hormone levels, the problem is not within the thyroid gland itself but rather is due to irregular hormonal feedback in the entire body as a result of high circulating levels of

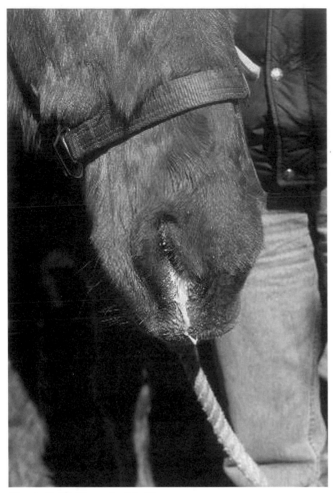

Figure 3-10 Chronic rhinitis.

corticosteroids.[5] At the current time, there is no approved treatment for this condition.

Thyroid Considerations

Thyroid disease is largely overdiagnosed in horses of any age. It is rare to see a horse with a primary thyroid deficiency. Many aged horses that appear to have thyroid dysfunction in fact are afflicted with ECD or peripheral Cushing's syndrome.[6] Other situations that may cause seemingly low thyroid levels in a euthyroid horse include high-energy diets; diets high in protein, zinc, or copper; fasting; ingestion of endophyte-infected fescue; or treatment with phenylbutazone or corticosteroids.[6] Some clinical signs of ECD are similar to a truly hypothyroid individual: Delayed shedding of the hair coat, decrease in appetite, and a blocky and boxy appearance of the face. A hypothyroid horse often has edema in the hind legs, is abnormally sensitive to the cold, and may have hair loss in symmetrical locations of the body. Fat horses are commonly accused of being hypothyroid when in fact all they may have wrong with them is access to an abundance of calories. In actuality, hypothyroid horses are not the obese ones with a fat, cresty neck; a hypothyroid horse has problems gaining weight, especially in conjunction with a poor appetite.

CANCER

Old horses develop a myriad of cancer issues of skin and internal organs. These do not necessarily pose an immediate threat to a horse's life, yet such cancer needs to be addressed and managed for continuing quality of life for the aged horse.

Melanoma

One study reported that more than 80 percent of gray horses past the age of 15 years have melanoma[7,8] (Fig. 3-11). Although this statistical probability may not necessarily be that high, many older gray horses do develop melanoma somewhere on their bodies. Common places to look include inside or along the sheath, under the tail, and around the anus and/or vulva in the area known as the perineum (Fig. 3-12). Less frequent but still common areas for melanoma include the lips and within the glandular tissues of the head, such as the area of the parotid salivary gland in the throatlatch (Fig. 3-13). Melanomas also occur as isolated nodules within the skin anywhere on a horse's body. Non-gray horses are not entirely immune; they just develop melanomas infrequently as compared to a gray horse.

Most times, it is best to leave the nodules alone unless they interfere with defecation or breeding or are located where the saddle, girth, bridle, or bit could further irritate them. Surgical excision sometimes "activates" a melanoma tumor, so it may regrow or sprout up in another location. The recent application of laser surgery as a treatment method enables complete excision of many of these tumors with the least possibility of metastasis. Also, chemotherapy with cimetidine has been reported to be effective in controlling the growth and spread of melanomas.[7]

Squamous Cell Carcinoma

Another common cancer of older horses is squamous cell carcinoma, mostly found at the mucocutaneous junctions around the eyes (Fig. 3-14), the lips, in the perineal area beneath the tail, and on the penis or prepuce of male horses (Figs. 3-15 and 3-16). Internal forms also occur in the stomach or esophagus. The external squamous cell carcinoma tumors are amenable to cryosurgery (freezing) and surgical excision, particularly if they are discovered early on. It is a good prevention to sedate a gelding or stallion once or twice a year to ensure a thorough examination of the penis and sheath to check for tumors, particularly in areas of nonpigmented tissue.

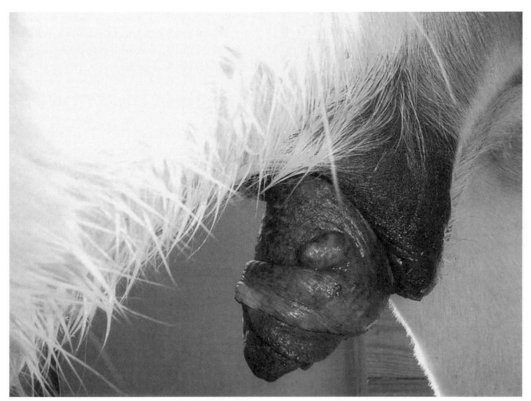

Figure 3-11 Melanoma of the penis.

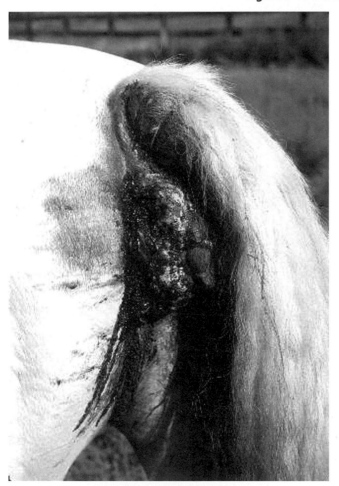

Figure 3-12 Invasive perineal melanoma.

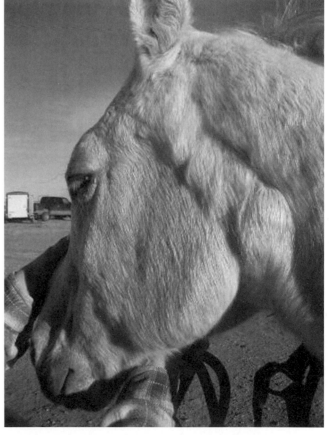

Figure 3-13 Multiple melanomas of the throatlatch.

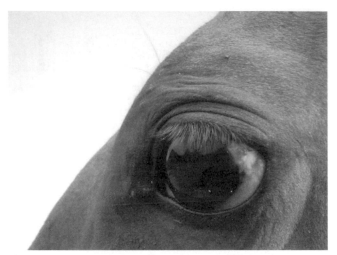

Figure 3-14 Squamous cell carcinoma of the eye.

Lymphosarcoma

Lymphosarcoma is another form of cancer that afflicts older horses. Sometimes it assumes a cutaneous form, with lumps popping up in various places beneath the skin. Biopsy of these lumps confirms the cancer. More commonly, lymphosarcoma arises in the internal organs. Although it is difficult to identify the internal or intestinal form, this should be considered in an older horse that experiences chronic weight loss or inability to gain weight or that is doing poorly. High lymphocyte counts may be evident on blood work.

BREEDING QUESTIONS ABOUT THE OLDER MARE OR STALLION

A common question that arises is that of whether it is safe or practical to breed an aged mare that is in her early to mid-20s. There is probably no harm in doing so as long as the owner goes into the enterprise understanding that fertility in the horse steadily declines after 14 years of age.[9] There is a greater possibility that an aged mare will remain barren despite reasonable uterine health as determined by a prebreeding examination work-up. An endometrial biopsy will determine the extent of age-related changes in the uterus and will provide a prognosis on her future breeding potential. The ovaries are not as active with functional follicles, and her hormones are not as stable to nurture or support conception. A mare with ECD may experience reduced ovarian follicular development due to increased production of androgens from the adrenal glands.[10] As a mare ages, sagging pelvic ligaments may change her reproductive conformation such that wind-sucking or urine pooling may be more likely. These structural changes place

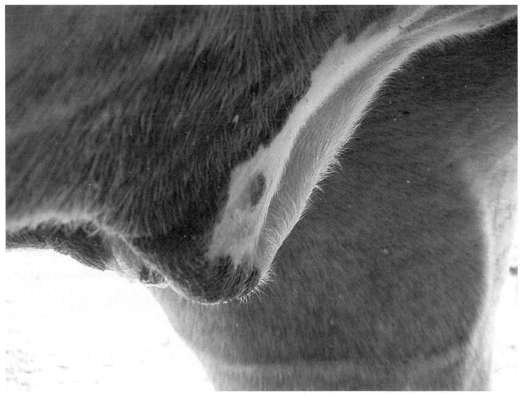

Figure 3-15 Squamous cell carcinoma of the sheath.

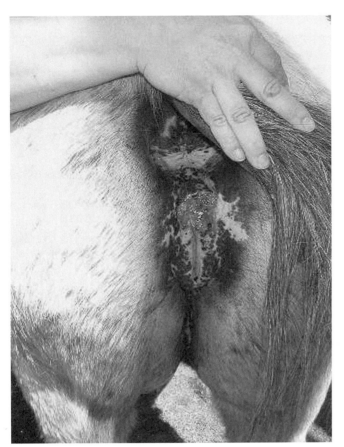

Figure 3-16 Squamous cell carcinoma of the vulva.

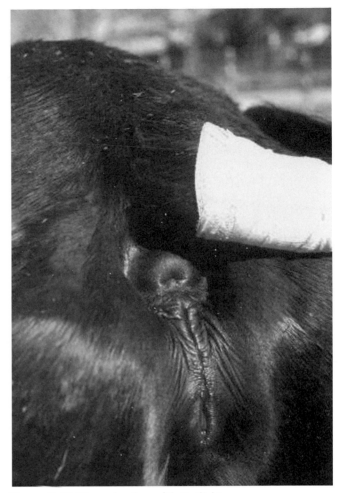

Figure 3-17 Tipped vulva with Caslick's surgery.

the uterus at increased risk of infection and subsequent scarring. Uterine abnormalities are identifiable with endometrial biopsy, culture, and cytology. A Caslick procedure should be performed on mares with a tipped vulva once uterine health is identified or regained (Fig. 3-17).

Following breeding of the cycling mare, it is valuable to perform ultrasonography on a mare as long as 5 to 7 days after breeding to ensure that the corpus luteum is functional rather than an anovulatory follicle incapable of producing sufficient progesterone.

In all cases, fertility is affected by nutrition. Fertility is diminished by poor body condition, weight loss, a low energy diet, and poor-quality feed. In one study, older mares that were fed a nutrient-dense and highly digestible feed such as a "senior" product ovulated 2 weeks sooner during spring transition than old mares fed a basic maintenance diet.[11] It is in everyone's best interest to introduce an older mare to the breeding season on a rising plane of nutrition and fed a balanced ration. Maintaining her body condition also minimizes the tendency for her to develop

a tipped vagina. If she becomes pregnant and foals uneventfully, there is no reason why the older mare cannot be an excellent mother. It is important to counsel the horse owner to keep breeding expectations realistic.

An older stallion may retain the enthusiastic desire to breed a mare, but it is likely that the quality of his semen has undergone an age-related decline. Before he is booked for an active breeding season, the quality of his semen and testicular function and anatomy should be evaluated in the spring so there are no disappointments on the part of mare owners in the months ahead.

REFERENCES

1. Ralston SL: Clinical nutrition of adult horses. Vet Clin North Am Equine Pract 6:339, 1990.
2. Lowder MQ, Mueller PO: Dental disease in geriatric horses. Vet Clin North Am Equine Pract 14:379, 1998.
3. Ralston SL, Nocckels CF, Squires EL: Differences in diagnostic test results and hematologic data between aged and young horses. Am J Vet Res 49:1387, 1988.

4. Johnson PJ, Slight SH, Ganjam VK: 11β-Hydroxysteroid dehydrogenase: Biomedical implications. In Proceedings of the Annual Meeting of the American College of Internal Medicine, Seattle, Washington, May 2000.

5. Johnson PJ: Laminitis, "hypothyroidism", and obesity: a peripheral cushingoid syndrome in horses? In Proceedings of the Bluegrass Equine Medical and Critical Care Symposium, Lexington, Kentucky, October 2001.

6. Messer NT: Thyroid disease (dysfunction). In Robinson NE, editor: Current Therapy in Equine Medicine, Philadelphia, WB Saunders, 1997, p 502.

7. Jegulum KA: Melanomas. In Robinson NE, editor: Current Therapy in Equine Medicine. Philadelphia, WB Saunders, 1997, p 399-400.

8. Johnson PJ: Dermatologic tumors. Vet Clin North Am Equine Pract 14:643, 1998.

9. Carnevale EM, Ginther OJ: Reproductive function in older mares. AAEP Proc 40:15, 1994.

10. McCue PM: Review of ovarian abnormalities in the mare. AAEP Proc 44:131, 1998.

11. Carnevale EM, Thompson KN, et al: Effects of age and diet on the spring transition in mares. AAEP Proc 42:146, 1996.

CHAPTER 4

Anesthetic Considerations for the Geriatric Equine

Lydia L. Donaldson

In approaching general anesthesia for any individual or population, it is important to consider whether they are at greater risk of complications or death. For geriatric people, in fact, there does appear to be an age-associated increase in the risk of a perianesthetic adverse event[1] (Fig. 4-1). Horses older than 12 years, although not all true geriatrics, were also found to have a significantly greater rate of mortality in a multicenter study that prospectively recorded outcomes of 6255 anesthesia procedures.[2] Thus forewarned, changes in anesthetic method that might reduce complications stemming from differences in physiology and pharmacology can be pursued. This chapter discusses the theoretic concerns related to anesthesia of geriatrics in general and the specifics of managing anesthesia for geriatric horses. Because there are few studies of the geriatric equine, the discussion will lean heavily on reports of anesthesia in aged humans and, to a lesser extent, small companion animal and laboratory species. It must be kept in mind that the aged equine does not resemble the often over-weight, sedentary human or dog, if for no other reason than that a horse must remain ambulatory to survive. There is, however, good evidence that decreased activity is a feature of aging regardless of the species,[3] and, there-fore, it may be expected that the aging horse experiences many of the physiologic changes identified in other mammals.

The clinically aged horse is often thin. Its ribs, scapular spine, tuber coxae, humerus, femur, and the outline of its cervical spine are often easily visible. Epaxial muscle atrophy accentuates the dorsal spinous processes of the thoracic and lumbar spine. The old horse walks deliberately, whether due to specific ortho-pedic or neurologic disease or to less specific aging changes. It may act vaguely annoyed at being asked to do something out of its routine and be slow to cooperate. Such a horse is usually 25 years or older, but some 18- to 20-year-olds fit this description. On the other hand, many 20-year-old horses may be ostensibly sound and robust yet will falter and resist when asked to perform to their 10-year-old level because of decreased muscle strength, coordination, flexibility, neuromuscular control, and cardiopulmonary reserve. Individual variability con-founds our ability to categorize "geriatric" to a given chronological age. An accepted definition of "geriatric" is older than 75 percent to 80 percent of the species' life expectancy.[1] Whereas the life span (the maximal obtain-able age) may be 40 years for a horse and 50 years for a pony, the life expectancy (average realistic maximum age) is probably more in the range of 25 and 30 years, respec-tively. Thus, people are considered elderly when over 65 years and horses and ponies considered so at 20 and 25 years, respectively. Consistent with this definition, pub-lished studies of aging horses, to date, have used 20 years of age in designating their geriatric populations.[4-6]

PHYSIOLOGY OF AGING PERTINENT TO ANESTHESIA

Agents used for equine general anesthesia and standing chemical restraint target the central nervous system and impinge on cardiovascular, respiratory, and neuromuscular

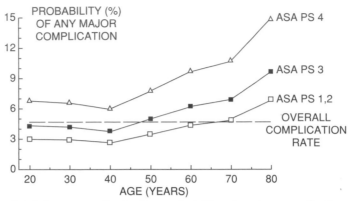

Figure 4-1 In geriatric human patients, the probability of major complications associated with anesthesia exceeds the overall rate. ASA PS indicates preoperative physical status as designated by the American Society of Anesthesiologists. A normal, healthy patient is ASA PS 1 and one with a severe, life-threatening disease is ASA PS 4.
(Adapted from Muravchick S: Anesthesia for the elderly. In Miller RM, editor: Anesthesia, 5th ed. London, Churchill Livingstone, 2000.)

function. Less overtly, hepatic, renal, endocrine, and immunologic function are also altered by anesthetics. The clinical effects of anesthetic drugs are influenced by the capacity of these critical organ systems to respond; the body's homeostatic mechanisms to adjust; and the drugs to be redistributed away from responsive tissues, metabolized, and excreted. In the mammalian species studied, normal aging modifies all of these factors. A summary of the physiologic changes pertinent to anesthesia is given in Table 4-1.

The human brain loses weight and volume with aging. Varying degrees of neuronal loss, neuronal shrinkage, and decreased dendritic density have been found in many, but not all, regions of the aged human brain.[1,7] Similar losses have been reported in areas of the central nervous system of laboratory and companion animals but have not been evaluated in the horse.[8] Of particular interest to anesthesiologists are the changes in neurotransmitter chemistry and receptors that have been identified in the aging human brain.[1,7] Circumstantial evidence would suggest that the equine brain does not suffer the same neuronal, neurochemical, or receptor changes demonstrated in the human brain in that the clinical manifestations of acetylcholine or dopamine depletion, in forms similar to Alzheimer- or Parkinson-like syndromes, have not specifically been recognized in the horse. Losses of α_2-adrenergic, β_1-adrenergic, serotonergic, and GABA-ergic receptors, as reported in the senescent human brain, would be even more difficult to identify in the aged horse, in whom our ability to distinguish changes in cognitive function and memory is limited. However, older horses do appear to respond to stimuli more slowly than do young horses. In human geriatrics, this is attributed to sensory deficits, delayed central processing, and reduced neuromotor structural and functional efficiency.[1,9] Geriatric horses do not apparently experience the

cognitive dysfunction that is reported in 10 percent to 25 percent of their human counterparts for days or months after anesthesia and surgery.[10] This may indicate relatively less attrition of neurons and networking in horses as they age but may also indicate our inability to recognize, associate, and report postoperative behavioral changes. Spatial learning, as determined by performance in a maze, was decreased for at least 3 weeks by exposure to isoflurane and nitrous oxide in old but not young rats.[11] Although the exact cause of postoperative confusion is not known, hypoxemia, hypotension, prolonged perioperative stress, and residual actions of anesthetic agents on a system that has lost a varying amount of its plasticity and neurochemical reserves have all been incriminated.[10] Certainly, hypoxemia, hypotension, and perioperative stress are features of equine anesthesia.[12,13] Atherosclerosis, a feature of the aging human cerebral vasculature,[7] undoubtedly contributes to altered cerebral perfusion during anesthesia. Although its clinical significance is unclear, mineralization of the intimal layer of blood vessels is reported to be a common finding in the cerebral arteries, capillaries, and veins of old horses.[14]

Apart from higher systolic systemic blood pressures, cardiovascular function at rest in healthy, aged people is not different from that of younger people. However, the cardiovascular response to exercise, an indicator of functional reserve, is reduced. Part of this reduced reserve may be due to a decrease in total body water.[1,15,16] Blood volume is not changed with aging, and the decrease in total body water is attributed to a contraction of the intracellular water compartment that is a reservoir for circulating volume. A decrease in ventricular and arterial compliance accompanies normal aging of the human cardiovascular system.[17] This results in an increased afterload and greater dependence of ventricular filling and stroke volume on preload. To a large extent, these age-associated

TABLE 4-1

Resting Heart Rates and Systolic, Diastolic, and Mean Blood Pressures among Young and Old Horses*

Age Group	n	Mean Age (years)	Heart Rate (bpm)	Indirect Blood Pressure (mm Hg)[†]		
				Systolic	Diastolic	Mean
<15 years	6	7.5 ± 3.3	34.6 ± 3.6	139.4 ± 10.6	74.8 ± 4.9	96.2 ± 4.5
>20 years	9	26.2 ± 3.1	40.5 ± 5.9	151.6 ± 17.3	69.8 ± 12.1	96.7 ± 10.2
P value		.00003	.056	.114	.139	.792

*As determined by indirect oscillometric measurement (Propaq Encore, Welch Allyn Protocol, Beaverton OR) with a cuff placed over the coccygeal artery.

[†]Pressure readings were corrected for cuff size and tail-to-shoulder distance as described by Perry et al.[22] Comparison of means was made using the unpaired Student *t*-test.

changes have been explained by increased connective tissue stiffness and reduced β-adrenergic receptor function.[17,18] Intimal thickening and hyaline deposits, not unlike the generalized structural modification of collagen and elastin credited to oxidative stress and glycosylation responsible for reduced compliance in old human and murine vasculature,[17,18] are also considered common in the small peripheral arteries of horses.[19] Ventricular stiffening in aging human hearts is attributed to structural changes in connective tissue proteins as well as hypertrophy of myocytes in an attempt to compensate for cellular attrition with time.[17] Equine hearts have not been studied as thoroughly, but fibrous scarring of the left ventricular apex is reported to occur in 60 percent of hearts from horses older than 20 years of age.[19]

Aged people are unable to attain the same increase in heart rate, cardiac output, and ejection fraction during exercise as younger people.[17] There appear to be no published, controlled studies investigating the exercise capacity of geriatric horses. In one work comparing the immune response of six older horses (mean age of 25.3 years) to that of six young horses (mean age of 7.5 years), the older horses were able to complete the exercise challenge to target heart rates of 160, 180, and 200 beats per minute. The speeds at which the two groups achieved these heart rates were not reported, nor was there note of the degree of exertion or distress.[20] A publication from 1919 reported the influence of age on the resting systolic and diastolic blood pressure in the coccygeal artery of healthy horses measured with a manually operated sphygmomanometer. Systolic blood pressure was higher in the "aged" group, which consisted of eight horses over the age of 12 years.[21] I have done a comparison of coccygeal artery blood pressure using an automated sphygmomanometer (Propaq Encore, Welch Allyn Protocol, Beaverton, OR) (Table 4-2). Although the mean heart rate of the older horses differed significantly from that of the younger horses, the mean systolic pressure of the older horses was higher but

not significantly different by unpaired Student *t*-test comparison. The data do suggest, however, that some old horses may very well be relatively tachycardic and hypertensive. This is different from the old person who is more likely to be bradycardic and hypertensive,[17] and it may reflect a shift of autonomic control at rest from the predominantly parasympathetic dominance of younger horses.[23]

A well-integrated autonomic nervous system is essential to cardiovascular homeostasis and is important to safe anesthesia. In addition, adrenergic and cholinergic receptors are distributed throughout the central nervous system, where the balance of receptor occupancy contributes to awareness, behavior, muscle tone and/or analgesia—that is, anesthesia. Peripheral β-adrenergic receptor dysfunction is manifested in human geriatrics by lower maximal heart rate (β_1) and less vasodilatation (β_2) during exercise, decreased rate of myocardial contraction (β_1), and attenuated baroreflexes.[1,17] Aged rats and dogs respond to isoproterenol (a nonspecific β-agonist) with smaller elevations in heart rate and blood pressure than do young animals.[24,25] The tendency of older people and perhaps horses to have higher systemic blood pressures suggests a change in the balance between vasoconstricting and vasodilating influences. Exactly how is unclear, as peripheral α-adrenergic vasoconstriction and endothelial-dependent relaxation, mediated by a host of endogenous agents, have been reported to be increased, decreased, or unchanged by aging depending on the species and tissue studied.[18] Of interest to the equine practitioner is the impact of these changes on responses, peripheral and central, to the sedative and vasoconstrictive actions of α_2-agonists (e.g., xylazine, detomidine) and the anxiolytic and hypotensive actions of phenothiazine neuroleptics (e.g., acepromazine, promazine).

Like the cardiovascular system, the ultrastructure of the aging human respiratory system suffers from oxidative stress. The result is an increase in collagen cross-linking,

TABLE 4-2

Physiological Changes of Aging That May Affect Anesthesia

	Change with Age	Consequence for Anesthesia	Evidence in Horses
Central Nervous System	Neuronal cell loss, decreased axon-dendritic complexity, receptor loss and/or signal transduction, decreased concentration of neurotransmitters	Altered pharmacodynamics, unpredictable responses to agents, increased sensitivity to some anesthetics	Sluggish responses to stimulation, careful gait
Peripheral Nervous System	Reduced afferent and efferent efficiency, slowed conduction and integration; cell, sensor, and receptor loss	Attenuated autonomic and neuromuscular reflexes, cardiovascular instability, higher pain threshold	Sluggish responses to stimulation, less parasympathetic dominance?
Cardiovascular System	Reduced ventricular and vascular compliance, decreased β-adrenergic receptor function	Increased dependence of cardiac output on venous return, decreased cardiac reserve, cardiovascular instability	Intimal fibrosis in small arteries, left ventricular scarring[19]
Respiratory System	Increased lung compliance, decreased thoracic compliance, decreased alveolar surface area, increased dead space	Decreased efficiency of gas exchange, decreased respiratory reserve, hypoxemia	Horses older than 20 years have lower Pao_2,[6] interstitial pattern on thoracic radiographs[28]
Skeletal Muscle	Myofiber loss, degeneration of neuromuscular junction	Weakness and less capacity to generate heat by shivering in recovery	Clinical appearance, careful gait
Body Composition	Decreased muscle mass, increased fat, decreased total body water	Altered pharmacokinetics: decreased volume of distribution and redistribution	Clinical appearance
Liver and Kidney	Cellular loss, decreased blood flow	Delayed metabolism and clearance, attenuated water and electrolyte balance	Right liver lobe atrophy[19]

a decrease in the ratio of elastin to collagen, and altered physiochemical properties of surfactant.[1,26] The lungs of geriatric people and dogs become more compliant and have less elastic recoil. Alveoli and intra-alveolar pores are large, and there is a loss of alveolar septa and pulmonary capillaries resulting in a reduced capacity for gas exchange.[27] Respiratory bronchioles and ducts are more dilated but less well supported by the surrounding interstitium than in younger lungs. The human chest wall becomes less compliant with aging as its cartilaginous components calcify and articulations degenerate.[1,26] This may be of less importance in the horse, since the adult equine thorax has limited compliance by design. However, the functional result of reduced lung recoil and a relatively rigid thoracic wall is a larger end-expired lung volume that potentially hinders effective ventilation. Once again, functional reserve is reduced with aging. The loss of respiratory muscle fibers and the central and

peripherally mediated reduction in concise control of ventilatory responses to changes in arterial oxygen or carbon dioxide or airway stimulation found in older people is likely to occur to some degree in older horses.[26] Whether the diffusing capacity of the aged equine lung is less than that of the lungs of young horses due to loss of gas exchange surface area, as has been seen in human and canine lungs, has not been investigated. The normal radiographic appearance of the lungs of healthy old horses is of an increased interstitial pattern.[28] This would be consistent with an increase in interstitial connective tissues adjacent to enlarged alveolar spaces as is described histologically in the lungs of geriatric people.[26]

A consequence of the age-associated structural changes in the lungs with age in people is a progressive decrease in resting arterial oxygen partial pressure (Pao_2), a widening alveolar to arterial oxygen gradient ($P[A-a]o_2$), uneven distribution of ventilation, greater dispersion of areas of ventilation/perfusion ($\dot{V}/\dot{Q}$) mismatch, and increased dead space and shunt.[26] Lower PaO$_2$ and a wider calculated P(A−a)O$_2$ were found in a group of awake, healthy horses older than 20 years of age when compared to a group of 3- to 8-year-olds.[6] Preoperative reduced pulmonary function is a particular concern for the equine anesthesiologist and surgeon in that, even in the healthiest of young horses, recumbency and current general anesthetic methods markedly compromise ventilatory mechanics and pulmonary gas exchange. In geriatric human patients under general anesthesia, P(A−a)O$_2$ and ($\dot{V}/\dot{Q}$) mismatch are greater than in young patients, but shunt and the area of atelectasis measured on thoracic computed tomography scan are not.[29] I am currently working on a retrospective comparison of the anesthetic management of geriatric horses with a matched group of younger horses. With first analysis, the mean PaO$_2$ from the horses older than 20 years of age appears to be higher and the P(A−a)O$_2$ smaller than that of the younger horses during anesthesia. This suggests that, at least in this group of old horses, gas exchange was maintained. To date, a breakdown of the results by subpopulations (e.g., exploratory laparotomy, recumbency) has not been done.

Muscle loss is an indisputable feature of aging. A generalized decrease in muscle mass in the anesthetized horse may mean that it will not have sufficient strength to stand upon regaining consciousness. In old people and rats, and most likely in old horses, decreased metabolic activity in the form of protein synthesis and cellular oxidative capacity result in myofiber atrophy.[30] The ability to stand after anesthesia may be further compromised by an age-associated loss of motor neuron units and neuromuscular junction complexity, which has been recognized in geriatric humans and rats.[9] Less efficient afferent sensory transduction and conduction delay as well as slowed spinal processing and basal ganglion dopamine depletion are components of aging in the human motor system.[1,7,9] The net effect of aging on neuromuscular function is of reduced contractile strength, proprioception, and coordination. Compounding the reduced neuromuscular efficiency are the osteoarthritic degenerative changes ubiquitous to aging joints. Periarticular degenerative disease of the axial skeleton may be sufficiently advanced to compromise spinal cord function in the horse.[19] Geriatric sarcopenia carries two additional ramifications for the anesthetized patient: compromised thermoregulation and altered pharmacokinetics. In the former, not only is the ratio of mass to surface area decreased, permitting more rapid heat loss, but also decreased muscle metabolic capacity limits the ability of the old body to generate heat by shivering. The impact on the pharmacokinetics of anesthetics will be discussed in the following section.

PHARMACOLOGY OF ANESTHETICS IN THE AGED

It is well accepted that geriatric people require smaller doses of anesthetics agents than do young people. To some extent, this may be due to decreased sensory acuity and decreased central neural reserve, but for the most part, it is the result of altered pharmacokinetics and/or agent-specific molecular mechanisms.[1,7,15] For anesthesia, drug distribution to and redistribution from the central nervous system is critical. These, in turn, depend on blood flow, the concentration of free drug in the blood, and the drug's ability to cross the blood-brain barrier. The pharmacological response to an anesthetic agent is dependent on both delivery to the brain and the functional integrity of its molecular mechanisms of action. In some cases, such as with thiopental, the decreased dose requirement in the aged subject appears to be a pharmacokinetic phenomenon in which, owing to a reduced volume of distribution and slower intercompartmental redistribution, the brain is exposed to a greater proportion of the injected dose.[15,31] In other cases, such as with the opioids and benzodiazepines, the increased sensitivity of older people is due to changes in agonist-receptor function.[15,32]

Access of anesthetics to the central nervous system is critically dependent on blood flow. Cerebral blood flow and its distribution within the brain of geriatric humans and rats appear to be associated with the regional decreases in metabolic activity that reflect neuronal loss and decreased cellular activity.[7] However, the relative fraction of cardiac output distributed to the brain compared to other tissues is no different in geriatric rats than in young rats.[16] Thus, the initial delivery of anesthetics may not be influenced by age; however, subsequent delivery to and clearance from the central nervous system may be slower in geriatrics in whom the cardiodepressant actions of anesthetics may be accentuated.[15] Although cerebral endothelial cells and the vascular basement membrane undergo recognized structural changes with aging, blood-brain barrier function is only subtly altered by age.[33] Binding of anesthetic drugs to plasma proteins also influences the concentration of drug molecules available for diffusion. Plasma albumin decreases and α$_1$-acid glycoprotein increases with age in people,[15] but total protein and albumin concentrations in several groups of horses older than 20 years of age have been reported to be similar to those of young horses.[4-6]

Distribution of anesthetic to muscle and adipose tissue contributes to both the initial concentration of drug that reaches the brain and the progressive reduction of blood and brain concentrations. The facility with which this occurs is dependent on blood flow to all tissues and the volume of the "reservoir" tissues. As mentioned earlier, muscle mass decreases and body fat increases with aging. In the awake geriatric subject, alterations in the regional distribution of blood flow are generally consistent with the proportional changes in body composition that accompany aging.[16] Thus, in the elderly, there is less muscle to take up anesthetic and it receives a relatively smaller fraction of cardiac output. This contributes to the initial higher concentration of anesthetic that reaches the brain and the slower early distribution of anesthetic away from the brain. Later redistribution to adipose tissue will also be slower in the geriatric compared with the young subject, despite the larger adipose compartment due, in part, to a relatively greater reduction in tissue perfusion in response to the anesthetic. Ultimately, the proportionally greater adipose tissue will be a larger reservoir of anesthetic to diffuse back into the blood for transport to sites of clearance by metabolism and excretion. Clearance of most anesthetics has been shown to be prolonged in the elderly.[1,15]

Although hepatic enzyme activity may be altered in some older individuals, this is not a necessary consequence of aging. In humans, hepatic volume and hepatic and renal blood flow decrease with age and are primarily responsible for reduced hepatic metabolism and drug clearance.[15] Age-associated atrophy of the right liver lobe, accompanied by compensatory hypertrophy of the left lobe, is a common finding in older horses.[19] Clinical liver and kidney disease are not commonly diagnosed in horses, regardless of their age, but some attrition of function with time would not be surprising. Renal creatinine clearance is progressively reduced in healthy geriatric people, whereas normal serum creatinine levels are maintained.[15] Thus, the fact that mean serum urea nitrogen, creatinine, albumin, several hepatic enzymes, and electrolytes of a group of 30 horses older than 20 years were found to be no different from those of a similar number of 5- to 12-year-olds[5] does not insure that there is no reduction in hepatic or renal functional reserve with the aging of horses.

ANESTHETIZING THE HEALTHY GERIATRIC HORSE

So, how do we anesthetize the geriatric horse? Fortunately, or unfortunately, we have a limited repertoire. Thus, it becomes a question of what we know about the use and actions of these few anesthetic agents in geriatrics and specifically the equine geriatric. Some known and hypothetical, age-associated changes to the pharmacokinetics and dynamics of anesthetic agents commonly used in horses are summarized in Table 4-3.

In general, having completed a physical examination and any blood work, radiographs, electrocardiography,

and echocardiography as well as having administered supportive measures, as deemed appropriate to the old horse's particular physical status and surgical condition, our choices for preanesthetic sedation are nothing, a phenothiazine, an α_2-adrenergic agonist, a benzodiazepine, some combination of these, or any of these with an opioid. Premedication is followed by induction to general anesthesia with ketamine, thiopental, or possibly propofol with our without guaifenesin or a benzodiazepine. Volatile inhalant anesthetics, repeated boluses or continuous infusion of some assortment of the induction agents and adjuncts, or a combination of inhalant and intravenous agents are used to maintain anesthesia. Padding and positioning of the recumbent geriatric horse may require extra attention to avoid compromising circulation or creating focal points of pressure beneath skeletal prominences. Monitoring of clinical signs of anesthesia, heart and respiratory rate, and blood pressure should be the minimum standard of care. The decision about whether to mechanically assist ventilation should take into consideration that aging reduces respiratory drive in response to increases in carbon dioxide and decreases in oxygen and reduces respiratory muscle mass. Finally, full recovery of horses from general anesthesia requires that they be able to stand and walk fairly soon after regaining consciousness. Preoperative nonsteroidal anti-inflammatory medication may attenuate postoperative pain.

There are no reports of the specific use of acepromazine, or any of the phenothiazines, in geriatric horses. The theoretic advantages are few and may consist solely of a reduction in afterload due to vasodilatation mediated by peripheral α_1-adrenergic blockade. The hypotension resulting from vasodilatation may be accentuated in geriatrics in whom circulating norepinephrine levels and resting vascular tone may be high and blood volume and cardiac reserves low.[1,17] Consistent with this theory, the risk of syncope has been reported to be greater in old people taking the neuroleptics aceprometazine or haloperidol.[34] The sedation produced by acepromazine is unpredictable in horses of any age. In an elderly horse with possibly marginal dopaminergic, serotoninergic, histaminergic, and cholinergic function, acepromazine might produce an unexpected degree of sedation and dyskinesia. Nevertheless, if a low dose of acepromazine, perhaps administered intramuscularly, would reduce the anxiety experienced by an old horse in a strange environment, it might enable other, more compromising sedatives and anesthetics to achieve a target level of sedation at smaller doses and in a more controlled fashion than if acepromazine had not been given. Acepromazine has been shown to decrease the minimum alveolar concentration (MAC) of halothane in young ponies[35] and to decrease

TABLE 4-3

Changes in Anesthetic Drug Pharmacodynamics or Pharmacokinetics with Age

Anesthetic Agent	Effect of Aging*
Phenothiazines: acepromazine, promazine, fluphenazine	Accentuated hypotension[†]
	Increased chance of dyskinesia?[†]
α_2-*Agonists*: xylazine, detomidine, medetomidine, romifidine	Less bradycardic[†]
	Increased sensitivity?[†]
Benzodiazepines: diazepam, midazolam	Increased sensitivity
	Decreased clearance
	Cardiovascular and pulmonary depression
Ketamine	Tachycardia and hypertension
	Decreased clearance
Hypnotics: Thiopental	Smaller initial volume of distribution
	Decreased clearance
Propofol	Increased sensitivity
Guaifenesin	Decreased clearance?[†]
Inhalants: halothane, isoflurane, sevoflurane, desflurane	Slowed uptake and elimination
	Increased sensitivity
Opioids: morphine, butorphanol, meperidine, fentanyl etc	Increased sensitivity
	Decreased clearance
Neuromuscular block: atracurium	None

* See text for details and references.
† indicates theoretic and/or clinical impression.

the anesthesia-associated risk of mortality in a large population of horses of all ages.[2]

The response of older horses to the α_2-adrenergic agonist sedatives xylazine and detomidine may be only slightly more predictable than that of acepromazine. On the one hand, the α_2-agonists may not produce as reliable sedation or analgesia as expected due to loss of α_2-receptors in the senescent central nervous system.[7,36] On the other hand, if all the regions of the brain show α_2-receptor attrition with age, the centrally mediated components of bradycardia and ataxia may also be less pronounced. This may be advantageous in old horses that are already unsteady on their feet and have decreased cardiovascular reserve. My clinical impression is that older horses become more sedate and ataxic at equivalent milligram per kilogram doses than do younger horses. They seem, as a group, to be more easily aroused from that sedation. The data from the populations compiled for my retrospective study of equine geriatric anesthesia seem to support this impression as well as to suggest that bradycardia and palpable arterial pulse deficits are less common in older than in younger horses after equivalent doses of xylazine.

Diazepam, the most frequently used benzodiazepine in equine anesthesia, is not a profound sedative in adult horses but has been shown to decrease MAC for halothane in ponies.[37] It is most often added to an induction regimen or as an adjunct to total intravenous

anesthesia in horses for this apparent synergism with other anesthetic agents and its muscle relaxant properties. Its fellow benzodiazepine, midazolam, is more potent, is water-soluble, and has a shorter and more predictable half-life.[38] Greater respiratory and cardiovascular depression and smaller dose requirements to achieve induction have been reported for both benzodiazepines with advancing age in people. Hepatic metabolic clearance of benzodiazepines is also slower in aged people[38,39]; thus, repeated or high single doses may be associated with prolonged recovery. The pharmacokinetic characteristics of benzodiazepines do not fully explain the increased sensitivity, and brain concentrations do not differ between young and old subjects despite more profound and prolonged pharmacological effects with increasing age.[15,39] In vivo cortical binding of the benzodiazepine clonazepam was less in older mice but was associated with greater ataxia. Thus, in the geriatric brain, the occupied benzodiazepine receptor may create a relatively greater hyperpolarization of the neuron and thereby a greater depression of neuronal activity.[32]

Ketamine has largely replaced thiobarbiturates as the drug of choice for inducing horses to inhalant and as a component of intravenous anesthesia. The impact of aging on the pharmacology of ketamine in the horse has not been studied. In fact, although documented to be safe in aged and high-risk human patients,[40] I was unable to find any direct comparisons of the pharmacology of ketamine in geriatric versus young adult people. As seen with the benzodiazepine receptor, binding of the channel protein associated with NMDA receptors, an important site of action for ketamine-mediated analgesia, is decreased with aging.[41] Whether this is associated with a change in clinical efficacy was not investigated. Some of the actions of ketamine are attributed to interactions with cholinergic, opioid, and GABA-ergic receptors, all of which are altered by aging.[7] Thus, it would be expected that ketamine would behave differently in the senescent central nervous system. Ketamine is lipid soluble, and redistribution to adipose tissue terminates its immediate clinical activity. Clearance of both ketamine and its active metabolite norketamine is delayed in older people,[40] consistent with an age-associated decrease in hepatic and renal blood flow. Elderly, critically ill people respond to the cardiovascular stimulatory effect of ketamine, attributed to an increase in sympathetic nervous activity, with a more pronounced tachycardia and hypertension than seen in younger people.[40]

Thiopental and the newer alkenol, propofol, are alternative agents to ketamine for induction or intravenous anesthesia in horses, although the latter is expensive and not marketed in a format that is easily adapted to equine anesthesia. For both of these hypnotic anesthetics, as much as a 50% smaller dose than that used in young people are needed to produce clinical anesthesia and electroencephalographic burst suppression in elderly people.[15,31,42] This is largely attributed to the pharmacokinetic behavior of these highly lipid soluble drugs, as they demonstrate smaller initial volumes of distribution and slower intercompartmental clearance rates. Both are also redistributed, metabolized, and excreted more slowly. A pharmacodynamic increase in sensitivity in older people has also been demonstrated for propofol.[42]

The third element of the traditional equine anesthetic induction or intravenous anesthetic regimen is guaifenesin. There are no reports of its use in old horses. Guaifenesin is cleared from the blood initially by redistribution and ultimately from the body by hepatic metabolism and renal excretion.[43] Therefore, it is likely to be influenced by many of the same pharmacokinetic factors discussed earlier. This would suggest that lower doses may be needed and a slower metabolism and excretion expected. In my retrospective study of old horse anesthesia, guaifenesin was given to effect for many of the inductions and it appears that there was no difference in the dose requirement to achieve recumbency in the two age groups.

Practically speaking, recognizing a reduction in the doses of induction agents for geriatric horses may be difficult because of the size of the patient and the need

to have it become recumbent safely. On the other hand, the use of combinations of α_2-agonists, guaifenesin or a benzodiazepine, or propofol and ketamine to create "total intravenous" anesthesia or these combinations in conjunction with inhalants to produce "balanced" or "multimodal" anesthesia have been advocated recently as methods that may be less physiologically compromising than inhalants alone.[44,45] In such situations, the possibility that lower dose and infusion rates may be required should be kept in mind. Infusion rates of thiopental, propofol, and midazolam needed to achieve anesthesia or sedation have all been shown to be lower in geriatric people as compared with younger adults.[15] Age-associated changes in metabolism and excretion, if not pharmacodynamics, could predict possible drug or active metabolite accumulation and suggest that smaller repeat doses or slower infusion rates during intravenous anesthesia would be appropriate.

Shortly after the introduction of the concept of MAC as a measure of inhalant anesthetic potency came the demonstration that MAC decreased with advancing age.[46] This is in part due to lower blood/gas solubility in aged people that may be partially explained by lower plasma albumin levels.[47] Because older people are not only maintained on lower concentrations for surgical intervention but also wake up at lower alveolar concentrations than do young people, it is believed that the decreased requirement has pharmacodynamic as well as kinetic mechanisms.[48] The pharmacokinetic behavior of inhalant anesthetics is highly dependent on the efficacy with which all gases are moved into alveoli (ventilation) and picked up by blood passing by alveoli (perfusion). As discussed earlier, in people, dogs, and horses, resting gas exchange becomes mildly less efficient with healthy aging, as manifested by lower Pa_{O_2} values.[6,24,25] The physiologic challenge of general anesthesia calls on respiratory and cardiovascular reserve function, which is likely to be less robust even in the healthy geriatric subject. In fact, the uptake of halothane, but not of isoflurane, has been found to be slower in older compared with younger people.[49] Halothane is the most soluble of the commonly available inhalants and therefore the one whose uptake is most retarded by decreases in effective alveolar ventilation and perfusion. Slower distribution and elimination of several inhalants, regardless of differences in their physicochemical properties, were found in a group of elderly human patients compared with a young group and attributed to decreased tissue perfusion and proportionally greater body fat.[50]

Elderly human patients do show greater cardiovascular depression and hemodynamic instability under inhalant anesthesia as compared with young patients.[17] In two groups of rats anesthetized with sufficient halothane to prevent response to tail pinch (0.78% for 28-month-olds and 0.95% for 4-month-olds), heart rate, blood pressure, and blood flow to the heart, brain, kidney, and small intestine were significantly lower in the older group.[51] The preliminary results of my retrospective comparison of geriatric to younger horses also seem to indicate that blood pressure is more labile in the aged equine. Cardiovascular instability and decreased tissue perfusion in the anesthetized horse contribute to less efficient gas exchange and hypoxemia and, perhaps, puts the geriatric equine at risk of tissue ischemia. Typically, people anesthetizing horses worry about muscle perfusion, since the potential consequences of severe myopathy are so profound. In the geriatric horse with marginally functional liver or kidneys, however, muscle may be only one of the tissues threatened. Hepatic metabolism of halothane and isoflurane produce reactively toxic molecules that are more tissue destructive under low-flow, hypoxic circumstances.[52] Hepatic insult due to halothane, which is 20 percent metabolized compared to the less than 1 percent metabolism of isoflurane and the approximately 5 percent metabolism of sevoflurane, may be a real concern in the geriatric horse and a valid reason to chose one of the other inhalants.

Opioids play a small but important role in equine anesthesia, play perhaps a more critical role in equine chemical restraint, and are increasingly being used in efforts to minimize pain in the awake patient. Adding intravenous butorphanol or morphine and, less frequently, meperidine to α_2-agonist, with or without acepromazine or diazepam, produces more profound and reliable sedation and contributes to analgesia. Plasma clearance of morphine is prolonged in elderly people but does not fully explain the decreased dose requirement reported for this and other α-agonists.[15,40,53] Thus, geriatric horses could be expected to experience better and longer analgesia with the small doses of butorphanol or morphine used to optimize standing chemical restraint. Anecdotally, the epidural morphine dose administered to effect and unmasked by a sedative to manage the pain of an infected hindleg tendon sheath in a 25-year-old horse was less than what I would have expected to administer to a younger horse. This would be consistent with both the age-associated increase in sensitivity to opioids and the reports, in people, that epidural dose requirements decrease linearly with age.[54] Also consistent with delayed elimination of opioids, this horse's return to non-weight-bearing lameness after discontinuing the morphine took longer than expected. Fortunately, when comparable doses of intravenous morphine were used to control acute postoperative pain in old and young human patients, no increase in frequency or intensity of adverse side effects was noted.[55]

To summarize, my approach to anesthetizing the healthy geriatric horse is not really very different from my approach to a young one. I may consider premedication with intramuscular acepromazine more seriously than I do for the average, moderately active young horse. Most often, xylazine is given intravenously to effect, starting at about 0.4 mg/kg. Additional xylazine or butorphanol is given to achieve a reasonable level of sedation. Guaifenesin and the benzodiazepines may cause venodilatation at higher doses, so the advantage of being able to administer guaifenesin to effect may avoid this additional hemodynamic challenge to a cardiovascular system that is preload-dependent. Ketamine, unless specifically contraindicated (any suspicion of increased intracranial pressure or severe corneal descemetocele), is given at a slightly lower dose than the traditional 2.2 mg/kg IV, but this is not different from the dose used in younger horses after adequate xylazine sedation and guaifenesin. Intubation has, on occasion, proven challenging due to difficulty opening the old horse mouth. Since these horses have been recumbent, well relaxed, and quiet, I have attributed this to craniomandibular degenerative joint disease but have no proof. Isoflurane or sevoflurane are my preferred inhalants for the geriatrics despite some evidence that the risk of death within 7 days is higher in older horses after isoflurane than after halothane.[56] Except for short procedures in lateral recumbency, old horses are mechanically ventilated. As mentioned earlier, monitoring should include, at a minimum, arterial blood pressure and an electrocardiogram and careful, repeated assessment of anesthetic depth and clinical indicators of cardiopulmonary function (capillary refill time, pulse quality, and rhythm). Managing hypotension in the geriatric horse, in my hands, does not differ from management of younger horses. This consists of appropriate volume support with a balanced electrolyte solution and inotropic support using dobutamine while repeatedly checking that anesthetic depth is not too great. Attenuated responses to the β-agonist dobutamine might be expected but, in the individual horse in whom dobutamine is administered as an infusion to effect, it might be difficult to distinguish the influence of age from that of any specific clinical situation. Arterial blood gases would be the next most important measurement for optimal patient care. In recovery, I expect these often-opinionated individuals to wake up annoyed and will give a small dose of xylazine to modify this. Manual restraint of old horses, to discourage premature efforts to stand, is often effective, as is assisting them to their feet with head and tail support. Age did not correlate with recovery score in a retrospective of 1314 equine anesthetic procedures.[57] However, in assessing the recovery of horses from inhalant anesthesia for ocular surgeries, it was noted that the average age of the horses with worse recoveries was greater than the average age of the entire study population.[58]

SPECIAL CONCERNS DUE TO AGE-ASSOCIATED PATHOLOGY

Age-associated disease may complicate the anesthetic management of the geriatric horse. The reader is referred to the other chapters of this book for more detail on these conditions. Truthfully, few old horses with significantly compromising medical conditions present for surgery and anesthesia. For example, unlike in humans and small companion animals, the diagnosis of heart failure is made infrequently in the horse and, in most instances, cardiac dysfunction is severe and the prognosis is poor. Thus, for both humane and economic reasons, the aged horse with severe cardiac disease is rarely a surgical candidate. The majority of heart murmurs in horses are incidental findings on physical examination, do not interfere with athletic performance, and are not age related.[59] The exception to this may be aortic insufficiency, which tends to be identified in middle age, and the consequent volume overload, regardless of magnitude, leads to progressive adaptations with aging as the heart works to maintain global blood flow. Thus, aortic insufficiency may become clinically significant but not yet life-threatening in older but not necessarily geriatric horses.[60] Likewise, atrial fibrillation is not specifically a condition of old age, but its occurrence in the older horse may carry a poorer prognosis. The concern with atrial fibrillation in the older horse is that the contribution of atrial contraction to cardiac output might be relatively more important in the geriatric cardiovascular system where stroke volume is more dependent on ventricular filling. In addition, the less precise autonomic control in older animals might precipitate greater extremes of heart rate and a greater risk of ventricular fibrillation or cardiac arrest. In all cases when a horse with identifiable cardiac disease is scheduled for surgery, full assessment of cardiac performance, including any history of exercise intolerance, should be undertaken before anesthesia.

The approach to general anesthesia for the horse with significant aortic insufficiency takes into consideration the fact that, because of diastolic regurgitation, effective net flow of blood out of the left ventricular is dependent on optimal forward flow and ventricular filling.[61] Lower aortic and peripheral arterial vascular resistance permit forward flow, and greater ventricular compliance, venous return, and diastolic duration encourage ventricular filling. Slower heart rates and a more compliant ventricle result in a longer, lower pressure diastole that may facilitate venous return. In the presence of aortic valve insufficiency, however, longer diastole allows more regurgitant flow and results in lower aortic root diastolic pressure, which may not be sufficient for myocardial perfusion. Thus, since, generally speaking, anesthetics decrease myocardial contractility, reducing afterload and encouraging venous return are important objectives. These goals become additionally challenging when the maintenance of mean blood pressure above 70 mm Hg is the traditional safety threshold for preventing postoperative myopathy. Choosing the less cardiodepressant inhalants, isoflurane or sevoflurane, with contractility and heart rate in mind, supporting venous return with aggressive fluid administration and maintaining blood pressure with inotropes rather than vasopressors are appropriate choices for the geriatric horse with aortic insufficiency but are also not unusual decisions when anesthetizing any horse. Combining small doses of acepromazine with reduced doses of xylazine for premedication would take advantage of their synergistic sedative effects while minimizing the cardiovascular effects of each.[62] The doses of xylazine and ketamine can also be reduced by adding either diazepam or guaifenesin to the induction regimen and thus limiting the vasoconstriction induced by either of these agents. The preemptive use of an anticholinergic to maintain higher heart rates is probably unwarranted, as higher heart rates per se in people with aortic insufficiency do not necessarily result in increased effective cardiac output.[61] Monitoring heart rate and blood pressure is essential. Ideally, capnography and pulse oximetry would provide indirect information about pulmonary and peripheral blood flow. Positive pressure ventilation compromises venous return and cardiac output and might be avoided if the position of the patient required for surgery does not profoundly interfere with ventilation. Proof of arterial oxygenation by blood gas analysis insures that the blood that is delivered to peripheral tissues is carrying oxygen.

Like aortic insufficiency, chronic obstructive pulmonary disease (COPD), also known as "heaves," is a diagnosis more often made in older, but not necessarily geriatric, horses.[63] Also like aortic insufficiency, COPD is a chronic, progressive condition that worsens with time. The recurrent cycle of small airway inflammation and spasm with secondary alveolar air trapping, inflammation, and septal destruction are followed by efforts to compensate and repair. Ultimately, with airway smooth muscle and pulmonary epithelia hypertrophy, there is a net loss of intra-alveolar septae and pulmonary capillaries with an increased number of intra-alveolar pores and deposition of collagen.[64] Pulmonary arterial pressure is increased and gas exchange is compromised in horses with COPD.[64,65] As the horse with COPD ages, many of the normal age-associated lung changes may be superseded by those produced by recurrent bouts of airway obstruction. Ultimately, a decrease in gas exchange area and an increase in end-expired lung volume are characteristics of both processes.

In my experience, anesthetizing horses with mild or moderate COPD has proven uneventful. By preference, elective surgeries are scheduled when the horse is not experiencing an acute episode and is managed preoperatively to avoid exposure to conditions that might trigger one. Medications used to modify airway resistance and responsiveness are not withheld preoperatively. This includes β_2-agonists despite concern that β-adrenergic-induced skeletal muscle tremor is well recognized in human medicine[66] and may contribute to shaky recoveries, particularly in older, muscle-poor horses.

The geriatric horse with severe COPD may not require anesthesia as often as mildly affected cases, but ensuring ventilation and gas exchange for these horses becomes a major objective. Anesthetized human patients with severe COPD experience greater ventilation/perfusion mismatch but less atelectasis than do normal volunteers.[67] The awake horse with severe COPD compensates for the increased resistance to expiratory flow and decreased alveolar elastic recoil by increasing the active, abdominal phase of expiration. Under anesthesia, this adaptive maneuver is lost and consequently the time for complete, passive expiration may be prolonged and return of the lung to its true end-expiratory volume may not be achieved. Attempts to accommodate full, passive expiration may result in respiratory rates and tidal volumes that are inadequate to meet oxygen requirements, carbon dioxide elimination, and inhalant anesthetic uptake. Repeatedly assisting inspiration before full expiration will eventually lead to alveolar hyperinflation, increased intrathoracic pressure, and decreased venous return, cardiac output, blood pressure, and tissue perfusion. For short surgical procedures performed on horses in lateral recumbency, allowing the horses to breathe spontaneously with an occasional manually assisted breath may be the least likely to worsen gas exchange. Fortunately, acepromazine, xylazine, ketamine, and the inhalant anesthetics are bronchodilators,[68-70] but these may be less helpful in horses with advanced, structure-altering pathology than they may be in preventing an acute bronchospastic episode in a hypersensitized COPD patient. Vaporizer settings may be higher than expected because inhalant uptake is decreased due to poor matching of ventilated to perfused alveoli. Longer, more involved surgeries with the horse in dorsal recumbency may necessitate more aggressive ventilatory assistance. Progressive hyperinflation of the lung due to insufficient expiratory time is less likely to occur with pressure-cycled than volume-cycled ventilators and may be recognized by observing that the bellows fails to return to its resting position at the end of expiration. Because hyperinflation will contribute to low cardiac output and blood pressure, it may be prudent to decompress the lung by disconnecting the expiratory limb of the breathing circuit during a breathing cycle if hypotension is a problem. Regardless of the method of supporting ventilation, these cases may be instances in which moderate hypercapnea is permissible as long as oxygenation is adequate.[70] Recovery of horses with COPD, particularly muscle-poor geriatrics, should include the ability to support ventilation and oxygenation as needed. The easiest means of doing this is with a demand valve.

Finally, hyperadrenocorticism and hypothyroidism often accompany aging in horses. The diagnosis of Cushing's disease has been reported to have an incidence of 0.5 percent and to be made in horses with an average age between 18.2 and 21.1 years.[71] Several of the typical features of equine Cushing's disease that are concerns for anesthesia, such as muscle wasting, fat redistribution, and lethargy, are accentuations of normal aging changes. Corticosteroid-induced hepatopathy, immunosuppression, and osteoporosis[71,72] may alter drug metabolism, pulmonary function secondary to pneumonia, and risk of fractures in recovery. Cushingoid horses may be tachypneic, tachycardic, and/or hypertensive.[72] Electrolyte abnormalities are not as recognized features of equine Cushing's disease as they may be in people,[73] but in horses with clinical signs consistent with secondary diabetes mellitus or insipidus, glucose, fluid, and electrolyte status should be evaluated. Hyperhidrosis may contribute to mild hypovolemia and hypokalemia.[72] Although there is some debate as to the incidence of hypothyroidism in the horse,[74] it may occur secondary to hyperadrenocorticism.[72] The physiologic effects of complete surgical thyroidectomy in horses included decreases in resting heart rate, cardiac output, respiratory rate, and body temperature and slight increases in plasma and blood volume. The heart rate increase in response to isoproterenol was less after thyroidectomy, which led the authors to conclude that β-adrenergic function had been altered.[75]

For elective surgeries, there is no excuse for old horses with these chronic endocrine diseases not to be fully evaluated and abnormalities corrected where possible. Thyroid supplements are available, and treatment of equine Cushing's disease with either a dopamine agonist or serotonin antagonist has met with considerable success.[76] Side effects of the dopamine agonists pergolide and bromocriptine have not been reported in horses, but the former may cause hypotension, agitation, and cardiac arrhythmias in people. Cyproheptadine, a serotonin antagonist, is also an antagonist at histamine and acetylcholine receptors and may cause sedation.[74]

Treated or untreated, geriatric cushingoid horses may be additionally sensitive to sedatives and anesthetics. The myocardium and diaphragm are spared the catabolic influence of corticosteroids as compared with skeletal muscle. Vascular smooth muscle may be more responsive to catecholamines.[73] Thus, the cardiovascular instability noted for geriatrics in general may be accentuated in hyperadrenocorticoid geriatrics. Vasoconstriction and hypovolemia result in reduced tissue perfusion, and it would be wise to volume-load these patients even if their apparent cardiovascular function is satisfactory as judged by arterial blood pressure. Supporting ventilation is a wise approach in these additionally sarcopenic animals and, likewise, being prepared to assist efforts to stand should be part of the anesthetic plan.

Enucleation and cataract removal are clinical situations in which anesthesia may be administered more often to older than younger horses. There are two peculiarities to ocular surgery and anesthesia that make these cases additionally challenging. The first is activation of vagally mediated bradycardia with ocular manipulation.[52] There is no indication that the oculocardiac reflex occurs any more or less frequently in old compared to young horses. The second is the use of neuromuscular blockade to immobilize the globe and reduce intraocular pressure. In horses, muscle paralysis is most commonly achieved with atracurium.[77] Despite what would seem to be less robust neuromuscular function,[9] the dose requirement and duration of action of atracurium in geriatric people has been shown to be minimally different from that of younger adults.[15,78]

SUMMARY

The losses of neuronal cells, axodendritic arrays, neurotransmitter, receptor, and signal transduction, cardiovascular structural and regulatory compliance, pulmonary gas exchange capacity, muscle mass, and hepatic and renal blood flow that accompany aging to some degree in all the mammalian species studied to date probably also occur in horses. The chronological age at which any of these may become clinically relevant is variable. In addition, age-associated diseases such as aortic insufficiency, COPD, and Cushing's disease further compromise the fragile balance and limited reserve of old age. In any case, it should be expected that the aged horse may require a lower dose than its young counterpart. However, unlike when anesthetizing a dog restrained on a countertop or a person on a gurney, the horse must proceed from a standing sedated state to a recumbent anesthetized position quickly to avoid injury to the horse or attending personnel. Ideally, this is achieved by the careful selection of a sequence of drugs given at just the necessary dose. It has been observed that the

anesthetic dose requirement in geriatric people has much greater individual variability than in young adults.[1,15] This is not surprising and is probably also the case with horses, since the geriatric population is not only a spectrum of genetic variation but also an accumulation of physiologically altering exposures. By the necessity of having to have this large animal lie down smoothly, a larger portion of the geriatric population of horses will be overdosed to ensure a safe induction. This may contribute to the greater cardiovascular instability that seems to be experienced by older horses under inhalant anesthesia. Ultimately, the horse must stand and walk out of the recovery stall, and getting these often quite feeble but opinionated horses to do so can be a challenge.

REFERENCES

1. Muravchick S: Anesthesia for the elderly. In Miller RM, editor: Anesthesia, 5th ed. London, Churchill Livingstone, 2000.
2. Johnston GM, Taylor PM, Holmes MA, et al: Confidential enquiry of perioperative equine fatalities (CEPEF-1): preliminary results. Equine Vet J 27:193, 1995.
3. Ingram DK: Age-related decline in physical activity: Generalization to nonhumans. Med Sci Sports Exercise 32:1623, 2000.
4. Ralston SL, Nockels CF, Squires EL: Difference in diagnostic test results and hematologic data between aged and young horses. Am J Vet Res 49:1387, 1988.
5. McFarlane D, Sellon DC, Gaffney D, et al: Hematologic and serum biochemical variables and plasma corticotropin concentrations in health aged horses. Am J Vet Res 59:1247, 1198.
6. Aquilera-Tejero E, Estepa JC, Lopez JC, et al: Arterial blood gases and acid-base balance in healthy young and aged horses. Equine Vet J 30:352, 1998.
7. Mrak RE, Griffin ST, Graham DI: Aging-associated changes in human brain. J Neuropath Exp Neurol 56:1269, 1997.
8. Summers BA: Neuropathology of aging. In Summers BA, Cummings JF, deLahunta A, eds: Veterinary Neuropathology. Baltimore, Mosby-YearBook, 1995.
9. Flanigan KM, Lauria G, Griffin JW, et al: Age-related biology and diseases of muscle and nerve. Neurol Clin North Am 16:659, 1998.
10. Dodds C, Allison J: Postoperative cognitive deficit in the elderly surgical patient. Br J Anaesth 81:449, 1998.
11. Culley DJ, Yukhananov, Baxter MG, et al: Spacial memory in young adult and aged rats 1 and 3 weeks after anesthesia. ASA Scientific Papers Abstracts. Available at: www.asa-abstract.com. Accessed 2000.
12. Grubb TL, Muir WW: Anesthetic emergencies and complications: Part 1. Equine Vet Educat 10:98, 1998.
13. Taylor PM: Stress responses in ponies during halothane or isoflurane anaesthesia after induction with thiopentone or xylazine/ketamine. J Vet Anaesth 18:8, 1991.
14. Fankhauser R, Luginbuhl H, McGrath JT: Cerebrovascular disease in various animal species. Annals NY Acad Sci 127:817, 1965.
15. Shafer SL: The pharmacology of anesthetic drugs in elderly patients. Anesth Clin North Am 18:1, 2000.
16. Delp MD, Evans MV, Duan C: Effects of aging on cardiac output, regional blood flow, and body composition in Fischer-344 rats. J Appl Physiol 85:1813, 1998.
17. Rooke GA: Autonomic and cardiovascular function in the geriatric patient. Anesth Clin North Am 18:31, 2000.
18. Marin J: Age-related changes in vascular responses: A review. Mechan Ageing Develop 79:71, 1995.
19. Rooney JR, Robertson JL: Equine Pathology. Ames, IA, Iowa State University Press, 1996.

20. Horohov DW, Dimock A, Guirnalda P, et al: Effect of exercise on the immune response of young and old horses. Am J Vet Res 60:643, 1999.

21. Schilling S: The blood pressure of the horse. J Am Vet Med Assoc 55:401, 1919.

22. Parry BW, McCarthy MA, Anderson GA: Survey of resting blood pressure values in clinically normal horses. Equine Vet J 16:53, 1964.

23. Hinchcliff KW, McKeever KH, Muir WW: Hemodynamic effects of atropine, dobutamine, nitroprusside, phenylephrine, and propranolol in conscious horses. J Vet Intern Med 5:80, 1991.

24. Simpkins JW, Field FP, Ress RJ: Age-related decline in adrenergic responsiveness of the kidney, heart and aorta of male rats. Neurobiol Aging 4:233, 1983.

25. Yin FCP, Spurgeon HA, Greene HL, et al: Age-associated decrease in heart rate response to isoproterenol in dogs. Mechan Age Develop 10:17, 1979.

26. Zaugg M, Lucchinetti E: Respiratory function in the elderly. Anesth Clin North Am 18:47, 2000.

27. Robinson NE, Gillespie JR: Pulmonary diffusing capacity and capillary blood volume in aging dogs. J Appl Physiol 38:647, 1975.

28. Butler JA, Colles CM, Dyson SJ, et al, eds: Clinical radiology of the horse, 2nd ed. Oxford, Blackwell Science, 2000.

29. Gunnarsson L, Tokics L, Gustavsson H, et al: Influence of age on atelectasis formation and gas exchange impairment during general anaesthesia. Br J Anaesth 66:423, 1991.

30. Welle S: Cellular and molecular basis of age-related sarcopenia. Can J Appl Physiol 27:19, 2002.

31. Stanski DR, Maitre PO: Population pharmacokinetics and pharmacodynamics of thiopental: the effect of age revisited. Anesthesiology 72:412, 1990.

32. Barnhill JG, Greenblatt DJ, Miller LG, et al: Kinetic and dynamic components of increased benzodiazepine sensitivity in aging animals. J Pharmacol Exp Ther 253:1153, 1990.

33. Mooradian AD: Effect of aging on the blood-brain barrier. Neurobiol Aging 9:31, 1988.

34. Cherin P, Colvez, Deville de Periere G, et al: Risk of syncope in the elderly and consumption of drugs: a case-control study. J Clin Epidemiol 50:313, 2001.

35. Doherty TJ, Geiser DR, Rohrbach BW: Effect of aceprotomazine and butorphanol on halothane minimum alveolar concentration in ponies. Equine Vet J 29:374, 1997.

36. Sastre M, Guimon J, Garcia-Sevilla JA: Relationships between β- and α-adrenoceptors and G coupling proteins in the human brain: effects of age and suicide. Brain Res 898:242, 2001.

37. Matthews NS, Dollar NS, Shawley RV: Halothane-sparing effect of benzodiazepines in ponies. Cornell Vet 80:259, 1990.

38. Reves JG, Fragen RJ, Vinik HR, et al: Midazolam: pharmacology and uses. Anesthesiology 62:310, 1985.

39. Macklon AF, Barton M, James O, et al: The effect of age on the pharmacokinetics of diazepam. Clin Sci 59:479, 1980.

40. Landrum AL: Use of intravenous techniques in the elderly. In White PF, editor: Textbook of Intravenous Anesthesia. Baltimore, Lippincott Williams & Wilkins, 1997.

41. Magnuson KR: Differential effects of aging on binding sites of the activated NMDA receptor complex in mice. Mechan Age Develop 84:227, 1995.

42. Schnider TW, Minto CF, Shafer SL, et al: The influence of age on propofol pharmacodynamics. Anesthesiology 90:1502, 1999.

43. Davis LE, Wolff WA: Pharmacokinetics and metabolism of glycerol guaiacolate in ponies. Am J Vet Res 31:469, 1970.

44. Taylor PM, Kerby JJ, Shrimpton DJ, et al: Cardiovascular effects of surgical castration during anaesthesia maintained with halothane or infusion of detomidine, ketamine and guaifenesin in ponies. Equine Vet J 30:304, 1998.

45. Yamashita K, Satoh M, Umikawa A, et al: Combination of continuous infusion using a mixture of guaifenesin-ketamine-medetomidine and sevoflurane in horses. J Vet Med Sci 62:229, 2000.

46. Gregory GA, Eger EI, Munson ES: The relationship between age and halothane requirement in man. Anesthesiology 30:488, 1969.

47. Lerman J, Gregory GA, Willis MM, et al: Age and solubility of volatile anesthetics in blood. Anesthesiology 61:139, 1984.

48. Katoh T, Suguro Y, Ikeda T, et al: Influence of age on awakening concentrations of sevoflurane and isoflurane. Anesth Analg 79:348, 1993.

49. Dwyer RC, Fee JPH, Howard PJ, et al: Arterial washing of halothane and isoflurane in young and elderly adult patients. Br J Anaesth 66:572, 1991.

50. Strum DP, Eger EI, Unadkat JD, et al: Age affects the pharmacokinetics of inhaled anesthetics in humans. Anesth Analg 73:310, 1991.

51. Hoffman WE, Miletich DJ, Albrecht RF: Cardiovascular and regional blood flow changes during halothane anesthesia in the aged rat. Anesthesiology 56:444, 1982.

52. Kenna JG, Jones RM: The organ toxicity of inhaled anesthetics. Anesth Analg 81:S51, 1995.

53. Kaiko RF, Wallenstein SL, Rogers AG, et al: Narcotics in the elderly. Med Clin North Am 66:1079, 1982.

54. Bromage PR: Ageing and epidural dose requirements. Br J Anaesth 41:1016, 1969.

55. Aubrun F, Monsel S, Langeron O, et al: Postoperative titration of intravenous morphine in the elderly patient. Anesthesiology 96:17, 2002.

56. Johnston GM, Eastment J, Taylor PM, et al: Perioperative risk in horses. World Congress Vet Anaesth 7:31, 2000.

57. Young SS, Taylor PM: Factors influencing the outcome of equine anaesthesia: a review of 1,314 cases. Equine Vet J 25:147, 1993.

58. Parvianen AKJ, Trim CM: Complications associated with anaesthesia for ocular surgery: a retrospective study 1989-1996. Equine Vet J 32:555, 2000.

59. Patteson M: Equine Cardiology. Oxford, Blackwell Science, 1996.

60. Reef VB, Spencer P: Echocardiographic evaluation of equine aortic insufficiency. Am J Vet Res 48:904, 1987.

61. diNardo JA: Anesthesia for cardiac surgery, 2nd ed. Stamford, CT, Appleton & Lange, 1998.

62. Muir WW, Skarda RT, Sheehan W: Hemodynamic and respiratory effects of a xylazine-acetylpromazine drug combination in horses. Am J Vet Med 40:1518, 1979.

63. Dixon PM, Railton DI, McGorum BC: Equine pulmonary disease: a case control study of 300 referred cases. Part 2: details of animals and of historical and clinical findings. Equine Vet J 27:422, 1995.

64. Robinson NE, Derksen FJ, Oleszewski MA, et al: The pathogenesis of chronic obstructive pulmonary disease of horse. Br Vet J 152:283, 1996.

65. Nyman G, Lindberg R, Weckner D, et al: Pulmonary gas exchange correlated to clinical signs and lung pathology in horses with chronic bronchiolitis. Equine Vet J 23:253, 1991.

66. Nelson HS: β-adrenergic bronchodilators. N Engl J Med 333:499, 1995.

67. Gunnarsson L, Tokics L, Lundquist H, et al: Chronic obstructive pulmonary disease and anaesthesia: formation of atelectasis and gas exchange impairment. Eur Respir J 4:1106, 1991.

68. Whatney GCG, Hall LW, Jordan C, et al: Effects of xylazine and acepromazine on bronchomotor tone of anaesthetized ponies. Equine Vet J 20:185, 1988.

69. Reich DL: Ketamine: An update on the first twenty-five years of clinical experience. Can J Anaesth 36:186, 1989.

70. Seigne PW, Hartigan PM, Body SC: Anesthetic considerations for patients with severe emphysematous lung disease. Int Anesthesiol Clin 38:1, 2000.

71. van der Kolk H: Diseases of the pituitary gland, including hyperadrenocorticism. In Watson TDG, editor: Metabolic and Endocrine Problems of the Horse. New York, WB Saunders, 1998.

72. Love S: Equine Cushing's disease. Br Vet J 149:139, 1993.

73. Lampe GH, Roizen MF: Anesthesia for patients with abnormal function of the adrenal cortex. Anesth Clin North Am 5:245, 1987.

74. Sojka JE: Hypothyroidism in horses. Compendium 17:845, 1995.

75. Vischer CM, Foreman JH, Constable PD, et al: Hemodynamic effects of thyroidectomy in sedentary horses. Am J Vet Res 60:14, 1999.

76. Beech J: Treatment of hypophysial adenomas. Compendium 16:921, 1994.

77. Martinez EA: Neuromuscular blocking agents. Vet Clin North Am Equine 18:181, 2002.

78. Kitts JB, Fisher DM, Canfell PC, et al: Pharmacokinetics and pharmacodynamics of atracurium in the elderly. Anesthesiology 72:272, 1990.

CHAPTER 5

Cardiac Disease in the Geriatric Horse

Celia M. Marr,

Mark Bowen

PREVALENCE AND CLINICAL SIGNIFICANCE OF CARDIAC DISEASE IN OLDER HORSES

Valvular heart disease is the most common form of cardiac disease in the horse; in a pathology survey, valvular heart disease was identified in 23 percent and nonvalvular lesions in 6 percent of a population of 1557 horses, 51 percent of which were 16 years of age or older.[1] Of the animals with valvular heart disease, aortic valve pathology was the most common, occurring in 82 percent of this group. There was a trend for all forms of valvular heart disease to increase with age, although the incidence of aortic regurgitation was highest in horses aged 15 to 20 years, with a lower incidence in horses older than 20 years. The lower incidence in this oldest subgroup is in contrast to findings in auscultatory studies. Cardiac murmurs are encountered commonly in older horses: in a survey of 1153 horses in Southeast England, with a median age of 14 years and age range from 1 to 45 years and therefore including a substantial proportion of older animals, cardiac murmurs were detected in 243 of the horses (21.1%; 95% CI, 18.7-23.5).[2] The prevalence of the various forms of murmur within this population is illustrated in Figure 5-1. Age was found to be a significant risk factor associated with the left-sided valvular insufficiencies, such as aortic and mitral insufficiency, occurring either alone or in combination, with an odds ratio of 1.07 (95% CI, 1.05-1.10). Thus, in that population the odds of having a left-sided valvular insufficiency

murmur increased by 0.05 to 0.1 for each additional year of life.[2]

Although aortic insufficiency and mitral insufficiency are the most common forms of underlying pathology that are found in horses that present with congestive heart failure (CHF), in many cases the valvular insufficiency is detected as an incidental finding. The population described above was evaluated over a 4-year period and, in a multivariable model, left-sided valvular insufficiency was not found to increase the risk of death, whereas, unsurprisingly, increasing age was associated with an increasing risk of death.[2] Survival rates and owner-reported causes of death or euthanasia within this population are displayed in Figure 5-2. Musculoskeletal and gastrointestinal problems were more common reasons for death or euthanasia than cardiovascular problems in all age groups. Cardiovascular deaths did not occur in the horses that were younger than 15 years of age, whereas the prevalence was 5.1 percent (95% CI, 2.3-7.9) in the 15- to 23-year-old group and 8.5 percent (95% CI, 5-12) in the 24-year-old and older group; however, this difference was not statistically significant in this study.[2] The majority of the animals included in this auscultatory survey had no other clinical signs of cardiac dysfunction. However, a variety of additional cardiac conditions should be considered when one is presented with an older horse with signs of cardiac compromise. Some are considered to be particularly prevalent in older horses, such as aortocardiac fistula and a variety of forms of neoplasia, whereas others, such as

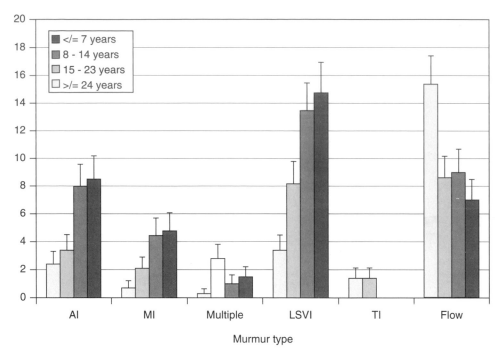

Figure 5-1 The prevalence of various types of murmur detected in a group of 1153 horses of mixed breed and age in Southeast England. AI, aortic insufficiency; Flow, physiologic flow murmurs; LSVI, left-sided valvular insufficiency such as aortic and mitral insufficiency either alone or in combination; MI, mitral insufficiency; multiple, more than one type of murmurs; TI, tricuspid insufficiency.

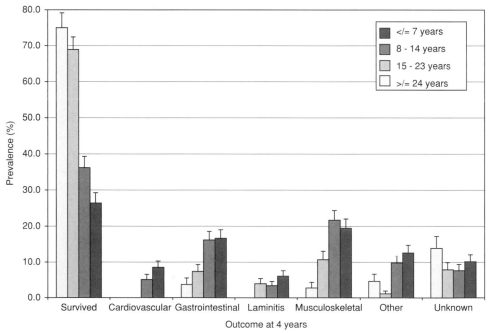

Figure 5-2 The survival rates and the owner-reported reasons for death or euthanasia in different age groups in a population of 773 horses followed over 4 years. By 4 years, 26% of the original study group of 1153 horses had been lost to follow-up.

myocardial disease and pericarditis, are not specifically associated with old age. It is also important to note that occasionally horses with congential lesions such as ventricular septal defect or patent ductus arteriosus[3] present with signs of heart failure in later years, having been asymptomatic until that point in life (Fig. 5-3).

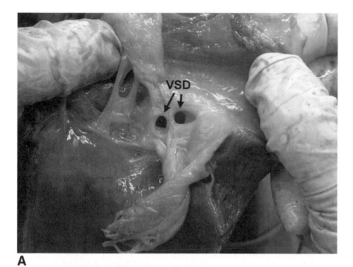

A

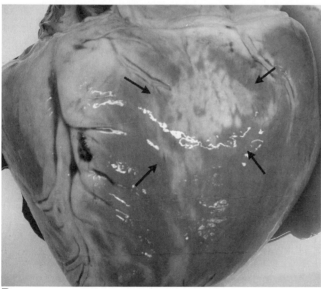

B

Figure 5-3 Pathologic specimens from a 16-year-old Thoroughbred broodmare. Ventricular septal defect (VSD) had first been diagnosed at 1 year of age. The mare was never trained but she had carried 10 foals with no major signs of ill health. Two days prior to euthanasia, her attendants had noted that she was slightly depressed and on the day of her death, she developed ventricular tachycardia, tachypnea, frothy nasal discharge, jugular distension, and ventral edema. **A,** The VSD consisted of a series of channels through the nonmembranous portion of the septum. **B,** There was extensive fibrosis within the myocardium that may have accounted for the arrhythmia. The case illustrates how a severe, long-standing cardiac pathologic condition can be remarkably well tolerated for prolonged periods.

CLINICAL ASSESSMENT AND MANAGEMENT OF CARDIAC DISEASES OF THE OLDER HORSE

Equine Aortic Valvular Insufficiency

Aortic valve regurgitation or insufficiency can be categorized into primary or secondary disease processes. In the horse, secondary aortic valve disease is undocumented, whereas in human beings, connective tissue disorders such as Marfan's syndrome can cause aortic regurgitation due to disorientation of collagen fibers within the valve.[4] Primary aortic valve disease can be infectious or noninfectious. Bacterial endocarditis[5] and aortitis[6,7] have been reported in the horse and cause significant valvular disruption. Although a bacterial cure can be brought about by antibiotic administration, the degree of fibrosis of the valve cusp will result in persistent and usually severe valvular regurgitation.[8] More commonly in the older horse population, aortic insufficiency is a noninfectious condition,[9] with a myxomatous noninflammatory infiltrate with fibrosis. A similar condition is documented in human beings of floppy aortic valve disease.[10] The origin of this form of pathology is unknown, although it has been postulated that a primary insult results in valvular insufficiency, and that the shear forces arising from regurgitant flow may perpetuate the fibrosis, leading to progression of the disease.[11]

One study has reported that the noncoronary cusp was most commonly diseased (44%), whereas lesions in the coronary cusps were evenly distributed and frequently more than one cusp was affected.[11] This distribution of disease is in contrast to the findings of another study in which pathology was identified most frequently in the left coronary cusp,[9] which is consistent with the two-dimensional echocardiographic appearance of the condition, in which the left and right coronary cusps are most commonly diseased.[12] The macroscopic pathology of aortic insufficiency can be classified as nodular and band-type lesions.[9,11] Nodular lesions are the most common form of pathology in horses with aortic insufficiency,[11] whereas band lesions are associated with a loss of elasticity and extend the entire length of the cusp.[9] The combination of band lesions with nodular thickenings results in severe distortion of the cusp.[9] Fenestration of the aortic valve is common but is not associated with regurgitant flow and can be seen in normal horses of all ages.[9,11] Fenestrations are usually located in the lunulae of the cusps, where there is considerable overlap between adjacent components of the aortic valve, explaining their lack of physiologic significance.

Microscopically noninfectious aortic valve pathologic condition is characterized by acid mucopolysaccharide and fibroblastic accumulations and elastic fiber disruption with an absence of inflammatory cells.[9-11] Band-type lesions involve all layers of the leaflet and are covered by an intact endothelium, whereas the nodular lesions involve endothelial loss with fibrin adhesion. Larger nodular lesions are associated with elastic fiber fragmentation. Populations of inflammatory cells are occasionally identified within the valve cusps, although they are not associated with the fibrous lesions.[11] Although their significance is unknown, they may represent a previous inflammatory or infectious process that has resulted in fibrosis and repair and thus an incompetent valve.

The diagnosis of aortic insufficiency can be confirmed by auscultation of characteristic diastolic murmurs,[13] with the use of Doppler echocardiography[14] or by the presence of subendocardial jet-lesions at postmortem examination.[1] Colour flow Doppler echocardiography can document regurgitant flow in the absence of an audible murmur (silent aortic regurgitation).[14,15]

The spectrum of clinical presentation relating to aortic insufficiency is varied. With mild valvular regurgitation without audible cardiac noises (silent aortic insufficiency), horses may present with diastolic cardiac murmurs of variable intensity with no clinical evidence of cardiac disease (incidental murmur) or with exercise intolerance and signs of CHF. No correlation has been demonstrated between the incidence of cardiac murmurs and race performance in young thoroughbreds.[16] This confirms that cardiac murmurs can occur without any compromise to cardiac function in most horses. However, the condition is not a static disease process, and animals with clinically irrelevant murmurs of aortic insufficiency may develop congestive heart failure with time. In a population of 57 predominantly older horses with aortic insufficiency, there was clinical progression of heart disease in 22.8 percent (95% CI, 11.9-33.7) over a 24-month period,[17] and it appears that this is more likely to happen in later years of life.

In aortic insufficiency cases, the characteristic findings on clinical examination are of a diastolic murmur with its point of maximal intensity over the left fourth intercostal space at the level of the point of the shoulder. The murmur is typically decrescendo in nature and frequently has a bussing or creaky quality that is thought to be due to vibration of intracardiac structures as they come into contact with the regurgitant jet. In some horses, the murmur is audible on the right side. The quality of the arterial pulses is a useful guide to severity as, with left ventricular volume overload and more severe regurgitant fraction, the pulses develop a bounding quality, and a wide pulse difference can also be documented using noninvasive sphygmomanometry via the coccygeal artery. Care should be taken to identify concurrent murmurs of mitral insufficiency, as the combination of aortic insufficiency and mitral insufficiency indicates more severe disease and warrants a slightly poorer prognosis.

Horses with aortic insufficiency appear to be at risk of developing both supraventricular and ventricular arrhythmias. These are rarely recognized on physical examination and require ambulatory and exercising electrocardiographic studies to document their presence. Jet lesions arising from aortic valve regurgitation consist of endocardial fibrosis, consisting of fibroblasts, fibrocytes, and ground substance that does not extend into the myocardium.[9] This is a finding in common with human beings with aortic insufficiency, in whom the degree of fibrosis is correlated with ejection fraction, clinical signs, and mortality.[18] Myofibrillar necrosis occurs adjacent to jet lesions in a proportion of affected horses,[9] extending 1 to 2 mm deep to the endocardium. The significance of the myofibril damage is unknown, but the association between aortic insufficiency and ventricular arrhythmias may be explained in part by areas of myocardial damage, as well as the proximity between the jet lesions and Purkinje fibers.[9] In human beings, myocardial fibrosis is reported in association with aortic valve regurgitation.[18-21] It is not clear whether this is a result of direct insult or activation of neurohormonal mechanisms of CHF. This is not a consistent feature in the horse and was not recognized in abattoir studies,[1,9] although myocardial fibrosis is occasionally observed in our laboratory in horses with chronic aortic insufficiency (unpublished observations).

Doppler echocardiography can be used to confirm the presence of aortic insufficiency. Regurgitant jets are generally most easily identified in long-axis images of the left ventricular outflow tract (Fig. 5-4). Subjectively, jets can be classified as very small (insignificant), small, moderate, and large. The length of the regurgitant jets is significantly longer when horses with aortic insufficiency murmurs and accompanying clinical signs at rest are compared to horses with aortic insufficiency murmurs without other clinical signs at rest, whereas the width at the base and maximal width of aortic regurgitant jets are not different between these two severity groups. The repeatability of these Doppler measurements of the aortic regurgitant jets has been evaluated in the authors' clinic and found to be poor; therefore, care should be taken in applying such measurements as tools with which to monitor patients over time. The M-mode measurements of the left ventricular diameter in diastole and systole appear to be more repeatable, and significant differences are present when horses with aortic insufficiency murmurs and accompanying clinical signs at rest are compared to horses with aortic insufficiency murmurs without other clinical signs at rest and with horses with no murmurs. Thus, these dimensions are more likely to be useful in assessing change over time, although their prognostic value has not yet been documented in a longitudinal study. The M-mode image

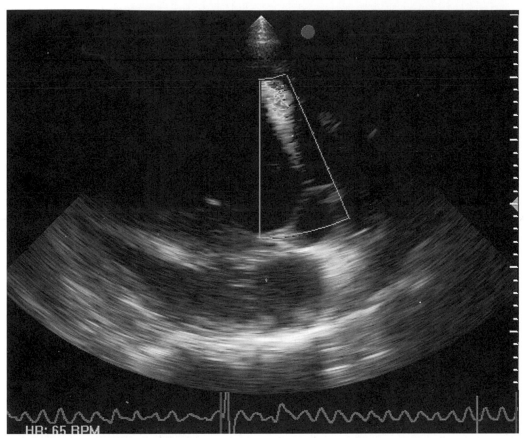

Figure 5-4 A left parasternal long-axis image of the left ventricular outflow tract from a 15-year-old Thoroughbred gelding demonstrating a jet of aortic regurgitation.

of the ventricles can also be used to assess the movement of the septum and left ventricular wall. In moderate and severe cases, exaggerated movement of the septum may be evident (Fig. 5-5). Common additional findings in cases of aortic insufficiency include nodular and diffuse thickenings of the aortic valve cusps, dilation of the aortic root, diastolic vibrations of the interventricular septum or mitral valve, and early closure of the mitral valve (Fig. 5-6).

Currently, objective studies addressing which clinical tools are the most reliable prognostic indicators in older horses with aortic insufficiency are limited. The prognostic value of the various echocardiographic indices has not been investigated critically. In a 2-year, field-based study of 57 horses with aortic insufficiency, 7 of which died and 6 of which progressed from having no signs of CHF to having CHF, the horses with ventricular arrhythmias at the outset of the study had the highest likelihood of progressing. The presence of supraventricular arrhythmias was not associated with a poor prognosis. There was a moderately increased likelihood of progression in horses with bounding pulses, multiple murmurs, and a pulse pressure of greater than 60 mm Hg.[17] Plasma norepinephrine and epinephrine concentrations were increased in aortic insufficiency cases compared to normal horses but did not appear to be useful prognostic indicators. Similarly, several

indices derived from heart rate variability studies support the conclusion that the sympathetic nervous system is activated in this disease, but were not useful prognostic tools.

Therapeutic options for older horses with aortic insufficiency are limited, although the renin-angiotensin-aldosterone system offers several options of pharmacological intervention. The angiotensin-converting enzyme (ACE) inhibitors are an important class of drug used for the control of cardiac disease in human beings and dogs. They have led to significant improvements in risk of mortality among symptomatic patients.[22,23] Despite an initial reduction in plasma aldosterone, chronic administration leads to "aldosterone escape" and a return to pretreatment values.[24] The combination of an ACE inhibitor with aldosterone receptor antagonists such as spironolactone or eplerenone enhances the benefits of ACE inhibition[25]; however, increased plasma aldosterone concentrations are not a consistent feature in heart disease in horses with aortic insufficiency (Bowen, Marr, Elliott, unpublished data). Similarly, in human beings and dogs with mitral valve prolapse, plasma aldosterone concentrations are low, whereas plasma renin activity is increased.[26-28] These studies document increases in plasma renin activity, despite reductions in plasma aldosterone concentrations. Several mechanisms can blunt or inhibit angiotensin II–mediated

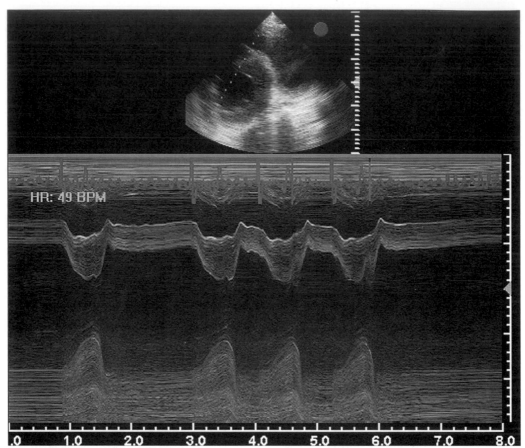

Figure 5-5 An M-mode echocardiograph of the right and left ventricles from a 15-year-old Thoroughbred gelding with moderately severe aortic insufficiency and mitral insufficiency. The accompanying two-dimensional image demonstrates the M-mode cursor placement. The movement of the septum is exaggerated due to left ventricular volume overload and the diameter of the ventricle is increased. Note: the superimposed electrocardiogram confirms that this horse has concurrent atrial fibrillation.

aldosterone secretion. Dopamine directly inhibits aldosterone secretion through D1, a receptor in the zona glomerulosa of the adrenal gland.[29] Adrenocorticotropic hormone augments angiotensin II–mediated aldosterone secretion; thus, in the absence of adrenocorticotropic hormone, plasma aldosterone secretion is reduced. It is unlikely that either of these factors would be increased in patients with cardiac disease. Atrial natriuretic peptide is produced by atrial myocytes in response to atrial stretch, as would occur in mitral valve regurgitation. It blocks both renin secretion and the actions of angiotensin II on aldosterone secretion.[30] This may explain the lack of increased plasma aldosterone in patients with mitral valve disease, although atrial stretch would not occur with aortic insufficiency and so would not occur in this condition. Activation of the renin-angiotensin-aldosterone system has not been documented in equine CHF and knowledge of renin-angiotensin-aldosterone system activation is essential prior to embarking on therapeutic intervention with any of these agents. Previously, use of the ACE inhibitor enalapril

was advocated[31]; however, recent pharmacokinetic studies on this drug have demonstrated that its oral bioavailability is poor and it was undetectable in plasma when administered orally at previously recommended doses.[32]

Mitral Insufficiency

Mitral insufficiency occurs in all age groups and is not specifically associated with the geriatric population. It was found to become increasingly prevalent in a group of young racehorses as they proceeded through the initial stages of training, although these horses show no overt signs of cardiac compromise associated with the phenomenon.[33] In a study of horses presenting with severe mitral insufficiency, the population had a mean ± SD age of 7.6 ± 8.1 years.[34] Nevertheless, murmurs of mitral insufficiency are increasingly prevalent in older horses (see Fig. 4-1), and the majority of horses presenting to the authors' clinics with noninfectious, noninflammatory disease are older than 10 years of age. Several forms of pri-

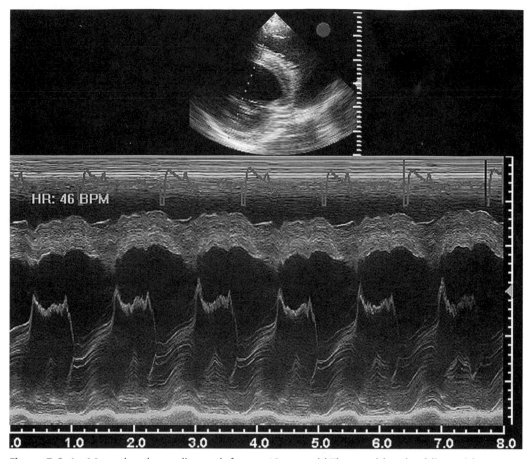

Figure 5-6 An M-mode echocardiograph from a 19-year-old Thoroughbred gelding with moderately severe aortic insufficiency illustrating marked diastolic vibration and early closure of the mitral valve. The accompanying two-dimensional image demonstrates the M-mode cursor placement.

mary pathology affect the mitral valve: the majority are fibrous thickenings that are either generalized diffuse lesions, localized or nodular lesions, or a combination of these types.[1] In cases in which valve lesions are severe, this is often accompanied by nodulation of the chordae tendineae,[1] and degenerative disease can predispose to rupture of the chordae tendineae, a condition that can also arise spontaneously and secondary to bacterial endocarditis.[34-36] Microscopically, in older horses mitral valve lesions are most commonly noninfectious and noninflammatory, with a histologic appearance similar to that described for degenerative aortic valvular disease.[11] In a substantial proportion of horses presenting with severe mitral insufficiency, there is concurrent myocardial fibrosis,[34] and in some of these individuals, the myocardial lesions are considered to be the primary disease leading to mitral insufficiency as a consequence of ventricular remodelling.[34] Severe mitral insufficiency commonly leads to pulmonary hypertension and pulmonary artery dilation, which in turn can be associated with pulmonary artery rupture.[34,37]

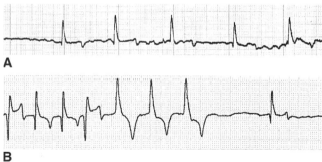

Figure 5-7 Electrocardiograph from a 13-year-old Hunter gelding with severe mitral insufficiency presenting with lethargy, ventral edema, and jugular distension of 5 days' duration. **A,** On initial presentation, rapid atrial fibrillation with a ventricular rate of around 60/min was detected (base-apex lead, 1 mV/cm; paper speed, 25mm/s). **B,** In a 24-hour ambulatory electrocardiogram, paroxysms of polymorphic ventricular tachycardia were present (modified base-apex lead). Postmortem examination confirmed that there was primary mitral valve disease accompanied by myocardial fibrosis.

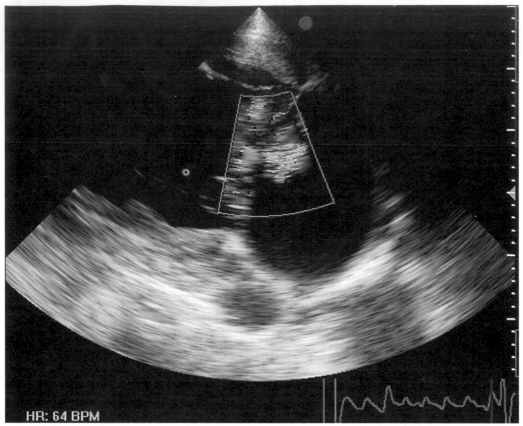

Figure 5-8 A left parasternal long-axis image of the left atrium and ventricle from a 15-year-old Thoroughbred gelding with moderately severe aortic insufficiency and mitral insufficiency. A jet from the mitral insufficiency is visible and the crosses indicate the calliper position for measurement of the left atrial diameter from this image.

With severe mitral insufficiency, common presenting complaints include exercise intolerance, depression, cough, weight loss, and peripheral edema.[34,38] Mitral insufficiency is associated with a mid-, holo-, or pansystolic murmur that is loudest over the left fifth intercostal space. Typically, it radiates to variable degrees in a caudodorsal or dorsal direction and may have a coarse, band-shaped quality. Prominent buzzing or musical tones are suggestive of a ruptured chorda tendinea. The presence of a loud third heart sound suggests that the mitral insufficiency may be severe and accompanied by left ventricular volume overload. Raised respiratory rate, coarse bronchovesicular sounds, and crackles on auscultation of the lungs are suggestive of pulmonary edema. Frothy nasal discharge is relatively uncommon and usually indicates an acute, severe onset, whereas signs consistent with right heart failure, ventral, preputial, and limb edema have often developed by the time of presentation. Horses with severe mitral insufficiency frequently have concurrent atrial fibrillation: this was noted in 24 of 43 horses (55.8%) in one report[34] (Figs. 5-5 and 5-7). Ventricular arrhythmias may also be noted, particularly if prolonged ambulatory electrocardiographic studies are conducted[34] (Fig. 5-7) and this may suggest concurrent myocardial disease. However, as noted earlier, many older horses have murmurs of mitral insufficiency and no other clinical signs of cardiac dysfunction, and mitral insufficiency, alone or in combination with aortic insufficiency, has not been shown to reduce life expectancy.[2]

The spectrum of echocardiographic findings that accompany severe mitral insufficiency have been well documented.[34] Thickening of the mitral valve can be generalized or nodular. Portions of the valve apparatus everting into the left atrium are suggestive of ruptured chordae tendineae. Mitral valve prolapse is often evident, although this can also be seen in younger horses with mild, nonprogressive mitral insufficiency.[15] Doppler echocardiography is used to semiquantitate the degree of regurgitation (Fig. 5-8), although the limitations with respect to measurement of jet sizes described in relation to aortic insufficiency are likely to apply to the mitral insufficiency also. The diameter of the left ventricle in systole and diastole is often increased (see Fig. 5-5). Left atrial enlargement can most readily be documented from a left parasternal long-axis image,[34] since, although the left atrium can also be measured in images made from the right side in normal horses, when the heart is enlarged, the full extent of the left atrium is often not present in the right-sided images when

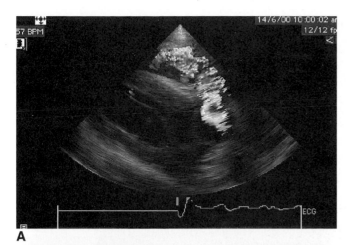

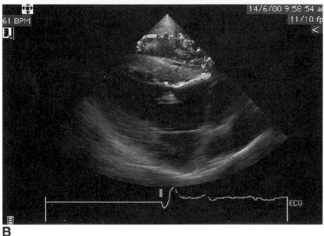

Figure 5-9 Right parasternal long-axis echocardiograms from a 13-year-old gelding with an aortocardiac fistula, presenting with exercise-intolerance, weight loss, and a loud continuous murmur on the right side. **A,** A turbulent jet is visible in the fistula between the aorta and the right ventricle. **B,** Blood flow is visible within a subendocardial hematoma dissecting through the interventricular septum.

cardiomegaly is present. Particular attention should be paid to measurement of the diameter of the pulmonary artery because enlargement is indicative of pulmonary artery dilation and warrants a poor prognosis.[34] In the presence of low cardiac output, the diameter of the aortic root is often decreased.[31,34]

Palliative therapy for cases of severe mitral insufficiency associated with CHF is aimed at reducing congestion and improving cardiac output. Although ACE inhibitors are theoretically useful in this setting, as noted earlier, the optimal drug and dosage regimen have yet to be determined. Digoxin can be useful for treatment of supraventricular tachycardia, and the recommended maintenance dose is 0.011 mg/kg orally twice daily.[39,40] Peak concentrations should be measured 1 hour after administration to ensure that therapeutic concentrations are maintained at 1 to 2 μg/mL. Furosemide is the most effective diuretic in horses. Unfortunately, the oral

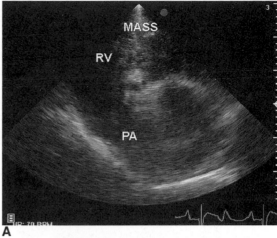

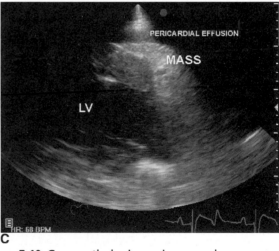

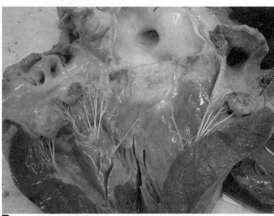

Figure 5-10 Gross pathologic specimens and echocardiograms from a 22-year-old mixed breed gelding presenting with a 1-month history of weight loss, intermittent colic, tachycardia, jugular distension, and loud coarse bilateral holosystolic murmurs due to generalized lymphosarcoma. **A,** In the right long-axis right inflow-outflow image, a mass associated with the tricuspid valve is visible. **B,** A gross specimen demonstrating that additional masses were found on all cusps of aortic and mitral valves. **C,** A left parasternal long-axis image of the left ventricle demonstrating a mass adherent to the epicardial surface and a pericardial effusion.

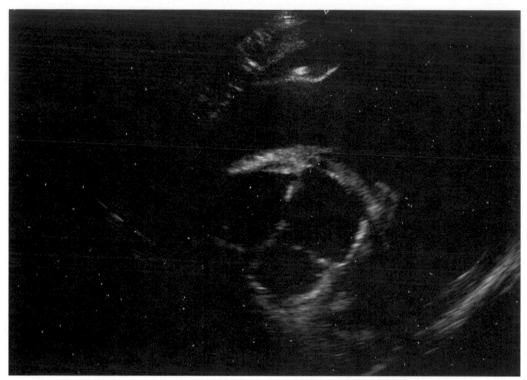

Figure 5-11 A right parasternal long-axis image of a 19-year-old polo pony that presented with weight loss, polydipsia, and polyuria associated with splenic lymphosarcoma and hypercalcemia of malignancy. Calcification of the aortic valves is evident.

absorption is poor[41] and therefore the intravenous or intramuscular routes are most appropriate, given at a dose of 1 to 2 mg/kg two or three times per day.

Aortocardiac Fistula

Aortocardiac fistula is not unique to the older horse population,[42,43] nor to males,[44] although this condition was first described as a disease of the older stallion.[45] The etiopathogenesis remains to be clarified, but it is thought that acquired degenerative changes in the media or a pre-existing sinus of Valsalva aneurysm precedes rupture.[42-45] On rupture, the fistula may enter the right atrium or ventricle, and such fistulas are frequently associated with a dissecting hematoma that tracks through the interventricular septum and disrupts the conduction tissue.[43] The rupture often occurs during exercise or breeding. Some horses die suddenly, whereas others exhibit signs of thoracic pain, with ventricular tachycardia and a continuous low-pitched murmur that is loudest on the right side. The diagnosis can be confirmed with echocardiography (Fig. 5-9). Unfortunately, the prognosis is hopeless, although affected horses can remain stable with a reasonable quality of life for periods as long as 12 months.[42-44]

Cardiac Neoplasia

Cardiac neoplasia appears to be uncommon in horses and, although in the authors' experiences older horses are

generally affected, neoplasia is not confined to older horses, occurring sporadically throughout all age groups. Lymphosarcoma, hemangiosarcoma, and metastatic carcinoma can affect the heart, and horses may present with loud murmurs and echocardiographic evidence of cardiac infiltration (Fig. 5-10). Hypercalcemia of malignancy has been reported in association with a wide range of forms of neoplasia, particularly lymphosarcoma.[46] Affected horses generally present with polydipsia and polyuria related to renal dysfunction. Cardiovascular signs are rarely prominent, but there can be systolic murmurs over the aortic valve associated with the calcification of the cardiac valves that is a common finding in this condition (Fig. 5-11).

SUMMARY

The existing pathologic and auscultatory studies on the prevalence of cardiac disease demonstrate that geriatric horses are at increased risk of developing left-sided valvular insufficiencies. Many are clinically well-tolerated and are not necessarily associated with an increased risk of death, but in a proportion of older horses, these and other forms of cardiac disease such as aortocardiac fistula and cardiac dysfunction can lead to signs of severe cardiac dysfunction. The approach to the geriatric horse with cardiac disease is similar to the approach to other cardiac patients. In horses, the main focus is on diagnosis, therefore careful clinical examination and echocardiography are the most important tools in this respect. Currently, our ability to manage cardiac failure effectively is somewhat limited, although palliative treatment in the short- or medium-term can be achieved. Many older horses with primary cardiac disease present before cardiac failure ensues, and studies that most effectively identify those individuals with a poor prognosis are emerging, although further work in this area is needed.

REFERENCES

1. Else RW, Holmes JR: Cardiac pathology in the horse: 1. Gross pathology. Equine Vet J 4:1, 1972.
2. Stevens KB, Marr CM, Horn JNR, et al: The effect of mitral and aortic valvular insufficiency on survival of a population of middle-aged and older horses. Equine Vet J, submitted, 2005.
3. Carmichael JA, Buergelt CD, Lord PF, et al: Diagnosis of patent ductus arteriosus in a horse. J Am Vet Med Assoc 158:767, 1971.
4. Missirlis YF, Armeniades CD, Kennedy JH: Mechanical and histological study of aortic valve tissue from a patient with Marfan's disease. Atherosclerosis 24:335, 1976.
5. Maxson AD, Reef VB: Bacterial endocarditis in horses: ten cases (1984-1995). Equine Vet J 29:394, 1997.
6. Reppas GP, Canfield PJ, Hartley WJ, et al: Multiple congenital cardiac anomalies and idiopathic thoracic aortitis in a horse. Vet Rec 138:14, 1996.
7. Diaz OS, Sleeper MM, Reef VB, et al: Aortitis in a Paint gelding. Equine Vet J 32:354, 2000.
8. Collatos C: Bacterial endocarditis. In Robinson NE, editor. Current Therapy in Equine Medicine. Philadelphia, W.B. Saunders, 1992, p 399-402.
9. Bishop SP, Cole CR, Smetzer DL: Functional and morphological pathology of equine aortic insufficiency. Vet Pathol 3:137, 1966.
10. Agozzino L, De Vivo F, Falco A, et al: Non-inflammatory aortic root disease and floppy aortic valve as cause of isolated regurgitation: a clinico-morphologic study. Int J Cardiol 45:129, 1994.
11. Else RW, Holmes JR: Cardiac pathology in the horse: 2. Microscopic pathology. Equine Vet J 4:57, 1972.
12. Reef VB, Spencer P: Echocardiographic evaluation of equine aortic insufficiency. Am J Vet Res 48:904, 1987.
13. Patteson MW, Cripps PJ: A survey of cardiac auscultatory findings in horses. Equine Vet J 25:409, 1993.
14. Blissitt KJ, Bonagura JD: Colour flow Doppler echocardiography in horses with cardiac murmurs. Equine Vet J Suppl:82, 1995.
15. Marr CM, Reef VB: Physiological valvular regurgitation in clinically normal young racehorses: Prevalence and two-dimensional colour flow Doppler echocardiographic characteristics. Equine Vet J Suppl 19:56, 1995.
16. Kriz NG, Hodgson DR, Rose RJ: Prevalence and clinical importance of heart murmurs in racehorses. J Am Vet Med Assoc 216:1441, 2000.
17. Horn JNR: Sympathetic nervous control of cardiac function and its role in equine heart disease. PhD Thesis, University of London, 2002.
18. Oldershaw PJ, Brooksby IA, Davies MJ, et al: Correlations of fibrosis in endomyocardial biopsies from patients with aortic valve disease. Br Heart J 44:609, 1980.
19. Liu SK, Magid NR, Fox PR, et al: Fibrosis, myocyte degeneration and heart failure in chronic experimental aortic regurgitation. Cardiology 90:101, 1998.
20. Maron BJ, Ferrans VJ, Roberts WC: Myocardial ultrastructure in patients with chronic aortic valve disease. Am J Cardiol 35:725, 1975.
21. Schwarz F, Kittstein D, Winkler B, et al: Quantitative ultrastructure of the myocardium in chronic aortic valve disease. Basic Res Cardiol 75:109, 1980.
22. Ettinger SJ, Benitz AM, Ericsson GF, et al: Effects of enalapril maleate on survival of dogs with naturally acquired heart failure. The Long-Term Investigation of Veterinary Enalapril (LIVE) Study Group. J Am Vet Med Assoc 213:1573, 1998.
23. Swedberg K, Kjekshus J, Snapinn S: Long-term survival in severe heart failure in patients treated with enalapril: ten year follow-up of CONSENSUS I. Eur Heart J 20:136, 1999.
24. McKelvie RS, Yusuf S, Pericak D, et al: Comparison of candesartan, enalapril, and their combination in congestive heart failure: Randomized evaluation of strategies for left ventricular dysfunction (RESOLVD) pilot study. The RESOLVD Pilot Study Investigators. Circulation 100:1056, 1999.
25. McMahon EG: Recent studies with eplerenone, a novel selective aldosterone receptor antagonist. Curr Opin Pharmacol 1:190, 2001.
26. Pedersen HD, Olsen LH, Arnorsdottir H: Breed differences in plasma renin activity and plasma aldosterone concentrations in dogs. J Vet Med Series A 42:435, 1995.
27. Pedersen HD, Olsen LH, Mow T, et al: Neuroendocrine changes in Dachshunds with mitral valve prolapse examined under different study conditions. Res Vet Sci 68:11, 1998.
28. Zdrojewski TR, Wyrzykowski B, Krupa-Wojciechowska B: Renin-aldosterone regulation during upright posture in young men with mitral valve prolapse syndrome. J Heart Valve Dis 4:236, 1995.
29. Aherne AM, Vaughan CJ, Carey RM, et al: Localisation of dopamine D1A receptor protein and messenger ribonucleic acid in rat adrenal cortex. Endocrinology 138:1282, 1997.
30. Lumbers ER: Angiotensin and aldosterone. Regul Pept 80:91, 1999.
31. Marr CM: Heart failure. In Marr CM, editor. Cardiology of the Horse. London WB Saunders, 1999, p 289-311.
32. Gardner SY, Atkins CE, Sams RA, et al: Characterisation of the pharmacokinetic and pharmacodynamic properties of the angiotensin-converting enzyme inhibitor, enalapril, in horses. J Vet Intern Med 18:231, 2004.
33. Young LE, Wood JL: Effect of age and training on murmurs of atrioventricular valvular regurgitation in young thoroughbreds. Equine Vet J 32:195, 2000.
34. Reef VB, Bain FT, Spencer PA: Severe mitral regurgitation in horses: Clinical, echocardiographic and pathological findings. Equine Vet J 30:18, 1998.
35. Brown CM, Bell TG, Paradis MR, Breeze RG: Rupture of mitral chordae tendineae in two horses. J Am Vet Med Assoc 182:878, 1983.
36. Holmes JR, Miller PJ: Three cases of ruptured mitral chordae tendineae in the horse. Equine Vet J 16:125, 1984.
37. Dedrick P, Reef VB, Sweeney RW, Morris DD: Treatment of bacterial endocarditis in a horse. Equine Vet J 193:339, 1990.
38. Miller PJ, Holmes JR: Observations on seven cases of mitral insufficiency in the horse. Equine Vet J 17:181, 1985.
39. Pedersoli WM, Belmonte AA, Purohit RC, Nachreiner RF: Pharmacokinetics of digoxing in the horse. J Equine Med Surg 2:384, 1978.
40. Sweeny RW, Reef VB, Reimer JM: Pharmacokinetic of digoxin administered to horses with congestive heart failure. Am J Vet Res 54:1108, 1993.
41. ACVIM furosemide oral abstract
42. Lester GD, Lombard CW, Ackerman N: Echocardiographic detection of a dissecting aortic root aneurysm in a Thoroughbred stallion. Vet Radiol Ultrasound 33:202, 1992.
43. Marr CM, Reef VB, Brazil TJ, et al: Aorto-cardiac fistulas in seven horses. Vet Radiol Ultrasound 39:22, 1998.
44. Roby KAW, Reef VB, Shaw DP, Sweeny CR: Rupture of an aortic sinus aneurysm in a 15-year-old broodmare. J Am Vet Med Assoc 189:305, 1986.
45. Rooney JR, Prickett ME, Crowe MW: Aortic ring rupture in stallions. Pathol Vet 4:268, 1967.
46. Marr CM, Love S, Pirie HM: Clinical, ultrasonographic and pathological findings in a horse with splenic lymphosarcoma and pseudohyperparathyroidism. Equine Vet J 21:221, 1989.

CHAPTER 6

Dentistry in the Geriatric Horse

Gordon J. Baker,

Keith J. Chandler

Dentistry is the branch of medical science that deals with the care of the teeth. It is recognized that abnormalities of the teeth and their supporting structures in the horse are influenced by conditions of wear. If an imbalance occurs between the rate of erupted crown attrition and the over- or super-eruption of the equivalent tooth or teeth in the opposing arcade, then the longer such imbalances exist without correction, the worse such abnormalities will become (Fig. 6-1). Consequently, the older horse may well present with extreme forms of such malocclusions as wave mouths, shear mouths, hooks, ramps, incisor malalignments, and periodontal diseases. Most elderly horses and ponies have some dental disease, and the degree of dysfunction and abnormalities present can be dramatic. Two elderly animals of a similar age, breed, and feeding regimen can present in contrasting body condition and the main difference between them will be inadequate dental care in one animal. Of all the regular care given to geriatric horses and ponies, dentistry is by far the most important. A failure to assimilate and digest food results in weight loss, and this is particularly evident in the winter months when the animals are fed a preserved diet. Veterinarians who mainly examine young equine athletes must be aware that the dentition is more important to the geriatric horse's welfare than may be the case in other age groups. The stress associated with a painful mouth and poor digestion may lead on to other problems, such as an increased susceptibility to infections.

Prior to evaluating the oral cavity, an accurate medical history should be obtained because many of the aged horses presented for correction of dental abnormalities have coexisting medical complaints. In addition, it is essential to obtain information on previous dental care, diet, appetite, and the presence of halitosis or quidding. Although quidding (spilling of masticated food) is a common sign of dental dysfunction, or oral pain, not all horses with dental disease display this sign and every geriatric horse should undergo a detailed and thorough oral examination with the use of an oral speculum. Examination of the oral cavity has been detailed elsewhere.[1]

AGE-RELATED CHANGES IN HORSES' TEETH

The timing of eruption of the permanent teeth of the horse is age-related, with some variation between individuals. The incisors erupt in sequence at 2.5, 3.5, and 4.5 years of age. The three deciduous premolar teeth in each row are replaced at approximately 2.5, 3, and 3.5 years. The true molar teeth numbers 9, 10, and 11 in the Triadan system erupt at 10 months to 1 year, 2 years, and 3.5 years of age, respectively.

As in other herbivores, the teeth of the horse erupt continuously; however, the teeth of hypsodonts such as the horse cease growing within a few years of erupting. In a study of the age-related morphology of equine mandibular cheek teeth, it was shown that even though the erupted crown is worn away during masticatory attrition, there is in fact an overall increase in tooth length during the first year after eruption.[2]

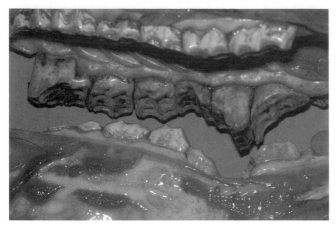

Figure 6-1 Fracture and loss of 410, overgrowth of 110, and reshaping of 109 and 111. (From Baker GJ, Easley J, editors: Equine Dentistry. St. Louis, W.B. Saunders, 1999.)

Overall tooth length is then maintained for 2 years. This discrepancy is caused by rate of production of the true roots faster than the rate of crown attrition immediately after eruption of the tooth. From 3 years after eruption, the loss of erupted crown due to wear exceeds the apical lengthening resulting from true root formation, and there is therefore a reduction in overall tooth length. While the crown and reserve crown length decrease each year from 0 to 8 years after eruption, the rate of tooth loss is also not constant. The rate of crown loss has been found to increase from 5 to 7 years after eruption. In studies, the rate of root formation was highest up until 5 years after eruption and then decreased. These results suggest that the cheek teeth of the horse undergo an increased rate of attrition, an increased rate of eruption, or both during the period of rapid root formation in the first 5 years after eruption. The variable rate of crown loss may be influenced by the rate of root formation, the rate of eruption of the reserve crown. It is also influenced by changes in "hardness" of the teeth as secondary dentin is formed in the pulp chamber to protect the pulp chamber from exposure to the oral cavity, thereby increasing the overall proportion of dentin in the tooth and hence the resistance to attrition. It is also probable that rates of crown attrition are influenced by the nature of the feedstuffs consumed.

It has been shown that the excursion (lateral movement) of the mandibles during the masticatory cycle is reduced when dry feeds are chewed as compared with grass.[3-5] Whether such reduction in lateral excursions affects the rate of crown attrition is unknown. It is known, however, that reduced or incomplete lateral excursions and occlusal surface contact does exacerbate the enamel points on the buccal edges of the maxillary cheek teeth and the lingual edges of the mandibular cheek teeth. In turn, these may create buccal mucosal

ulcers, scars, and indurations. Such areas are sensitive to cheek pressure on palpation and mouth opening and tend to compound the problems of tooth wear and irregularities.

It has been noted that the teeth of the horse function as integrated units. Two sets of incisor teeth made up of six individual teeth and four rows of cheek teeth each made up of six individual teeth. The integrity of each row is created by the deposition of peripheral coronal cementum such that there are minimal interproximal spaces between the teeth. With age, as the reserve crowns are erupted, it will be seen that there is a change in the shape of each tooth component as they taper toward the roots. A combination of events therefore starts a trend in which interproximal (interdental) pockets enlarge with age.

Maturation is also accompanied by continuous rostral movement and flattening of the incisor bite plane. As the reserve crowns erupt, the maxillary paranasal sinus cavities enlarge and there is slight rostral movement of the cheek teeth. As the teeth wear away, there are subtle changes in the architecture of the occlusal surfaces of the cheek teeth. Pulp chamber exposure is protected by the production of secondary dentin and, in the upper cheek teeth, the infundibular or cement lakes are worn away. This process has been described as "cupping out" or "cupped out" (Fig. 6-2). It follows that, since the first upper molars (108 and 208) erupt at some 8 months of age, they are subject to up to 3.5 more years of wear than their associates in the cheek tooth masticatory unit. Dentine and cementum are both softer than enamel and, as a consequence, the surfaces flatten and become

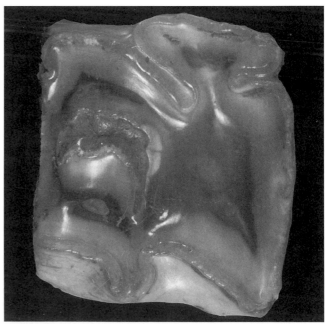

Figure 6-2 Occlusal surface of 108 showing cupping out after attrition of the cement lakes.

smoother as the infundibula are lost. It has been suggested that this phenomenon is the cause of the onset of wave mouth formation.[3]

DENTAL PATHOLOGIC CONDITIONS IN THE GERIATRIC HORSE

Periodontal Disease

Most geriatric horses have a degree of periodontal disease. Periodontal disease is the presence of disease and loss of tissue in those structures that surround the tooth or teeth. *Periodontium* means "around the tooth" and in that sense is confined to the bony socket. In clinical practice, the periodontium includes the alveolus (bony socket) cement, the periodontal ligament, and the gingiva.

Classification of various periodontal diseases is difficult, as nearly every case begins as a minor localized disturbance, which, unless adequately treated, gradually worsens until the alveolar bone is resorbed, the periodontal ligament becomes compromised, and the tooth loosens and is eventually exfoliated. This means that a variety of causative stimuli may produce similar end-stage pathologic conditions and so the true etiopathogenesis may not be clear.

Periodontal inflammation has been recognized for years as being important in the horse. It was suggested that quidding was a pathognomonic sign of periodontal disease or alveolar periostitis.[6] In those observations, it was noted that the lesions start primarily in the interproximal (interdental) areas of the teeth and the caudal mandibular spaces were most affected. In an examination of the teeth and gums of 218 and 446 skulls, it was found that the incidence of periodontal disease changed with age. There was a 40 percent prevalence in horses 3 to 5 years of age; this fell in horses 5 to 10 years of age and then increased to 60 percent in horses older than 15 years of age.

Gingival hyperemia, edema, ulceration, deepening periodontal pockets, and packing of feed material into these spaces are the classic pictures of periodontal disease (Figs. 6-3 and 6-4). The presence of diastema enables food entrapment and its subsequent degradation, which results in gingivitis. It is necessary, of course, to carry out a detailed examination of the mouth to detect such conditions at an early stage. There may be both supra- and subgingival plaque and calculus deposits associated with these lesions. Periodontal disease in the horse has been divided into four categories based on evaluation of the severity of the lesion (Box 6-1).

Horses with grades 1 and 2 periodontal disease may not show overt signs of oral discomfort. The careful owner may notice some excess salivation and sensitivity to cold water. Halitosis is the pathognomonic sign for

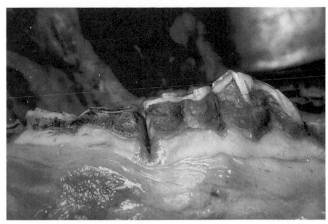

Figure 6-3 Gingival hyperemia and edema. (From Baker GJ, Easley J, editors: Equine Dentistry. St. Louis, W.B. Saunders, 1999.)

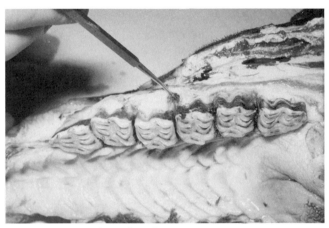

Figure 6-4 Periodontal pocketing.

severe periodontal disease in the horse, and for this reason the use of disposable gloves is recommended when examining the oral cavity of the horse.

The role of normal dental work in maintaining the health of periodontal structures has been documented in most mammals. It therefore is not surprising that abnormalities of wear associated with tooth eruptions in young horses and arcade irregularities in older horses are the most common initiating factors in the pathogenesis of

---

Box 6-1

The Four Categories of Periodontal Disease

1. Local gingivitis with hyperemia and edema
2. Erosion of gingival margin 5 mm and periodontal pocket
3. Periodontitis with loss of gum
4. Gross periodontal pocketing, lysis of alveolar bone, loosening of bone support

periodontal disease in the horse. Detection of periodontal changes and dental procedures to prevent deterioration may be particularly important in preventing or delaying chronic, irreversible changes.

Other factors influence the development and progression of periodontal disease, and it is commonly described as being a multifactorial infection. Some of these factors include plaque, oral microflora, and calculus as well as age, general health, chewing patterns, breed, immune status and local irritants (e.g., grass awns).

Plaque is an organic matrix made up of salivary glycoproteins and it contains oral bacteria as well as inorganic material derived from feed materials. Bacterial fermentation within this layer releases free radicals and material that results in injury to the gingiva and within the gingival sulcus. Aerobic bacteria are more prevalent in supragingival plaque, and facultative anaerobes live in the sulcus. Bacterial numbers and types change in the presence of initial gingival inflammation and initiate the "domino" cycle (Fig. 6-5).

In cases of advanced disease, there is significant loss of alveolar bone. Periodontal inflammation may result in attempted repair with the production of excess cementum over the surface of the reserve crown. In some cases, this may progress to a form of hypercementosis and the production of nodules of cementum.

Treatment

The horse is no exception to the general rule of periodontists that prevention is better than treatment. Once gum recession and loss have occurred, it is not possible to undertake a treatment regimen that will result in reattachment of gum and a reduction of gingival pocket size in the horse. Consequently, the equine clinicians' role is to eliminate irregularities of wear, oral ulcers, and other conditions that may initiate the progressive process of periodontal pathology.

In horses with major irregularities of wear and advanced periodontal pocketing, treatment is aimed at restoring, as closely as possible, normal or near-normal occlusion. Loose teeth should be extracted and periodontal pockets irrigated and opened where possible—that is, enlarged so as to discourage food impactions in these areas.

In the management of cases with large diastemal pockets, it is recommended that, in addition to introducing a program of regular arcade balancing, the pockets be irrigated, sterilized, and packed with protective coatings, such as impressions material. The use of systemic antibiotics and local packing with antimicrobial eluting materials (Doxyrobe Gel, Pharmacia and Upjohn, Kalamazoo, MI) have also been advocated.[7]

Although periodontal disease affects the cheek teeth most commonly, the incisors can also be affected, particularly if substantial diastemata are present, although these teeth rarely become so diseased as to need extracting. Incisor diastemata are usually not associated with severe clinical signs, but they can be enlarged using a rotary saw or a diastema burr, and this prevents build up of food material. However, daily brushing (with a soft nail brush, for example) of the incisors is easy to perform and can become a part of the animal's daily grooming routine.

Diastema

A *diastema* is defined as an abnormal, detectable space between the teeth. These normally arise as a result of tooth narrowing with age and the interproximal (interdental) space enlarging. In addition, it has been proposed that diastemata also develop as a result of interdental wear and lack of rostrocaudal compression.[8] Although easy to visualize in the incisors, they are more difficult to appreciate in the cheek teeth, and it has been suggested that the use of a flexible or rigid endoscope orally, or palpation with a fingernail, is used to chart the presence of a diastema.[8] As a primary problem, they are commonly found between fourth and fifth cheek teeth and often as a result of cheek teeth displacements or rotations (Fig. 6-6). Although these displacements may occur developmentally in the young horse, displacements tend to affect the caudal cheek teeth—that is, the molars of the maxilla and more commonly the mandibular molars—in geriatric horses. Large opposing

Inflammation → Plaque build up → Hyperemia

↑

Loss of tooth ↓

↑

Bone loss ← Loss of support ← Edema
                              tissue

Figure 6-5 The "domino" cycle.

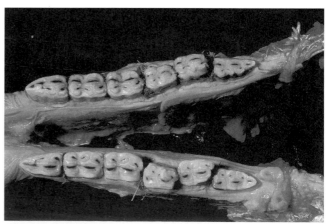

Figure 6-6 Diastema formation and tooth rotation.

overgrowths are sometimes present and a diastema is found on either side of the displacement, often with concomitant periodontal disease.

Treatment

Diastemata are a significant cause of oral pain and quidding associated with food pocketing and periodontal disease or gingivitis. Removing dental overgrowths and sharp enamel points can result in an improvement; in advanced cases, some animals respond well to tooth reduction or removal even where significant periodontal disease is present.[8] Daily oral lavage appears to help some animals by removing food debris from diastema, and this also helps the associated periodontal disease that many of these animals have. Feeding soft feed or grass and avoiding hay appears to help reduce food build-up in some cases. Judicious use of nonsteroidal anti-inflammatory drugs can alleviate some oral discomfort.

Malocclusions

Abnormalities of wear may lead in some older horses to bizarre occlusal patterns. Large hooks on 106, 206, 311, and 411 exacerbate wave formations and, with the loss of rostrocaudal and caudorostral compression, there may be rotation of affected teeth as diastemal pockets enlarge. Loss of teeth in one unit will result in apparent super-eruption of the opposing tooth. Such overgrowths may be pronounced (see Fig. 6-1). Invariably, advanced forms of periodontal disease, often with loosening of teeth, accompany such overgrowths. Incisor malocclusions are often linked to cheek tooth malocclusion but may also occur from primary incisor tooth disease[9,10] (Fig. 6-7). However, many horses with incisor brachgnathism do not appear to have cheek tooth malalignment, suggesting that the growth abnormality is in the incisive bone or rostral mandible. Old horses with untreated "parrot" mouths may have palatine trauma as a result of the lack of occlusal attrition of the erupting mandibular incisors. These lower incisors impact into the hard palate caudal to the upper incisors.

Treatment

All loose and decayed teeth in association with malocclusions should be extracted. Major overgrowths, hooks, ramps, and steps should be reduced. The use of power dental equipment, sedation, head supports, and good lighting greatly facilitates such work. It is important that the equine veterinary dentist keeps in mind that major malalignments have not occurred over a short period. Because of the dangers of thermal injury and pulp exposure associated with misuse of mechanical burrs, it is best to correct major anomalies in stages.[11]

Care must be taken in the use of molar cutters in old horses. It is quite easy to fracture overgrown teeth

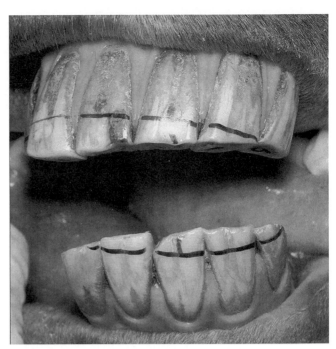

Figure 6-7 Incisor malalignment following loss of 403. Markings indicate line of incisor reduction for correction.

longitudinally when trying to cut overgrowths. Such accidents may create pulp exposures and subsequent dental decay and abscessation. Modern mechanical tools have rendered such instruments largely obsolete.

It is not appropriate to restore a normal occlusal shape (in the rostrocaudal plane) in advanced cases of wave mouth because this may remove occlusal contact between parts of the cheek teeth rows for a prolonged period, resulting in an exacerbation in masticatory difficulties.[12] It is better to remove focal overgrowths and sharp points and reduce the extremes of the wave mouth step by step. In addition, because of the short reserve crowns in aged horses, preservation of the tooth should always be the aim.

All major dentistry in geriatric horses should be supported with analgesic/anti-inflammatory drugs and, when indicated, antibiotics.

Smooth Mouth

Smooth mouth is the absence of enamel on the occlusal surface of the cheek teeth. As the enamel wears out, the dentin and cement are exposed, resulting in rapid wear of these teeth. It is easy to identify, as the affected teeth are extremely smooth on the occlusal surface and have lost all the enamel in-folding and ridges. All the cheek teeth can be affected progressively, although this condition tends to begin in the maxillary cheek teeth. As certain teeth lose their enamel, these teeth wear rapidly, and the opposing tooth can become overgrown, resulting in wave mouth (Figs. 6-8 and 6-9). Smooth mouth is the precursor of complete tooth loss through wear, and little

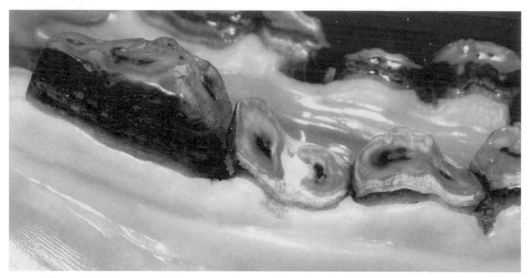

Figure 6-8 Wave mouth in an aged pony. Note food trapping in the diastemata.

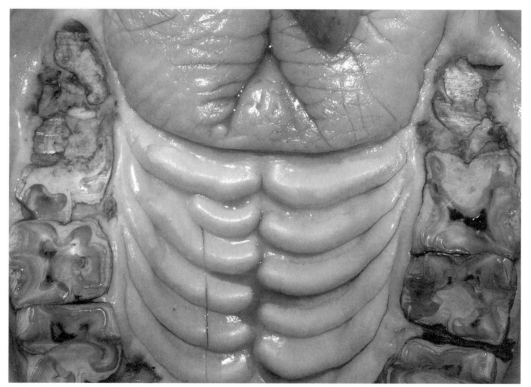

Figure 6-9 Smooth mouth: the penultimate state before complete tooth loss in aged equine animals. Note the food trapping between 208 and 209.

can be done to help these animals, apart from dietary management (see below) and the reduction of opposing overgrowths.

Dental Caries

Caries is the disease and dissolution of the inorganic portion of the tooth and is associated with an increased prevalence with advancing age,[13] although apical abscesses are more common in horses 2 to 7 years of age.[14] The cause is unclear, although pulpal exposure due to infundibular caries or failure of secondary dentine deposition in the pulp cavity as the tooth erupts has been suggested. Parasagittal fractures communicating with one or more pulp cavities have also been identified (Dacre I, personal communication). Cemental hypoplasia may be a developmental disorder, or dissolution may be the consequence of continued infundibular food impaction. Many apparently idiopathic longitudinal fractures of maxillary molars—particularly of 109, 110, 209, and 210—can be the result of a preexisting caries lesion, although the pathogenesis is currently unclear. Although in many cases the condition is apparently not painful in the early stages, advanced caries resulting in apical pulpal necrosis and abscessation is associated with alveolar remodelling and dental sinusitis if the caudal maxillary teeth are involved. Parasagittal cheek tooth fractures can be associated with lateral displacement of the lateral fragment, allowing severe overgrowths of the opposing tooth that contributes to impaction of food in the fracture line. Currently, the only treatment for severely necrotic teeth or those with advance caries is tooth removal by extraction, repulsion, or lateral buccotomy. Some attempts to perform endodontic root canal treatments in early cases are currently being attempted.[15] Chronic cases of dental sinusitis in geriatric horses can be frustrating to treat and may also be associated with Cushing's disease. Such cases can be refractory to treatment and carry a more guarded prognosis

SUMMARY

The classic picture of the older horse with dental disease is a thin, slow-eating horse with improperly digested feed in the feces. There may be quidding and halitosis. It has been emphasized that disease of the support struc- tures of the teeth—periodontal disease—is the single most important contributor to impaired dental function in the geriatric horse. The equine dental veterinarians may well be presented with conditions for which only palliative treatment is necessary. For that reason, it is now possible to supplement any treatments with custom designed feed materials and calorie additives (corn oil or canola oil) to restore and maintain body condition in old horses. Cases have been reported in which horses with totally smooth mouths or mouths with minimal erupted crown (Fig. 6-10) material are able to thrive on soaked senior equine feed materials and/or corn oil and soaked alfalfa cubes.

Geriatric horses should have their mouths examined at least twice a year, to enable early detection of potentially serious abnormalities, and have appropriate dental treat- ments applied. Not every loose cheek tooth should be removed, as many will re-attach if other dental abnormali- ties are attended to. In addition, these animals should be current on vaccinations, worm control programs, and hoof care, and a thorough examination of the animal for any predisposing intercurrent disease should be performed.

The objective of all dentistry in geriatric horses is to document the nature of the dental problems and to ini- tiate a treatment program or programs that will arrest the progression of the disease process and to restore bal- ance in the masticatory machinery.

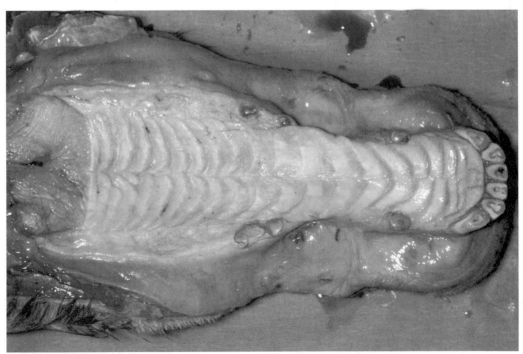

Figure 6-10 Upper jaw of a 35-year-old horse. This horse was euthanized because of a fractured humerus. It had been maintained on Equine Senior (Purina) for 5 years.

REFERENCES

1. Easley J: Dental and oral examination. In Baker GJ, Easley J, eds: Equine Dentistry. St. Louis, W.B. Saunders, 1999, p 107-127.
2. Kirkland KD: The Morphology of the Endodontic System Reserve Crown and Roots of Equine Mandibular Cheek Teeth. M.S. thesis, University of Illinois, 1994, p 24-102.
3. Leue G: [Relationship between tooth anomalies and digestive disorders in equids.] Veterinary Medicine Dissertation, Hanover, 1941.
4. Baker GJ: Dental physiology. In Baker GJ, Easley J, eds: Equine Dentistry. St. Louis, W.B. Saunders, 1999, p 29-34.
5. Bonin SJ: Three Dimensional Kinematics of the Equine Temporomandibular Joint. M.S. Thesis, Michigan State University, 2001.
6. Little WM: Periodontal disease in the horse. J Comp Pathol Therap 24:240, 1913.
7. Greene SI, Basile TP: Recognition and treatment of equine periodontal disease. Proc AAEP 48:463, 2002.
8. Dixon PM, Tremaine WH, Pickles K, et al: Equine dental disease. Part 2: a long term study of 400 cases: disorders of development and eruption and variations in position of the cheek teeth. Equine Vet J 31:519, 1999.
9. Wilewski K, Basile T, Pence P: Geriatric horse dentistry. In Pence P, editor: Equine Dentistry, A Practical Guide. Philadephia, Lippincott Williams & Wilkins, 2002, p 169-189.
10. Lowder MQ, Mueller POE: Dental disease in geriatric horses. Vet Clin North Am 14:365, 1998.
11. Baker GJ, Allen ML: The use of power equipment in equine dentistry. Proc AAEP 48:438, 2002.
12. Dixon PM, Tremaine WH, Pickles K, et al: Equine dental disease. Part 3: A long term study of 400 cases: disorders of wear, traumatic damage and idiopathic fractures, tumors and miscellaneous disorders of the cheek teeth. Equine Vet J 32:9, 2000.
13. Baker GJ: Some aspects of dental disease. Equine Vet J 2:105, 1970.
14. Dixon PM, Tremaine WH, Pickles K, et al: Equine dental disease. Part 4: a long-term study of 400 cases: apical infections of cheek teeth. Equine Vet J 32:182, 2000.
15. Baker GJ: Dental decay and endodontic disease. In Baker GJ, Easley J, eds: Equine Dentistry. St. Louis, W.B. Saunders, 1999, p 79-85.

CHAPTER 7

Endocrine Dysfunction in the Aged Horse

Nat T. Messer IV

The function of the endocrine system changes in the aged horse both as a normal process of aging as well as with various pathologic disorders resulting in endocrine dysfunction. Our understanding of equine endocrine disease has made significant advances in the past few years, making it apparent that past clinical impressions and extrapolation of findings from other species to horses must be discarded in some instances and embraced in others in lieu of new discoveries.

THYROID DYSFUNCTION

The normal equine thyroid gland is located dorsal to the trachea in the most proximal portion of the trachea. The two lobes of the thyroid gland are joined by an isthmus and in the normal state are not visible but can be easily palpated. Approximately 90 percent of the hormone secreted by the thyroid gland is thyroxine (T4), with the remainder being triiodothyronine (T3). A considerable portion of the secreted T4 is converted to T3 in peripheral tissues by 5′-monodeiodinase. The functions of these two hormones are qualitatively the same, but they differ in rapidity and intensity of action, with T3 being four times as potent as T4 but persisting in blood for a much shorter period of time.

The thyroid gland is composed of large numbers of follicles filled with a secretory substance called *colloid* and lined with cuboidal epithelial cells that secrete into the interior of the follicles. The major component of colloid is a large glycoprotein called *thyroglobulin*, which contains the thyroid hormones. This extracellular stor-age of hormone within an endocrine gland is unique to the thyroid gland, allowing the thyroid gland to have a large reserve capacity. For secretion of thyroid hormones to take place, the thyroglobulin-thyroid hormone complex must enter the apical portion of the thyroid follicular cell where digestive proteinases digest the thyroglobu-lin molecules and release T3 and T4, which then diffuse through the base of the thyroid cell and enter the circula-tion. The thyroid gland is estimated to have a blood flow equal to five times the weight of the gland each minute, which is as rich a blood supply as any other area of the body with the possible exception of the adrenal gland.

The most important regulator of thyroid activity is thyroid stimulating hormone (TSH), or thyrotropin. TSH secretion is regulated by levels of thyroid hormone by way of negative feedback inhibition of the synthesis of thyrotropin-releasing hormone (TRH) at the level of the hypothalamus (long-feedback loop) and by inhibi-tion of the activity of TSH at the level of the pituitary gland (short-feedback loop) (Fig. 7-1).

In adult euthyroid horses, there is a slight but progres-sive decrease in thyroid hormone levels with age.[1] Other disorders of thyroid gland function in horses are uncom-mon and, in most cases, misunderstood or misdiag-nosed.[2-4] Hypothyroidism accounts for most cases described in horses. Hypothyroidism indicates that there are low serum levels of biologically active thyroid hor-mones and is classified as primary, secondary, or tertiary, depending on the cause. Primary hypothyroidism, caused by intrinsic thyroid gland disease, is very rare in horses. Secondary hypothyroidism, caused by inadequate

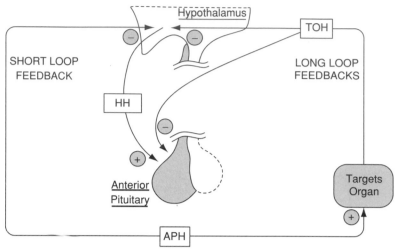

Figure 7-1 Regulation of anterior pituitary hormone (APH) secretion by hypophysiotropic hormones (HH), short-loop negative feedback, and long-loop negative feedback by target organ hormones (TOH). Plus signs indicate stimulation, and minus signs indicate inhibition. (From Hedge GA, Colby HD, Goodman RL: Clinical Endocrine Physiology. Philadelphia, W.B. Saunders, 1987, p 78.)

production and/or release of thyrotropin (TSH), may be the most common form of hypothyroidism in horses but is currently difficult to definitively diagnose because of the lack of readily available specific equine TSH assays. Tertiary hypothyroidism, caused by inadequate production and/or release of TRH, has not be described in horses.[3] Hyperthyroidism, characterized by high serum levels of biologically active thyroid hormones, has recently been described in association with thyroid gland neoplasia[5,6] (Fig. 7-2).

A number of nonthyroidal factors can affect serum levels of thyroid hormones in horses with normal thyroid glands, that is, euthyroid horses. These factors exert their effects through disruption of the normal hypothalamic-pituitary-thyroid axis or by affecting peripheral thyroid hormone action or metabolism.[7] The effect of phenylbutazone on serum levels of thyroid hormone is a good example.[3,8,9] Since phenylbutazone is highly protein bound, it tends to displace thyroid hormones from protein binding sites, effectively increasing levels of free hormone, which then decreases TSH release via negative feedback, resulting in decreased production of thyroid hormones by the thyroid gland. Other nonthyroidal factors that have been shown to cause low serum levels of thyroid hormones in horses with essentially normal thyroid glands include high-energy diets,[10] high-protein diets,[11] diets high in zinc and copper,[11] diets high in iodine,[11,12] diets with a high carbohydrate-to-roughage ratio,[13] conditions associated with glucocorticoid excess,[14] food deprivation,[14] level of training,[15] stage of pregnancy,[16,17] and ingestion of endophyte-infected fescue grass (Boosinger, 1995). There are undoubtedly other factors, as yet unidentified, that could potentially affect thyroid hormone levels in euthyroid horses.

Clinical Signs

A variety of clinical signs and conditions have been attributed to low serum levels of thyroid hormones in horses. Such things as obesity, "cresty" necks, laminitis, and infertility have all been attributed to low levels of thyroid hormones in clinical practice. However, the clinical signs resulting from surgical thyroidectomy, in

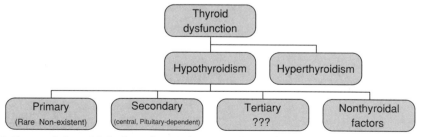

Figure 7-2 Types of thyroid dysfunction. In horses, primary hypothyroidism is rare, if not nonexistent; secondary hypothyroidism appears to be common; tertiary hypothyroidism has not been described; and there are numerous nonthyroidal factors resulting in low levels of thyroid hormones.

which serum levels of thyroid hormone are typically undetectable, are considerably different than those usually associated with "hypothyroidism" in clinical practice (Fig. 7-3). Thyroidectomized horses are more sensitive to cold temperatures and have coarse hair coats, mild alopecia, delayed shedding of hair coat, thickened facial features, edema in the hind legs, decreased feed consumption, decreased weight gains, lower rectal temperature, lower heart rate, decreased cardiac output, and exercise intolerance.[18-20] Thyroidectomized mares continue to cycle, become pregnant, and subsequently deliver normal foals.[21] Thyroidectomized stallions show reduced libido, but fertility is normal.[22]

A possible explanation for this discrepancy is that low serum levels of thyroid hormones occur as a result of another disease process or endocrine abnormality and are inappropriately attributed to thyroid gland dysfunction. The underlying disease or abnormality is actually what is responsible for causing the clinical signs observed and not the low thyroid hormone levels. Many of the clinical signs associated with low serum levels of thyroid hormones in clinical practice are nonspecific and have been shown to occur in horses with other diseases or endocrine abnormalities.[3]

In the cases of reported hyperthyroidism associated with thyroid gland neoplasia having high serum levels of thyroid hormones, clinical signs similar to those seen in other species with hyperthyroidism were present, including enlargement of the thyroid gland, weight loss, hyperexcitability, tachycardia, and polyphagia. These clinical signs disappeared after surgical removal of the tumor.[5,6]

Evaluation of Thyroid Dysfunction

Most cases of hypothyroidism are inappropriately diagnosed based on atypical and unreliable clinical signs, measurement of serum levels of thyroid hormones (total T3 and T4), and response to therapy with thyroid hormone supplementation.[2,3,23] As discussed earlier, clinical signs frequently associated with hypothyroidism have not been recognized in thyroidectomized horses; thus, clinical signs other than those seen in thyroidectomized horses may not be reliable diagnostic criteria. Serum thyroid hormone levels, when used alone are insensitive and often misleading, frequently resulting in the misdiagnosis of hypothyroidism in horses.[2,3,23,24] Measurement of free forms of thyroid hormones does reflect levels of biologically active thyroid hormones, but in horses it does not appear to provide additional useful information in assessing thyroid dysfunction.[23] A favorable response to therapy with thyroid hormone supplement is commonly cited as evidence of hypothyroidism, but since thyroid hormone supplementation improves overall metabolism, it may help horses affected with a variety of nonthyroidal illnesses and not be indicative of hypothyroidism.[3]

Accurate diagnosis of hypothyroidism must depend on the use of additional diagnostic tests to determine whether the function of the hypothalamic-pituitary-thyroid axis is normal.[25] Horses with a normal hypothalamic-pituitary-thyroid axis should not be referred to as hypothyroid. Ideally, the use of specific equine TSH assays combined with either TSH- or TRH-stimulation tests are required to accurately differentiate primary from secondary hypothyroidism and to differentiate both from other conditions resulting in low serum thyroid hormone levels in otherwise euthyroid horses.[2,3,25] Unfortunately, these additional tests are used less frequently in horses because of expense, limited availability, safety issues, and the potential for spurious results. Validated assays for equine TSH are not yet readily available for routine testing. Commercially available TSH and TRH for injection are both expensive and occasionally unavailable. Reagent grade TRH is being utilized for

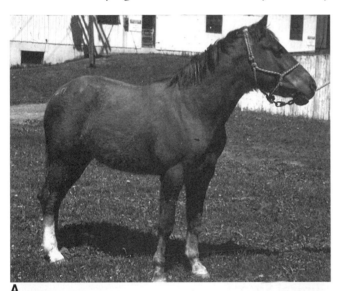

A

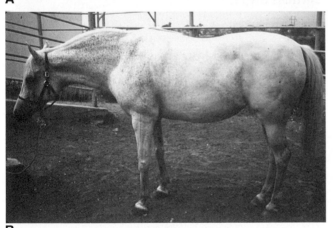

B

Figure 7-3 The horse on the top (A) has been thyroidectomized and is truly "hypothyroid," whereas the horse on the bottom (B) is obese, has a "cresty neck" and chronic laminitis, but is not "hypothyroid," as traditional dogma would suggest. (A, Courtesy of Dr. J.E. Lowe.)

diagnostic testing in research applications and by some clinically, but it is not packaged for sterile injection and should thus be used with caution. In some forms of secondary hypothyroidism, in which there is abnormal TSH release or TRH-induced TSH release, as might occur in states of glucocorticoid excess or during long-term supplementation with exogenous thyroid hormone, there may be minimal response to TRH stimulation resulting in the misdiagnosis of primary hypothyroidism.[3]

The TRH stimulation test is currently the only means of evaluating the status of the hypothalamic-pituitary-thyroid axis.[26,27] (Sojka, 1985). To perform this test, collect a serum sample just prior to testing, administer 1 mg of TRH intravenously and then collect serum samples 2 and 4 hours after administration of TRH. Serum levels of T3 and T4 in normal horses will be at least twice baseline levels after 2 and 4 hours, respectively. This test will not distinguish primary hypothyroidism from other forms of hypothyroidism and does have the limitations mentioned previously in this chapter. Since validated assays for equine TSH are not yet readily available for routine testing, naturally occurring thyroid dysfunction in adult horses remains difficult to characterize.

Treatment

Thyroid hormone supplementation should be implemented when horses have clinical signs similar to those observed in thyroidectomized horses, persistently low serum levels of thyroid hormones, and an inadequate response to TRH stimulation testing and when known nonthyroidal factors affecting thyroid function, mentioned previously in this chapter, have been ruled out as an underlying cause.[3] Thyroid hormone supplementation in horses with low serum levels of thyroid hormones due to things other than primary hypothyroidism have unknown benefit and may, in some instances, be detrimental.

A number of thyroid hormone replacement therapies are commercially available for use in horses. Treatment protocols should follow the label recommendation of the manufacturer and be accompanied by regular measurement of serum thyroid hormone levels to evaluate the effectiveness of the treatment.

In cases of hyperthyroidism associated with thyroid gland neoplasia, surgical removal of the thyroid tumor resulted in a return to normal thyroid hormone levels.[5,6]

PITUITARY PARS INTERMEDIA DYSFUNCTION

Pituitary pars intermedia dysfunction (PPID) in the horse is a slowly progressive disorder with a characteristic clinical picture (Fig. 7-4). Affected horses are usually older (>15 years) obese animals with a thick, "cresty"

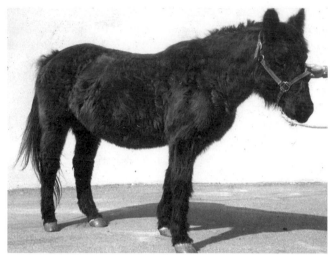

Figure 7-4 Horse with PPID demonstrating the classic sign of hirsutism: a long, shaggy hair coat that fails to shed in the spring.

neck and a long, curly hair coat (hirsutism) that fails to shed normally in the summer months.[28,29] Many of the horses have signs of chronic laminitis, polydipsia, polyuria, infertility, and chronic infections and are frequently hyperglycemic. In the end stages of this disease, horses tend to lose weight and muscle mass. Also referred to as equine Cushing's disease because of some similarities to Cushing's disease in human beings, this disorder may occasionally occur even when these characteristic clinical features are inapparent.[30]

The anterior lobe of the pituitary consists of three parts: pars distalis, pars intermedia, and pars tuberalis. The main secretory products of the corticotropes, located in the pars distalis, are adrenocorticotropic hormone (ACTH) and β-endorphin–related peptides, whereas the main secretory products of the melanotropes, located in the pars intermedia, are melanocyte-stimulating hormone and β-endorphin–related peptides. Both corticotropes and melanotropes synthesize the same precursor hormone, pro-opiomelanocortin, but cleave it into different hormones. Under normal circumstances, adrenocortical steroidogenesis is maintained by corticotrope secretion of ACTH and corticotropes are inhibited via negative feedback of glucocorticoids.

Historically, this condition has been considered to be neoplastic ("pituitary tumor," "pituitary adenoma"). Recent investigations indicate that PPID is more likely due to hypertrophy and hyperplasia of cells in the pars intermedia caused by loss of hypothalamic dopaminergic innervation.[31] Pars intermedia tumors in horses contain markedly reduced amounts of dopamine compared to normal pars intermedia tissues, and immunohistochemical methods show increased expression of type 2 dopamine receptors on pars intermedia melanotropes from horses with PPID.[32]

In horses with PPID, hypertrophy and hyperplasia of melanotropes result in a marked increase in pro-opiomelanocortin synthesis, with release of large amounts of melanocyte-stimulating hormone and β-endorphin–related peptides as well as comparatively small, but increased, amounts of ACTH.[31,33] The melanocyte-stimulating hormone and β-endorphin–related peptides are capable of inducing a six-fold increase in the steroidogenic properties of ACTH.[34] Therefore, a small increase in ACTH coupled with a large increase in potentiating peptides is sufficient to stimulate adrenocortical steroidogenesis resulting in an increase in plasma cortisol levels and, even more importantly, loss of the circadian pattern of cortisol secretion.[30] The insensitivity of melanotropes to glucocorticoids has diagnostic implications that permit differentiation of melanotrope-maintained steroidogenesis in affected animals from corticotrope-maintained steroidogenesis in normal animals by use of the dexamethasone suppression test.

Diagnosis

The dexamethasone suppression test (Box 7-1) is considered the "gold standard" endocrinologic test for PPID by many equine clinicians. In a study comparing endocrinologic test results in a large group of horses with both clinical and pathologic evidence of PPID with results in normal horses, 43 of 43 horses with PPID had plasma cortisol levels greater the 1 μg/dL 19 hours after dexamethasone administration, as compared with 18 control horses who had plasma cortisol values less than 1 μg/dL.[30] Dexamethasone administration must precede the normal diurnal increase in release of ACTH (early morning hours), and the post-dexamethasone blood sample must be collected after the normal time of increased ACTH release.[7] Prolonged suppression of ACTH by dexamethasone is dose-related, with 40 μg of dexamethasone per kilogram body weight causing maximal blockade and therefore maximal suppression of plasma cortisol.[30]

Box 7-1

Overnight Dexamethasone Suppression Test

1. Begin test between 4 and 6 pm.
2. Collect a baseline (pre-dexamethasone) sample into a heparinized container.
3. Administer dexamethasone (40 μg/kg or 2 mg/45 kg) IM between 4 and 6 pm.
4. Collect post-dexamethasone samples into heparinized containers at 12 pm the following day (approximately 19 hours after dexamethasone administration).

The heparinized containers should be centrifuged immediately after collection and the plasma harvested and either refrigerated or frozen depending on the time between collection and analysis. Samples are analyzed to determine plasma cortisol concentration; normal horses will have less than 1 μg/dL cortisol 19 hours after dexamethasone administration using the overnight protocol.

A variety of other tests have been recommended for evaluating pituitary-adrenocortical dysfunction in horses, including plasma cortisol levels, ACTH levels, ACTH stimulation tests, combined dexamethasone suppression/ACTH stimulation tests, glucose and insulin tolerance tests, insulin levels, TRH stimulation test alone or in combination with a dexamethasone suppression test, and the "cortisol rhythm" test. None of these tests show any greater sensitivity or specificity than the dexamethasone suppression test and are frequently less convenient to perform and/or are more expensive. However, because of the purported infrequent association between corticosteroid administration and an increased risk for the development of laminitis, tests that do not rely on the administration of glucocorticoids are frequently used in place of the dexamethasone suppression test.

The convenience, safety, and recent increase in the availability of plasma ACTH assays validated for the horse have made this test more widely utilized.[35,36] The reported sensitivity of plasma ACTH levels in the diagnosis of PPID is 84% to 100%, making it nearly as sensitive as the dexamethasone suppression test without the attendant, albeit small, risk of causing laminitis.[36,37] This test may potentially provide false-positive results where overlap of values between stressed normal horses and those early in the course of PPID can occur.[32] Also, because plasma ACTH is under ultradian rhythm and levels can change more than 50% during a peak or trough, horses that have a high clinical suspicion of PPID and have normal values would benefit from a repeat sample.[37,38]

Measurement of glucose levels and insulin levels are only 64% and 77% sensitive, respectively, whereas measurement of cortisol and evaluation of cortisol diurnal rhythm are not reliable diagnostic tests for PPID.[29,36]

Treatment

Treatment of horses with PPID can be difficult because of the age of the animal and the frequent occurrence of multiple problems in a given animal. The most effective treatment is often strict attention to management (housing, exercise, and feeding practices) and routine health care.[32,39] Two types of drugs have been used in affected horses with variable success. Anecdotal reports from practitioners are more favorable than the few controlled studies that have been performed in horses. None of the drugs are approved for use in horses.

Pergolide is a dopaminergic agonist that has been shown to produce significant reductions in concentrations of pro-opiomelanocortin and ACTH in horses affected with PPID.[33,36,37] Treated horses "improved clinically," but results of dexamethasone suppression tests in one study remained abnormal in two thirds of the patients.[40] Since ACTH does appear to decrease significantly in horses with PPID treated with pergolide and actually return to normal in a significant number of affected horses, measurement of ACTH levels provides a better way of monitoring the effects of pergolide treatment than the dexamethasone suppression test.[35-37] The recommended dose of pergolide (1.7–5.5 µg/kg) varies considerably, with the higher doses being utilized in the more advanced cases or those refractory to treatment at a lower dose.[41]

Cyproheptadine (Periactin), a serotonin antagonist, used in human beings for the treatment of certain allergies, has resulted in "clinical improvement" and in some cases lowering of blood glucose and ACTH levels in horses affected with PPID. The exact mode of action of cyproheptadine on the equine pars intermedia is unknown. It may take several weeks of therapy for any signs of improvement to be recognized. Recent studies suggest that pergolide is superior to cyproheptadine for the treatment of PPID based on the ability of pergolide to lower ACTH levels and improve clinical signs.[36,40]

Numerous other treatments for PPID have been proposed, including certain herbal remedies and trace mineral supplementation (chromium, magnesium). A recent study using one of the herbal products containing extracts from Vitex agnus castus, which supposedly has dopaminergic activity, has shown there was no significant effect on plasma ACTH levels or clinical signs of disease in horses with PPID.[41] The remainder of the treatments remains empirically derived, testimonially justified, and largely speculative.

EQUINE METABOLIC SYNDROME (PERIPHERAL CUSHING'S SYNDROME)

There has long been a clinical association made between the development of obesity in older horses or ponies and the risk of developing laminitis. Obesity-associated laminitis has been linked to such conditions as hypothyroidism, insulin resistance in ponies, and most recently, "peripheral Cushing's syndrome."[42] Traditionally, obesity in horses has most often been inappropriately attributed to "hypothyroidism" in horses, despite the fact that neither obesity nor laminitis is seen in horses that have undergone surgical thyroidectomy.[18] In addition, appropriate diagnostic testing for disease of the thyroid gland

invariably fails to identify hypothyroidism in obese horses, and pathologic changes in thyroid glands from affected horses are absent.[4,43]

Likewise, results of testing these obese, laminitic horses for pituitary pars intermedia dysfunction are normal.[29] The pituitary and adrenal glands of affected horses, examined at necropsy, are normal, even though these horses do exhibit some clinical signs suggesting that they may have been affected by increased glucocorticoid effects, including such things as abnormal distribution of adipose tissue, elevated circulating insulin, glucose intolerance, elevated plasma lipids, predisposition to laminitis, and infertility.[4] Excluding laminitis of course, these signs are seen in humans affected with a syndrome that is quite similar to that which occurs in horses and which has had several pseudonyms applied to it (central obesity syndrome, omental Cushing's syndrome, syndrome X, and metabolic syndrome).

Horses affected with equine metabolic syndrome are usually obese or, at least, generally overweight. They have abnormal accumulation of fat in areas such as the crest of the neck, over the rump adjacent to the base of the tail, in the sheath of stallions and geldings, and in the omentum[4] (Fig. 7-5). They are typically younger than

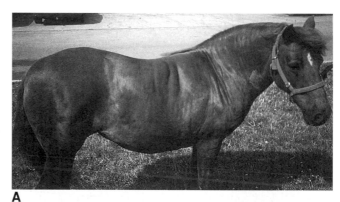

A

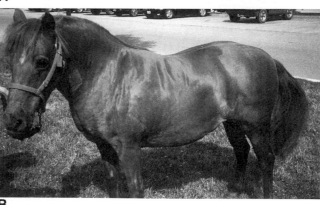

B

Figure 7-5 An obese horse with "cresty neck," abnormal accumulation of subcutaneous fat, and chronic laminitis typical of horses with metabolic syndrome and frequently misdiagnosed as "hypothyroidism." (Courtesy of Dr. Philip Johnson, University of Missouri.)

horses affected with PPID ranging in age from 5 to 15 years. There does not appear to be any sex predilection, but certain breeds appear to be over-represented. Attempts by the owner to reduce their weight through dietary restrictions are frequently unsuccessful and they are commonly referred to as "easy keepers." Affected mares may have abnormal estrous cycles and have difficulty conceiving and maintaining pregnancy.

Obesity is frequently associated with insulin resistance and glucose intolerance in humans,[44] and it appears this may be the case in horses as well. Horses with obesity-associated laminitis (metabolic syndrome) are commonly glucose intolerant and refractory to the effects of insulin. Pony breeds, which tend to become obese more frequently than horses, have been described as glucose intolerant compared to horses.[45,46] Adipocytes, particularly the intra-abdominal omental adipocytes, can no longer be considered to be just simple fat storage depots, but rather important cells in the production of numerous factors involved in the regulation of energy balance in the body, including such substances as leptin, resistin, free fatty acids, 11-β-hydroxysteroid dehydrogenase-1 (11-β-HSD-1), and cortisol.[4] As an example, leptin is an important regulator of energy metabolism that acts in the hypothalamus to suppress appetite in normal individuals, thereby regulating the accumulation of adipose tissue in the body. There exists a strong association between body fat mass and elevated plasma leptin levels in humans, suggesting that leptin resistance, rather than leptin production, may contribute to the development of obesity and associated disorders.[47] A similar association between body fat mass and elevated plasma leptin levels has recently been described in obese ponies, suggesting that leptin resistance might play a role in the development of obesity in horses and ponies as well.[48-51] In addition, overexpression of 11-β-HSD-1 in omental adipose tissue results in the conversion of cortisone to cortisol and represents an important molecular mechanism in which local cortisol production could contribute to the development of visceral obesity and insulin insensitivity.[52] Interestingly, increased 11-β-HSD-1 activity has recently been demonstrated in integumentary tissues from obese horses affected with laminitis, suggesting that tissue-specific glucocorticoid dysregulation may play a role in the cause or effect of laminitis.[42]

The development of laminitis in horses with metabolic syndrome is usually different than what occurs in the typical case of alimentary-induced laminitis. The onset of laminitis is more insidious and by the time it becomes clinically apparent, there are usually chronic changes present such as rotation of the third phalanx within the hoof and abnormal patterns of hoof growth. This pattern of development suggests that repeated episodes of subclinical damage takes place, eventually leading to sufficient damage to the laminar tissues to cause clinical signs. One plausible explanation for this gradual onset may be the fact that the insulin resistance and glucose intolerance in obese individuals results in persistent elevations in blood glucose (glucotoxicity). Persistent hyperglycemia, in turn, results in attenuated release of nitric oxide (a potent endogenous vasodilator) and increased release of endothelin-1 (a potent endogenous vasoconstrictor) from endothelial cells resulting in a state of relative vasospasticity. Increased vascular tone and impaired endothelial function have been associated with other effects of glucotoxicity, including increased formation of reactive oxygen species, increased lipid oxidation, decreased prostacyclin synthesis, increased production of vasoconstrictor eicosanoids, increased adhesion molecule expression, hypertension, and vascular remodeling.[53] Endothelial dysfunction therefore represents an important link between hyperglycemia and vascular complications. Recently, endothelin-1 levels have also been shown to be elevated in hoof lamellar tissues from horses affected with laminitis, suggesting that increased expression of endothelin-1 and vasoconstriction could contribute to reduced lamellar blood flow and laminitis.[54] In addition, treatment of ponies with nitric oxide donors was shown to result in clinical improvement, suggesting that impaired nitric oxide production could be important in some forms of laminitis.[55,56] Thus, the association between the risk for laminitis and obesity and the concurrent presence of insulin resistance strongly implies that, in these cases, laminitis arises as a vascular manifestation of disordered glucose regulation and not, as popularly advocated, hypothyroidism.[4]

The development of obesity and obesity-associated laminitis in mature horses and ponies is potentially genetically determined to some degree, based on the fact that certain breeds appear to be overrepresented, and this deserves further investigation. Most pony breeds, domesticated Spanish Mustangs, Morgans, Peruvian Pasos, Paso Finos, and some European warmbloods all anecdotally appear to be more prone to developing metabolic syndrome than other breeds. In addition, the common practice of feeding diets that are rich in soluble carbohydrates and have a high glycemic index to young growing horses whose physical activity is typically much less than that which would utilize the energy provided by such diets further predisposes both normal and genetically prone horses to obesity later in life. Therefore, treatment and preventative strategies for horses that have developed or are prone to developing metabolic syndrome must involve, first and foremost, limiting dietary carbohydrate intake and providing sufficient exercise to ensure that energy expenditure is equal to or greater than energy intake.[46]

Other potential treatments for the metabolic syndrome in horses that should be investigated include the use of antioxidants, enhancing endothelial nitric oxide effect, reversing vasoconstrictive effects of endothelin-1, antidiabetic (insulin sensitizing) and antiglycemic drugs used in humans for treatment of adult onset (type II) diabetes, inhibitors of the biosynthetic pathways for cortisol, and supplementation with certain trace minerals.

REFERENCES

1. Chen CL, Riley AM: Serum thyroxine and triiodothyronine concentrations in neonatal foals and mature horses. Am J Vet Res 42:1415, 1981.
2. Messer NT: Thyroid dysfunction in horses. Proc Annu Conv Am Assoc Equine Pract 40:649, 1994.
3. Frank N, Sojka J, Messer NT: Equine thyroid dysfunction. Vet Clin North Am Equine Pract 18:305, 2002.
4. Johnson PJ: The equine metabolic syndrome/peripheral Cushing's syndrome. Vet Clin North Am Equine Pract 18:271, 2002.
5. Alberts MK, McCann JP, Woods PR: Hemithyroidectomy in a horse with confirmed hyperthyroidism. J Am Vet Med Assoc 217:1051, 2001.
6. Ramirez S, McClure JJ, Moore RM, et al: Hyperthyroidism associated with a thyroid adenocarcinoma in a 21-year-old gelding. J Vet Intern Med 12:475, 1998.
7. Sojka JE: Factors which affect serum T3 and T4 levels in the horse. Equine Pract 15:15, 1993.
8. Morris DD, Garcia M: Thyroid-stimulating hormone response test in healthy horses, and effect of phenylbutazone on equine thyroid hormones. Am J Vet Res 44:503, 1983.
9. Ramirez S, Wolfsheimer KJ, Moore RM, et al: Duration of effects of phenylbutazone on serum total thyroxine and free thyroxine concentrations in horses. J Vet Intern Med 11:371, 1997.
10. Glade MJ, Reimers TJ: Effects of dietary energy supply on serum thyroxine, triiodothyronine, and insulin concentrations in young horses. J Endocrinol 104:93, 1985.
11. Swinker AM, McCurley JR, Jordan ER, et al: Effects of dietary excesses on equine serum thyroid hormone levels. J Anim Sci 65(Suppl 1):255, 1989.
12. Drew B, Barber WP, Williams DG: The effect of excess dietary iodine on pregnant mares and foals. Vet Rec 97:93, 1975.
13. Powell DM, Lawrence L: Thyroid hormone. Equine Dis Q 6:3, 1997.
14. Messer NT, Johnson PJ, Refsal KR, et al: Effect of food deprivation on baseline iodothyronine and cortisol concentrations in healthy, adult horses. Am J Vet Res 56:116, 1995.
15. Bayly W, Andrea R, Smith B, et al: Thyroid hormone concentrations in racing Thoroughbreds. Pferdeilkunde 12:534, 1996.
16. Symonds ME: Thyroid hormones and nutrient supplementation during pregnancy. Equine Vet Educ 7:246, 1995.
17. Flisinka-Bojanowska A, Komosa M, Gill J: Influence of pregnancy on diurnal and seasonal changes in cortisol, T3 and T4 levels in the mare blood serum. Comp Biochem Physiol 98A:23, 1991.
18. Lowe JE, Baldwin BH, Foote RH, et al: Equine hypothyroidism: the long term effects of thyroidectomy on metabolism and growth in mares and stallions. Cornell Vet 64:276, 1974.
19. Frank N, Sojka JE, Latour MA, et al: Effect of hypothyroidism on blood lipid concentrations in horses. Am J Vet Res 60(6):730-733, 1999
20. Vischer CM, Foreman JH, Constable PD, et al: Hemodynamic effects of thyroidectomy in sedentary horses. Am J Vet Res 60:14, 1999.
21. Lowe JE, Foote RH, Baldwin BH, et al: Reproductive patterns in cyclic and pregnant thyroidectomized mares. J Reprod Fert Suppl 35:281, 1987.
22. Lowe JE, Baldwin BH, Foote RH, et al: Semen characteristics in thyroidectomized stallions. J Reprod Fert Suppl 23:81, 1975.
23. Sojka JE, Johnson MA, Bottoms GD: The effect of starting time on dexamethasone suppression test results in horses. Domest Anim Endocrinol 10:1, 1993.
24. Beech J: Disorders of thyroid gland function. In Watson T, editor. Metabolic and Endocrine Problems of the Horse. Philadelphia, W.B. Saunders, 1998, pp 69-74.
25. Breuhaus BA: Thyroid-stimulating hormone in adult euthyroid and hypothyroid horses. J Vet Intern Med 16:109, 2002.
26. Beech J, Garcia M: Hormonal response to thyrotropin-releasing hormone in healthy horses and in horses with pituitary adenoma. Am J Vet Res 46:1941, 1985.
27. Chen CL, Li OW: Effect of thyrotropin releasing hormone (TRH) on serum levels of thyroid hormones in thoroughbred mares. Equine Vet Sci 6:58, 1986.
28. van der Kolk JH: Diseases of the pituitary gland, including hyperadrenocorticism. In: Watson TD, editor. Metabolic and endocrine problems of the horse. London: W.B. Saunders, 1998, p 41-59.
29. Schott HC: Pituitary pars intermedia dysfunction: equine Cushing's disease. Vet Clin North Am Equine Pract 18:237, 2002.
30. Dybdal NO, Hargreaves KM, Madigan JE, et al: Diagnostic testing for pituitary pars intermedia dysfunction in horses. J Am Vet Med Assoc 204:627, 1994.
31. Millington WR, Dybdal NO, Dawson R, et al: Equine Cushing's disease: differential regulation of β-endorphin processing in tumors of the intermediate pituitary. Endocrinology 123:1598, 1988.
32. Levy M, Sojka J, Dybdal NO: Diagnosis and treatment of equine Cushing's disease. Compend Contin Educ Pract Vet 21:766, 1999.
33. Orth DN, Holscher MA, Wilson MG: Equine Cushing's disease: plasma immunoreactive proopiolipomelanocortin peptide and cortisol levels basally and in response to diagnostic tests. Endocrinology 110:1430, 1982.
34. Seger M, Bennett H: Structure and bioactivity of the amino-terminal of proopiolipomelanocortin. J Steroid Biochem 25:703, 1986.
35. Couëtil L, Paradis MR, Knoll J: Plasma adrenocorticotropin concentration in healthy horses and horses with clinical signs of hyperadrenocorticism. J Vet Intern Med 10:1, 1996.
36. Donaldson MT, LaMonte BH, Morresey PM, et al: Treatment with pergolide or cyproheptadine of pituitary pars intermedia dysfunction (equine Cushing's disease). J Vet Intern Med 16:742, 2002.
37. Perkins GA, Lamb S, Erb HN, et al: Plasma adrenocorticotropin (ACTH) concentrations and clinical response in horses treated for equine Cushing's disease with cyproheptadine or pergolide. Equine Vet J 34:679, 2002.
38. Cudd TA, Leblanc M, Silver M, et al: Ontogeny and ultradian rhythms of adrenocorticotropin and cortisol in the late-gestation fetal horse. J Endocrinol 45:271, 1995.
39. van der Kolk JH: Equine Cushing's disease. Equine Vet Educ 9:209, 1997.
40. Schott HC, Coursen CL, Eberhart SW, et al: The Michigan Cushing's project. Proc Annu Conv Am Assoc Equine Pract 47:22, 2001.
41. Beech J, Donaldson MT, Lindborg S: Comparison of Vitex agnus castus extract and pergolide in the treatment of equine Cushing's syndrome. Proc Annu Conv Am Assoc Equine Pract 48:175, 2002.
42. Johnson PJ, Slight SH, Ganjam VK: Laminitis, "hypothyroidism," and obesity: a peripheral Cushingoid syndrome. Proc Am Coll Vet Int Med 192, 1999.
43. Graves EA, Schott HC, Johnson PJ, et al: Thyroid function in horses with peripheral Cushing's syndrome. Proc Annu Conv Am Assoc Equine Pract 48:178-180, 2002.
44. Ferrannini E, Natali A, Bell P, et al: Insulin resistance and hypersecretion in obesity. J Clin Invest 100:1166, 1997.
45. Jeffcott LB, Field JR, McClean JG, et al: Glucose tolerance and insulin sensitivity in ponies and Standardbred horses. Equine Vet J 18:97, 1986.
46. Freestone JF, Beadle R, Shoemaker K, et al: Improved insulin sensitivity in hyperinsulinemic ponies through physical conditioning and controlled feed intake. Equine Vet J 34:187, 1992.
47. Chu NF, Spiegelman D, Yu J, et al: Plasma leptin concentrations and four-year weight gain among US men. Int J Obes Relat Metab Disord 25:346, 2001.
48. Buff PR, McFadin-Buff EL, Morrison CD, et al: Growth and plasma leptin in yearling mares fed a high-fat diet [abstract]. J Anim Sci 79(Suppl 2):21, 2001.

49. Buff PR, Morrison CD, McFadin-Buff EL, et al: Diurnal and fasting effects on plasma leptin concentrations in pony mares [abstract]. Proc Eq Nutrit Physiol Soc Symp 41, 2001.

50. Buff PR, Morrison CD, McFadin-Buff EL, et al: Effects of melatonin implants on plasma concentrations of leptin and body weight in obese pony mares [abstract]. J Anim Sci 79(Suppl):209, 2001.

51. Buff PR, Whitley NC, McFadin-Buff EL, et al: Dose dependent decrease in feed intake following intravenous injection of urocortin into pony mares [abstract]. J Anim Sci 78(Suppl):149, 2000.

52. Tomlinson JW, Bujalska I, Stewart PM, et al: The role of 11-β-hydroxysteroid dehydrogenase in central obesity and osteoporosis. Endocr Res 26:711, 2000.

53. Taylor AA: Pathophysiology of hypertension and endothelial dysfunction in patients with diabetes mellitus. Endocrinol Metab Clin North Am 30:983, 2001.

54. Katwa LC, Johnson PJ, Ganjam VK, et al: Expression of endothelin in equine laminitis. Equine Vet J 31:243, 1999.

55. Hinckley KA, Fearn S, Howard BR, et al: Glyceryl trinitrate enhances nitric oxide mediated perfusion within the equine hoof. J Endocrinol 151:R1, 1996.

56. Hinckley KA, Fearn S, Howard BR, et al: Nitric oxide donors as treatment for grass induced acute laminitis in ponies. Equine Vet J 28:17, 1996.

SUGGESTED READING

Beech, J: Evaluation of thyroid, adrenal, and pituitary function. Vet Clin North Am Equine Pract 3:649, 1987.

Beech J, Donaldson MT, Linndborg S: Comparison of Vitex agnus castus extract and pergolide in treatment of equine Cushing's syndrome. Proc Annu Conv Am Assoc Equine Pract 48:175, 2002.

Breuhaus BA: Thyroid stimulating hormone in euthyroid and hypothyroid horses. In Proceedings of the 17th American College of Veterinary Internal Medicine Forum, Chicago, 1999, p 71.

Foreman JH: Cardiovascular effects of equine hypothyroidism. In Proceedings of the 15th American College of Veterinary Internal Medicine Forum, Lake Buena Vista, 1997, p 374.

Harris P, Marlin D, Gray J: Equine thyroid function tests: a preliminary investigation. Br Vet J 148:71, 1992.

Held JP, Oliver JW: A sampling protocol for the thyrotropin-stimulation test in the horse. J Am Vet Med Assoc 184:326, 1984.

Messer NT: Thyroid disease (dysfunction). In Robinson NE, editor: Current Therapy in Equine Medicine 4. Philadelphia, W.B. Saunders, 1998, p 502.

Messer NT, Ganjam VK, Nachreiner RF, et al: Effect of dexamethasone administration on serum thyroid hormone concentrations in clinically normal horses. J Am Vet Med Assoc 206:63, 1995.

Mooney CT, Murphy D: Equine hypothyroidism: the difficulties of diagnosis. Equine Vet Educ 7:242, 1995.

Morris DD, Garcia M: Effects of phenylbutazone and anabolic steroids on adrenal and thyroid gland function tests in healthy horses. Am J Vet Res 46:359, 1985.

Sojka JE: The effect of oral iodine administration on equine thyroid hormone concentrations. In Proceedings of the 15th American College of Veterinary Internal Medicine Forum, Lake Buena Vista, p 106.

Sojka JE: Hypothyroidism in horses. Compend Contin Educ Pract Vet 17:845, 1995.

Sojka JE, Johnson MA, Bottoms GD: Serum triiodothyronine, total thyroxine, and free thyroxine concentrations in horses. Am J Vet Res 54:52, 1993.

Sojka JE, Levy M: Evaluation of endocrine function. Vet Clin North Am Equine Pract 11:415, 1995.

CHAPTER 8

Aging and How It Affects the Response to Exercise in the Horse

Kenneth Harrington McKeever

According to Hintz and others, the number of horses older than 20 years of age is increasing every year, and many of those animals are still performing various athletic activities well into their 20s.[1-4] As with older humans, older horses that remain active continue to perform in athletic events for a variety of reasons, including genetics, better health care, and greatly improved nutritional management.[1-8] Studies of older humans show that the ability to perform strenuous work decreases with age, with much of the decline in aerobic capacity and anaerobic power attributed to the effects of aging on physiologic function.[9-15] However, debate in the literature focuses on how much of that decline is due to actual physiologic aging versus disease processes related to inactivity.[9-12,14,15] Disease and inactivity result in a decline in function that may be preventable, and studies of aged humans have shown that both dynamic and resistance exercise training forestalls or even reverses some of the decline in cardiopulmonary performance and muscle function.[9-16] This information illustrates the fact that some of the decline in exercise capacity in older individuals is related to a general decline in physical activity rather than to physiologic aging.[9-12] These facts have led to better exercise prescriptions for the older human athlete that prevent the potentially dangerous effects of excessive work.[10-12] The results are new and improved programs to promote fitness for the growing population of older adult humans.[10-14,17-20]

Limited data have been published regarding the exercise capacity of the aged horse.[2,6,21-30] The rationale for these studies has been the fact that more horses are living into their 20s.[1,2,4] Nutritional studies have resulted in the development of complete rations specifically tailored to the unique nutritional needs of the older horse.[7,8] Other studies have demonstrated that insulin-like growth factor-1 concentrations decline with age in the horse,[5] and that aging appears to alter metabolic control, immune function, and endocrine function in horses, both at rest and after exercise.[2,6,21-30a]

The older horse also undergoes significant changes in body composition, with some older horses exhibiting an obese phenotype and some having a thin old mare appearance.[23,24] Importantly, the thin old horses have a smaller muscle mass, a pattern that is also seen in aged humans, whereas the obese old horses tend to have 50% more fat mass than their younger counterparts.[23,24] However, as with other organ systems, the question remains as to whether this is due to inactivity or aging.[23,24] Interestingly, old horses, like old humans, undergo a change in muscle fiber type distribution away from a more aerobic profile that fits with their less active lifestyle and decline in aerobic capacity.[23,24] Functional studies have demonstrated that maximal heart rate (HR_{max}) and maximal aerobic capacity (VO_{2max}) appear to decline with age,[2,6,21] similar to the decrease in cardiovascular function seen in humans.[10-15] As with old humans, older equine athletes (i.e., horses older than 20 years) have the ability to continue to perform in athletic events. Unfortunately, many horse owners continue to train their older animals with using exercise training protocols that, while appropriate for a younger or middle-aged animal, may not be appropriate for the older equine athlete. This chapter reviews how aging affects the major physiologic systems that would be expected to alter exercise ability.

Aging-Induced Changes in Respiratory Function That Can Affect Exercise

It is well recognized that factors affecting lung health can have a cumulative effect in the horse.[31] Over a lifetime, older horses can be exposed to many pathogens and allergens that ultimately can lead to small airway disease.[31] Pathologic conditions such as hyper-reactive airway disease, chronic obstructive pulmonary disease, or exercise-induced pulmonary hemorrhage tend to be more prevalent in older animals.[31] Furthermore, those conditions can negatively affect respiratory function during exertion.[31] Unfortunately, there are no published studies of the effects of aging by itself on the respiratory response to exercise in healthy older horses. In humans, however, aging appears to have a significant effect on lung function during exercise, and one would expect similar changes to occur in the horse.[32]

A recent review article[9] suggests that there are several alterations in pulmonary function that can limit respiratory capacity in older individuals. Studies reporting flow-volume loops suggest that an expiratory flow limitation occurs at lower work intensities in older individuals.[9] Dempsy and Seals[9] also point out that the elastic recoil of the lung is altered with aging, a change negatively affecting expiratory flow rates.[9] Older humans also have a greater dead space that affects the dead space-to-tidal volume ratio.[9] All together, these age-related changes affect the work of breathing during exertion. Lung hemodynamics are also affected by aging-induced decreases in arteriolar compliance, a detrimental change that may lead to capillary stress failure.[9] The latter may have implications for the horse as capillary stress fractures are part of the cause of exercise-induced pulmonary hemorrhage.[9] Finally, Dempsey and Seals[9] report that despite all of these aging-related changes in lung physiology, "alveolar to arterial gas exchange and pulmonary vascular hemodynamics are only slightly modified by aging." The normal young equine lung is not built large enough to handle the demands of high intensity. Thus, data are needed to determine whether patterns of aging-induced change in the horse are similar to those in humans.[31] Data are also needed to determine whether there are cumulative damaging effects on lung health associated with lifelong problems caused by dust, mold, and other pollutants affecting stall air quality. From a clinical standpoint, repeated small airway inflammation and disease, chronic obstructive pul-

monary disease, multiple bouts of exercise-induced pulmonary hemorrhage, and other chronic problems may account for more of any age-related decline in lung function. Good management practices and environmental cleanliness thus become an important consideration for the care of the older horse.

Age-Related Changes in the Cardiovascular Response to Exercise

Many papers have been published on the effects of aging on cardiovascular function in healthy older humans.[9-16,18-20,33] Aging has profound effects on the cardiovascular system, with resulting decreases in maximal heart rate (HR_{max}), changes in baroreceptor sensitivity, decreased vascular compliance, and hypertension in species such as rats, dogs, and humans.[9-16,18-20,33] Data are mixed regarding the effect of age on stroke volume, with some studies demonstrating a decline and others suggesting that fit aged humans make up for the lower HR_{max} by increasing stroke volume.[9-16,18-20,33] In very old individuals, however, there appears to be a decrease in both HR_{max} and stroke volume that certainly results in a decline in maximal cardiac output in humans.[9,11,13-15] The decline in HR_{max} and maximal cardiac output most likely contributes to the decline in maximal oxygen uptake and exercise capacity seen both in older humans and in older horses.[6,9-13,21]

Mechanistically, decreases in HR_{max} with age appear to be due to several mechanisms, including aging-induced changes in the number of pacemaker cells in the sinoatrial node, increases in the elastic and collagenous tissue in all parts of the conduction system, and the deposition of adipose tissue around the sinoatrial node.[13] In humans, aging also alters autonomic tone with a resulting down-regulation of sensitivity to the sympathetic nervous system. This appears to influence the ability to increase heart rate during exercise.[13] The horse appears to use similar autonomic mechanisms to control heart rate, and indirect evidence suggests that the horse may also undergo aging-induced changes in the neuroendocrine control of cardiovascular function.[6,34,35]

The decrease in heart function can also affect the ability to perform aerobic exercise. Maximal aerobic capacity is the product of the ability to deliver oxygen (i.e., central limitations—cardiac output) and the ability to utilize oxygen (peripheral factors limiting the distribution of blood flow and actual factors within the muscle limiting utilization). Data are mixed regarding the contribution of central (heart) and peripheral cardiovascular (blood vessel) factors in the decline in exercise performance seen in horses, dogs, and humans.[6,9,11,13,14,21,36] In humans and other species, an age-related decline in the ability of the heart to pump blood accounts for some of the observed decrease in VO_{2max}. However, decreased muscle mass, alterations in muscle capillary density, and decreased vascular compliance may also limit exercise capacity by limiting blood flow to working muscles.[31] Thus, some of the decline in aerobic capacity is also due to changes in peripheral mechanisms affecting the ability to utilize oxygen. This makes sense as increases in muscle mass through resistance exercise improve aerobic capacity as well as strength in old humans. Unfortunately, these data have been extrapolated from submaximal studies of humans, and the debate continues on whether age-related declines in maximal cardiovascular capacity in humans are predominated by central or peripheral mechanisms.

Older horses undergo a decline in maximal aerobic capacity (VO_{2max}), similar to that seen in healthy older humans. Such was the case in a study by McKeever and Malinowski[6] that demonstrated an age-related decrease in VO_{2max} as well as the amount of work needed to reach VO_{2max}.[6] There was also a decline in the capacity to tolerate high-intensity anaerobic exercise in older horses.[6] Those observations were similar to well-documented, age-induced decreases seen in humans.[9,11,13-15] In terms of physiologic age, the older horses mentioned above were analogous to humans ranging from 60 to 80 years of age.[6] Interestingly, compared to other species, the older mare has a tremendous innate aerobic capacity.[6] For example, maximal aerobic capacity in moderately fit, healthy, postmenopausal women averages 22 mL/kg/min,[11,14] whereas elite, female, Olympic-caliber, human athletes typically have maximal aerobic capacities ranging from 60 to 80 mL/kg/min.[10] The average mass specific VO_{2max} of 90 mL/kg/min seen in old mares is well below that of their fit equine counterparts (145-200 mL/kg/min) but still above levels reported for young, fit, elite human athletes.[6]

There are practical considerations to the above-mentioned data. When one looks closely at the data, submaximal oxygen consumption was similar in young and old horses subjected to an incremental exercise test. That observation suggests that there is no difference in the metabolic efficiency of sound old and young horses of similar body weights. Thus, in theory, during slow exercise at the same speed, old horses and young horses should have the same metabolic cost for moving each kilogram of body weight from point A to point B. In other words, if a young horse and an old horse were similar in weight, free from orthopedic problems affecting efficiency, and walked side by side, then they would have the same absolute rate of oxygen consumption (e.g., 70 mL/kg/min). However, the important point to consider if one is using an older horse for pleasure rides or other activities is this: Even though the two horses are walking

at the same absolute work intensity, they are in reality exercising at dramatically different relative work intensities. How can this be? If the maximal aerobic capacity of the young horse is 140 mL/kg/min and the cost of walking is 70 mL/kg/min, then that horse is walking at a submaximal intensity of 50% VO_{2max}. If, for example, the older horse had a VO_{2max} of 90 mL/kg/min, then the older horse would be walking at much higher relative work intensity (78%). Because most of the acute responses to exercise are more closely related to the relative work intensity, the older horse in the example given above would have more demand placed on all of its physiologic systems to keep up with the younger animal. Fortunately, recent studies performed in the Equine Exercise Physiology Laboratory at Rutgers University demonstrate that moderate training can reverse some of the decline in cardiopulmonary capacity seen in old horses.

Another benefit of the greater aerobic capacity seen in younger horses is a delay in the need to increase the rate of anaerobic glycolysis to fuel higher intensity exercise.[6] Younger horses must work harder to reach their "anaerobic threshold." This is the point where one observes the onset of blood lactate accumulation, conventionally marked by a blood lactate concentration of 4 mMol/L.[6] At this point, there is a curvilinear increase in blood lactate concentration indicating that lactate production by the working muscles has exceeded lactate utilization throughout the rest of the body.[6] This variable is important, because the velocity to produce a blood lactate concentration of 4 mMol/L (V_{LA4}) coincides with changes in several important physiologic processes. Older horses appear to reach the V_{LA4} at both a lower speed and a lower relative work intensity,[6] suggesting a possible central limitation on the ability to perform work.[6] However, the older mares were also not able to run as long or as hard (V_{max}) before reaching fatigue, suggesting a reduction in factors affecting peripheral mechanisms associated with general exercise tolerance. More work is needed to determine the relative role of central versus peripheral limitations in the decline of the ability to transport and utilize oxygen during exercise in older horses.

Until recently, data on the effects of age on central cardiovascular function, cardiac output, HR_{max}, and stroke volume have been lacking in horses. However, a recent study by Betros et al.[21] attempted to determine whether there were age-related declines in HR_{max} and whether any of the changes in cardiovascular function were reversed with training.[21] That study found that HR_{max} (218 vs. 213 beats/min), VO_{2max} (116 vs. 109 mL/kg/min), maximal oxygen pulse (OP_{max}) (0.55 vs. 0.52 mL/kg/beat) velocity at HR_{max} (9.0 vs. 9.3 m/s) or velocity at VO_{2max} (8.8 ± 0.2 m/s vs 8.8 ± 0.2 m/s) was similar in young and middle-aged horses.[21] However, there appeared to be a breakpoint once a horse was older than 20 years of age. Old horses had a lower HR_{max} (193 beats/min), VO_{2max} (95 mL/kg/min) and OP_{max} (0.43 mL/kg/beat) and reached those maximal values at lower velocities compared to young and middle-aged horses.[21] Interestingly, the authors found that training resulted in substantial improvements in VO_{2max} and OP_{max} but did not alter HR_{max} in young, middle-aged, or old horses.[21] Two important findings of that study include the observation of an age-related decline in HR_{max} and maximal stroke volume in the horse.[21] This observation may be important to horse owners who use heart rate monitoring to judge the physiologic intensity of the work their horses are performing. Secondly, training can partially reverse some of the decline in cardiovascular function in the older horse.[21] A more recent study demonstrated that older horses experience a similar beneficial training-induced decrease in resting heart rate. This bradycardia allows for a greater cardiac reserve (the difference between rest and maximal values) that ultimately may explain why older horses can improve cardiovascular function even though they undergo a permanent decline in maximal heart rate.

Age-Related Changes in Thermoregulation and Fluid and Electrolyte Balance

The horse's athletic capacity can be considered elite among mammalian species, but its ability to dissipate heat during exercise is limited due to a relatively small surface area-to-mass ratio.[38] During high work intensities, the rate of heat production of the horse can exceed basal levels by 40- to 60-fold.[38] If the excess metabolic heat generated during exercise is not dissipated, life-threatening elevations in body temperature may develop, and the horse's athletic performance will be adversely affected.[38] The adverse effects of hyperthermia on the health and performance of horses can develop during all exercise intensities and weather conditions. Failure to dissipate metabolic heat can cause a continuous and excessive rise in internal body temperature.[38,39] If heat loss mechanisms are impaired by aging, then the only way that a horse would be able to decrease its body temperature would be to decrease the rate of heat gain by decreasing the intensity of the exertion.[38]

Studies comparing the thermoregulatory responses of older and younger men and women during exercise in the heat have shown that age influences thermoregulatory function during exercise.[40-42] Suggested reasons for this age-related decline in the ability to thermoregulate properly during exercise in humans include lower cardiovascular capacity due to the age-related decrease in

cardiac output, alterations in mechanisms associated with the control of skin blood flow, and a possible state of hypohydration in the elderly.[41,42] Data are mixed on the role of each of these factors alone and in combination in exercising older humans.[41,42] In research performed specifically on humans, lower stroke volumes and cardiac outputs have been seen in older men when compared to younger men during upright exercise. These differences are also present when skin venous pooling is augmented by the imposition of an additional heat stress.[41,42] In studies of older men and women, it has been demonstrated that older individuals have lower cardiac outputs than younger subjects, even though they were exercising at the same absolute low-intensity workload.[19,41,42]

The are many papers reporting data on thermoregulation in young horses.[39,43] However, only a few studies have addressed effects of age on the thermoregulatory response to exercise in the horse.[40,46] Exercise is a costly endeavor energetically, and the generation of adenosine triphosphate fuels work but also generates a great deal of heat that must be dissipated. If one presumes that two horses are the same weight and have similar mechanical efficiencies, then the cost of the activity for any given submaximal activity should be similar. Thus, old and young horses running at the same submaximal speed should generate a similar amount of metabolic heat that must be dissipated. The ability to deal with that heat was tested in a study by McKeever and coworkers.[2,28] In that experiment, the authors exercised young and old horses at the same submaximal absolute work intensity of 1625 watts until the horses reached a core body temperature of 40°C. Old horses reached a core temperature of 40°C in almost half the time required by the younger mares.[2,28] Heart rates were substantially greater in the older mares compared to the younger mares when they reached 40°C. However, both groups had similar heart rates and core temperatures by 10 minutes after exercise.[2,28] This suggested that older mares were not able to thermoregulate as effectively as younger mares during exercise. The greater heart rate seen in the older mares suggested that their hearts had to work harder to muster sufficient cardiac output to accommodate the combined exercising demand of increased blood flow to the organs and muscles as well as to the skin for thermoregulation.[2,28] Even with the more rapid heart rate, older horses were still unable to dissipate the heat generated from exercise as quickly as younger mares, therefore leading to a faster increase in core temperature after the onset of exercise. Interestingly, both groups had similar core temperatures and heart rates 10 minutes after exercise.[2,28] The authors interpreted this to suggest that the old mares could handle the demands of thermoregulation alone but not the combined demand of exercise and thermoregulation.[2,28]

Human studies may shed light on mechanisms causing the impairment of thermoregulation with age. During exercise, delivery of oxygen to active muscle involves a local decrease in vascular resistance, which in turn creates a challenge to blood flow delivery that is met by both increases in cardiac output and adjustments in vascular resistance in nonactive tissues.[41,42] Increasing cardiac output during exercise helps meet the dual demand for increased blood flow to working muscle and the skin, especially when coupled with the redistribution of blood flow from visceral organs to augment perfusion of skin and active muscle vascular beds.[41,42] In aged horses and humans, cardiac output is limited and thus there is blood flow to sufficiently support flow to the both the working muscles and skin blood flow. This leads to a compromise of the ability to dissipate heat and defend against hyperthermia.[41,42] In the older horse, there may have been an aging-related decrease in maximal cardiac output, which in turn led to compromised thermoregulatory capacity during exercise.

Aging-related alterations in fluid and electrolyte balance can also impair thermoregulatory capacity in older individuals. Older humans commonly have lower total body water, plasma volume, and reserves of fluid for sweating.[11,41,42] Data are mixed, however, as to whether older humans are chronically hypohydrated.[41,42] Interestingly, changes in the above-mentioned markers of fluid status suggested that fluid shifts were of a similar relative magnitude in young and old horses.[41,42] However, another study revealed that older horses have a substantially lower pre-exercise plasma volume as compared with younger animals.[27] Thus, while the relative reduction in plasma volume during exercise was similar, the older horses started off with a significantly lower absolute plasma volume. This would lead to lower venous return, stroke volume, and cardiac output and a compromise of thermoregulatory stability. Unfortunately, new unpublished data document that, unlike young horses, old horses cannot increase plasma volume in response to training. This suggests that caution should be taken when training and exercising older animals, as they do not appear to be as adaptive as the younger horse.

Skin blood flow was not measured in the above-mentioned horse studies; however, studies of humans have demonstrated that aging impairs the skin blood flow response to exercise.[41,42,44] The paradoxical inability to keep cool despite an increase in the sweat rate in older horses is consistent with an impairment of skin blood flow as observed in humans. While pure speculation, the mechanism for an age-related decline in skin blood flow during exercise could involve alterations in the sensitivity of mechanisms affecting vascular tone. Recognizing that older horses have a decreased ability to thermoregulate during exercise should lead to improved monitoring practices for heat stress and therefore a decreased occurrence of exercise-induced hyperthermia during equine athletic activities. The increased susceptibility of older horses to overheating exemplified by this study will enable veterinarians, owners, and riders of horses to identify certain horses as more likely than others to develop hyperthermia during exercise so that exercise regimens and athletic events can be designed to prevent heat stress.

Effects of Age on Body Composition and Muscle Fiber Type

Another measure that may have an important bearing on the ability to perform exercise is a horse's body composition and more importantly, total fat-free mass (FFM).[45-47] Older humans exhibit substantial decreases in muscle mass and in many cases increases in fat mass that affect the ability to perform exercise.[15,48-50] Data from recent work in horses suggest that they may undergo similar aging-induced changes.[23-25] That study found that old horses could be divided into two groups by appearance.[23,24] Some horses were either very lean or very fat.[23,24] The "skinny" old mares had significantly smaller rump fat thickness, lower percentage of body fat, and less fat weight than both the fat old mares and the young mares.[23,24] The skinny old mares had significantly less body weight than the fat old mares but not compared to the young mares.[23,24] They also had greater lean body weight than the young mares, but there was no significant difference in this parameter when compared to the old fat mares.[23,24] In turn, the old fat group had a significantly larger rump fat thickness, percentage of body fat, and fat weight when compared to the young mares.[23-25] Those data suggest that as mature horses gain weight, they gain fat mass at a rate faster than FFM. This is indicated by an increase in percentage of fat per given body weight.

The larger fat mass seen in some older horses may be detrimental to performance[24] and may lead to other complications in older horses, such as insulin resistance.[25] The observed morphometric differences may have resulted from some of the same factors at play in aged humans.[15,48,49,50] For instance, aged horses exhibit similar clinical metabolic and endocrine disorders as those seen in aged humans, including hyperinsulinemia and hyperglycemia, pituitary and thyroid adenomas, Cushing's disease, decreased somatotropin concentrations, and so on.[2,25]

Although old horses appear to retain muscle mass, one must ask whether that is functional muscle mass. There are many studies that have documented muscle fiber type, enzymatic activity, and substrate storage and utilization patterns in the horse.[51-57] However, only limited studies have examined peripheral changes associated with aging in the horse and those studies have focused on changes in fiber type associated with aging.[23,24,53] We are aware of only two papers that have attempted to present data grouped by age.[23,24,53] Riviero[53] examined muscle fiber type distribution in a number of horses; however, the mean age of the oldest age group in that study was only 15 years, an age at which many horses are still in their prime athletically and physiologically, analogous to 40-year-old and older humans.[53] A more recent study, on the other hand, compared young and very old horses and found that older horses had less type I and IIA fibers than the young mares.[23,24] Old horses had more type IIX fibers than the young horses.[23,24] Type I and IIA fibers are the fibers recruited to perform endurance exercise, whereas type IIX fibers are those recruited to perform sprint/anaerobic exercise. On a functional level, this suggests that the older horse undergoes a switch in fiber type population away from that which would be favorable to endurance exercise. This may, in part, explain the decrease in $\dot{V}O_{2max}$ documented in other studies.[6]

On a cellular level, aging appears to alter muscle structure and function.[23,32,54,58-61] Studies of other species (rats and humans) demonstrate that connective tissue content in the muscle is altered, with evidence of significant amounts of collagen—changes that would tend to interfere with normal contractile function.[15,62,63] Other studies have reported changes in skeletal muscle blood capillarity and decreases in blood flow in older men.[11] Oxidative capacity, glucose utilization, GLUT-4 activity, insulin insensitivity, insulin-regulatable glucose transporter, and glycogen depletion/repletion patterns in skeletal muscle appear to be altered by age in rats and humans.[11,13,62-64] Unfortunately, no data have been published that have examined the effect of exercise on muscle enzyme concentrations or glycogen depletion and repletion patterns in the old horse. More work is needed to determine whether there are other aging-related differences in the metabolic profile of horse muscle at both the cellular and the molecular level.

Aging-Related Alterations in the Endocrine Response to Exercise

Exercise involves the integration of multiple organ systems that communicate via neural and endocrine pathways. Humans undergo substantial alterations in neural control mechanisms, with primary alterations in sympathetic nervous system responsiveness.[11,20,49,65] No such information exists for the horse. Aging also alters the endocrine response to exercise, with reported changes in hormones associated with the control of cardiovascular function, stress hormones, and endocrine/paracrine factors related to the control of metabolic function and substrate utilization.[11,20,65]

A recent study reported on the effect of aging on four of the hormones related to the control of cardiovascular function in the horse.[29] The authors reported similar resting concentrations of the various hormones involved in the control of cardiovascular and renal function, including atrial natriuretic peptide (ANP), arginine vasopressin (AVP), plasma renin activity (PRA), aldosterone (ALDO), and endothelin-1 in healthy old and young horses. Similar observations have been reported for normal healthy humans and other species.[41,42,66] Old and young horses had directionally similar exercise-induced alterations in plasma renin activity, ANP, AVP, and ALDO.[29] However, the major finding of this investigation was an aging-related change in the magnitude of the response to exertion.[29] Although old horses had different concentrations of these hormones, the observed concentrations were still within the range of normal for maximally exercised horses and other species.[33,41,42,66] Interestingly, plasma concentrations of the vasoconstrictor endothelin-1 were not affected by exercise in either group of horses, a phenomenon previously reported for young horses and humans.[2] Aging-related differences in PRA and the plasma concentrations of the ANP, AVP, and ALDO may reflect differences in sensitivity in the regulation of blood pressure and blood flow during exertion. Younger horses were observed to have greater plasma concentrations of the vasodilator ANP. Functionally, this ANP-induced vasodilation would aid in the redistribution of blood flow during exercise.[33,66] ANP also inhibits PRA and the production and release of antagonistic hormones such as AVP and ALDO.[33,66] Thus, greater concentrations of plasma ANP in younger animals may enhance the ability to optimally vasodilate blood vessels in the periphery, especially in the working muscles.

McKeever and Malinowski[29] also reported that older horses had greater PRA at speeds eliciting $\dot{V}O_{2max}$. This change may be physiologically important as part of the defense of blood pressure during exercise and defense of fluid and electrolyte balance after exercise. Increases in circulating plasma angiotensin I and II aid in the vasoconstriction in non-obligate tissues that is part of the redistribution of blood flow.[33,66] Furthermore, increases in PRA and angiotensin also act to stimulate thirst and cause an increase in the synthesis and release of aldosterone.[33,66] Mediation of this neuroendocrine defense of blood pressure involves the integrative actions of both the low- and high-pressure baroreceptors.[33,66] However, aging appears to alter baroreceptor sensitivity and the normal feedback loop that integrates cardiovascular control.[20] One might speculate then that reported differences in ANP and PRA reflect an age-related difference in baroreceptor sensitivity to the challenge of exercise. It may also reflect differences in autonomic control and input from the sympathetic nervous system and other stimuli that affect the control of central and peripheral cardiovascular function. This may be important, as increases in renal sympathetic nerve activity and the stimulation of the juxtaglomerular apparatus is the primary stimulus for renin release during exertion. A recent study of humans suggests that aging-induced changes in PRA may also affect renal function and may indirectly contribute to possible alterations in skin blood flow.[41,42] The latter speculated that aging-induced change could be important, as it potentially could alter the ability to thermoregulate in humans. It would also be important to horses, because they are the only other athletic species that sweat to thermoregulate.[33] Any age-related difference in blood volume, HR_{max}, and vascular tone may have also influenced the integrative neuroendocrine defense of blood pressure.

Surprisingly, younger horses appear to have a greater vasopressin response during exercise. Plasma AVP concentration increases when the cardiopulmonary baroreceptors sense that cardiac filling pressure is inadequate, when the high pressure baroreceptors sense that mean arterial blood pressure is too low, or when hypothalamic osmoreceptors sense that plasma osmolality is too high.[33,66] Vasopressin causes vasoconstriction in nonobligate tissues during exercise. It also facilitates the uptake of water and electrolytes from the large intestine, another important action during exercise.[33,66] Post-exercise AVP causes a retention of solute free water by the kidney and stimulates thirst and drinking.[33,66] Studies are needed to explore the role of aging in these functions, as some studies suggest that aged humans do not drink as much and many times are hypohydrated.[41,42] Suppression of thirst and drinking is an important consideration for people concerned with post-event care of the horse.

It is well recognized that older horses have lower plasma concentrations of the thyroid hormones, somatotropin, and insulin-like growth factor (IGF)-1 compared with young animals, suggesting an age-related decline in somatotropic axis in horses that is similar to that observed in other mammalian species.[5] This may be linked to aging-induced changes, including decreases in cardiopulmonary function, decreased aerobic and exercise capacity, decreased immune function, impaired nutrient utilization, decreased nitrogen retention, and decreased lean body mass.[5] Similar changes have been observed in other species and comparative physiological data from rats, dogs, and humans.[10,11,15] have shown that there is a causal relationship between plasma concentrations of somatotropin and what has been termed the "aging phenotype."

Endorphins and cortisol have been utilized as markers of the degree of physiologic stress during exercise.[67] The release of these two hormones is a normal response to exercise; however, the direction and the magnitude of their response differentiates between what one can consider a normal response to the physiologic challenge of exertion and a true stress response. Increases in these hormones are linked to duration and intensity, and their release may provide protection from the physiologic challenge of exertion.[67,68] Beta-endorphin functions as a natural opiate, forestalling the central mechanisms that would induce fatigue.[67,68] Cortisol functions as a metabolic hormone during exercise, influencing glucose metabolism.[67,68] After exercise, cortisol exerts anti-inflammatory and immunosuppressive activity, possibly aiding in the repair of tissue altered by exertion and protecting against the inflammation associated with overexertion.

We are aware of only one study that has attempted to determine whether training and age affected the plasma β-endorphin, cortisol, and immune function responses to acute exercise in unfit Standardbred mares.[67] Unfortunately, β-endorphin and cortisol were measured at rest and at 5, 10, 20, 40, 60, and 120 minutes after a graded exercise test but not during exercise. The authors reported that cortisol rose by 5 minutes after the graded exercise test in young and middle-aged mares before and after training.[67] However, there was no rise in cortisol in the old mares after the graded exercise test either before or after training.[67] Before training, plasma β-endorphin increased by 5 minutes post-exercise in all mares.[67] After training, β-endorphin was higher compared to pre-training in all three age groups; however, the peak in the old mares occurred later than in the other groups.[67]

Aging substantially alters metabolic function in humans[33,49,62,63,65,69] and is frequently associated with glucose intolerance and insulin resistance in both humans and horses.[8,33] Participation in regular exercise activity may elicit a number of favorable responses that contribute to healthy aging.[33] Only one study has attempted to examine the effects of aging and training on the glucose and insulin response after acute exertion in horses.[67] The primary finding of that study was that old horses required greater concentrations of insulin to successfully manage their response to an oral glucose tolerance test.[67] The authors also reported that there was an aging-related effect on the glucose and insulin responses to acute exercise both before and after 12 weeks of exercise training.[67] Interestingly, 12 weeks of exercise training resulted in a post–graded exercise test increase in insulin in all age groups.[67] The authors concluded that the resultant hyperinsulinemia post-exertion after training may have been related to an increased need for glycogen repletion in the muscle after exercise.[67]

Interestingly, this post-training response was highest in the oldest horses, quite possibly because of a greater need to replenish muscle glycogen.[67] The authors also reported that exercise training altered the insulin responses more in the old horses and that it did not affect the glucose response of any of the horses, regardless of age.[67] This was interpreted to suggest an improvement in insulin sensitivity in the older animals.[67] The exact mechanisms to explain the age-related difference in glucose and insulin metabolism are unknown, but published papers from studies of rats and humans suggest that it may be related to differences in fuel utilization, mitochondria respiration rates, and skeletal muscle content of GLUT-4 transporters.[59,60,62,63]

Alterations in the Immune Response to Exercise

Studies of humans have demonstrated that aging alters the immune response in general and more importantly the immune response to the challenge of exercise.[43,70] Two studies have reported on the effect of aging on the immune response to acute exertion in horses.[22,67] Horohov and coworkers[22] reported that there were differences in the immune system of young and old horses both before and after exertion. Interestingly, acute exercise caused a decrease in the lymphoproliferation response in the younger horses but not the old mares.[22] Old horses also exhibited a lower proliferative response to mitogens, suggesting an aging-related alteration in T-cell-mediated function and an immunosenescence that the authors suggested may have been related to a lower cortisol response to exertion in the old horses.[22] A more recent experiment examined the effects of aging and training by measuring immune responses to a graded exercise test performed before and after 12 weeks of training.[67] The older horses had lower monocyte counts post–graded exercise test after training.[67] Age also affected the lymphocyte response to acute exercise before and after training, suggesting a degree of immunosenescence.[67] Together, these studies suggest that special preventative care may be needed for the older athletic horse.

Renal, Gastrointestinal, and Other Systems

Research using humans has suggested that many of the observed changes in renal function seen with aging are not inevitable and are the combined effect of pathologic conditions coupled with the aging process. We are aware of only limited data on the effect of age on the renal response to acute exercise in humans.[41,42,71] Those studies have primarily focused on the effect of aging on the normal reduction in blood flow seen with acute exertion.[41,42,71] Functionally, older individuals have smaller reductions in renal blood flow and smaller increases in skin blood flow compared with younger humans.[41,42,71] This may alter renal function as well as thermoregulatory capacity, because the redistribution of blood flow away from nonobligate tissues toward the working muscles and skin are important responses to exertion.[41,42,71] No work has been performed in the horse. More work is also needed to determine whether aging alters mechanisms affecting the glomerular filtration rate and tubular function both during exercise and afterwards. The latter may be important, as long-term control of total body water, plasma volume, and fluid and electrolyte balance appear to be altered in humans and horses.

In other species, the gastrointestinal tract, bones, and ligaments as well as the integumentary system are altered with age.[11,12] Changes in the gastrointestinal tract, from wear-down of teeth to decreased absorptive capability, all influence the uptake of water and nutrients and have the potential to alter the ability to perform exercise. Bone pathology ranging from osteoarthritis to demineralization certainly can alter the ability of the old horse to perform exercise. Changes in the skin have the potential to alter sweating and thermoregulation. We are unaware of any data on the effects of age on these organ systems in the horse.

Conclusions

Surveys indicate that equine population in the United States older than 20 years of age is growing larger.[2,4,71] As with humans, these geriatric equine athletes have the ability to continue to perform in athletic events. Unfortunately, many horse owners continue to train their active older animals with using exercise training protocols that, while appropriate for a younger animal, may not be appropriate for the older equine athlete. Studies of aged humans have led to a fine-tuning of exercise prescription for the older human athlete to prevent the adverse and potentially dangerous effects of excessive work. Published results have led to new and improved programs to promote fitness for the growing population of older adult humans. Future studies of the effects of aging on exercise capacity in equine athletes should have similar goals.

Acknowledgments

This work was supported by funds from New Jersey Agricultural Experiment Station and the New Jersey State Special Equine Initiative. The author thanks Jennifer McKeever for her help editing the manuscript.

REFERENCES

1. Hintz HF: Nutrition of the geriatric horse. In Proceedings of the Cornell Nutrition Conference, Cornell University, 1995, p 195-198.

2. McKeever KH: Exercise physiology of the older horse. Vet Clin North Am Equine Pract 18:469, 2002.

3. McKeever KH: Aging and how it affects the physiological response to exercise in the horse. Clinical techniques in equine practice: sports medicine/exercise physiology series. 2:258, 2003.

4. Rich GA: Nutritional and managerial considerations of the aged equine. In Proceedings of Advanced Equine Management Short Course, Colorado State University, 1989, p 121-123.

5. Malinowski K, Christensen RA, Hafs HD, Scanes CG: Age and breed differences in thyroid hormones, insulin-like growth factor-I and IGF binding proteins in horses. J Animal Sci 74:1936, 1996.

6. McKeever KH, Malinowski K: Exercise capacity in young and geriatric female horses. Am J Vet Res 58:1468, 1997.

7. Ralston SL, Breuer LH: Field evaluation of a feed formulated for geriatric horses. J Equine Vet Sci 16:334, 1996.

8. Ralston SL: Effect of soluble carbohydrate content of pelleted diets on post prandial glucose and insulin profiles in horses. Pferdeheilkunde 112, 1992.

9. Dempsey JA, Seals DR: Aging, exercise, and cardiopulmonary function. In Lamb DR, Gisolfi CV, Nadel E, eds: Perspectives in Exercise and Sports Medicine, Vol 8. Exercise in Older Adults. Carmel, IN, Cooper Publishing, 1995, p 237-304.

10. Haskell WL, Phillips WT: Exercise training, fitness, health, and longevity. In Lamb DR, Gisolfi CV, Nadel E, eds: Perspectives in Exercise and Sports Medicine, Vol 8. Exercise in Older Adults. Carmel, IN, Cooper Publishing, 1995, p 11-52.

11. Holloszy JO, Kohrt WM: Exercise. In Masoro EJ, editor: Handbook of Physiology, Section 11. Aging. New York, Oxford University Press, 1995, p 633-666.

12. Holloszy JO: Exercise, health, and aging: a need for more information. Med Sci Sports Exerc 15:1, 1993.

13. Lakatta EG: Cardiovascular system. In Masoro EJ, editor: Handbook of Physiology, Section 11. Aging. New York, Oxford University Press, 1995, p 413-474.

14. Raven PB, Mitchell JH: Effect of aging on the cardiovascular response to dynamic and static exercise. In Westfeldt ML, editor: The Aging Heart: Its Function and Response to Stress. New York, Raven Press, 1980, p 269-296.

15. Stamford BA:. Exercise and the elderly. In Pandolf KB, editor: Exercise and Sport Science Reviews, Vol 16. New York, MacMillan Publishing Company, 1988, p 341-380.

16. Ekelund LG, Haskell WL, Johnson JL, et al: Physical fitness in the prevention of cardiovascular mortality in asymptomatic North American men. N Engl J Med 319:1379, 1988.

17. Ready AE, Naimark B, Ducas J, et al. Influence of walking volume on health benefits in women post-menopause. Med Sci Sports Exerc 28:1097, 1996.

18. Seals DR, Reiling MJ: Effect of regular exercise on 24-hour arterial blood pressure in older hypertensive humans. Hypertension 18:583, 1991.

19. Seals DR, Hagberg JM, Hurley BF, et al: Endurance training in older men and women: I. Cardiovascular responses to exercise. J Appl Physiol 57:1024, 1984.

20. Seals DR: Influence of aging on autonomic-circulatory control at rest and during exercise in humans. In Gisolfi CV, Lamb DR, Nadel E, eds: Perspectives in Exercise Science and Sports Medicine, Vol 6. Exercise, Heat, and Thermoregulation. Dubuque, IA, W.C. Brown, 1993, p 257-297.

21. Betros CL, McKeever KH, Kearns CF, et al: Effects of aging and training on maximal heart rate and VO2max. Equine Vet J 34:100-105, 2002.

22. Horohov DW, Dimock AN, Gurinalda PD, et al: Effects of exercise on the immune response of young and old horses. Am J Vet Res 60:643, 1999.

23. Lehnhard RA, McKeever KH, Kearns CF, et al: Aging-related changes in fat free mass and myosin heavy chain in Standardbred mares. Vet J 167:59-66, 2002.

24. Lehnhard RA, McKeever KH, Kearns CF, et al: Myosin heavy chain is different in old versus young Standardbred mares. Med Sci Sports Exerc 33:S13, 2001.

25. Malinowski K, Betros CL, Flora L, Kearns CF, McKeever KH: Effect of training on age-related changes in plasma insulin and glucose. Equine Vet J Suppl 34:147, 2002.

26. McKeever KH, Kearns CF, Antas LA: Endothelin response to exercise in horses. Vet J 164:41, 2002.

27. McKeever KH, Kearns CF: Aging-induced alterations in plasma volume in horses. Med Sci Sports Exerc 33:S257, 2001.

28. McKeever KH, Eaton TL, Geiser S, Kearns CF: Thermoregulation in old and young horses during exercise. Med Sci Sports Exerc 32:S156, 2000.

29. McKeever KH, Malinowski K: Endocrine response to exercise in young and old horses. Equine Vet J Suppl 30:561, 1999.

30. McKeever KH, Malinowski K, Christensen R, Hafs HD: Chronic equine somatotropin administration does not affect aerobic capacity or indices of exercise performance in geriatric horses. Vet J 155:19, 1998.

30a. Ralston SL, Nockels CF, Squires EL: Differences in diagnostic test results and hematologic data between aged and young horses. Am J Vet Res 49:1387, 1988.

31. Lekeux P, Art T: The respiratory system: anatomy, physiology, and adaptations to exercise and training. In Hodgson DR, Rose RJ, eds: The Athletic Horse: Principles and Practice of Equine Sports Medicine. Philadelphia, WB Saunders, 1994, p 79-128.

32. Davies CTM, Thomas DO, White MJ: Mechanical properties of young and elderly muscle. Acta Med Scand Suppl 711:219, 1988.

33. Reaven GM: Insulin resistance and aging: modulation by obesity and physical activity. In Lamb DR, Gisolfi CV, Nadel E, eds: Perspectives in Exercise and Sports Medicine, Vol 8. Exercise in Older Adults. Carmel, IN, Cooper Publishing, 1995, p 395-428.

34. Goetz TE, Manohar M: Isoproterenol-induced maximal heart rate in normothermic and hyperthermic horses. Am J Vet Res 51:743, 1990.

35. McKeever KH, Hinchcliff KW: Neuroendocrine control of blood volume, blood pressure, and cardiovascular function in horses. Equine Vet J Suppl 18:77, 1995.

36. Haidet GC, Parsons D: Reduced exercise capacity in senescent beagles: an evaluation of the periphery. Am J Physiol 260:H173, 1991.

37. White T: Skeletal muscle structure and function in older mammals. In Lamb DR, Gisolfi CV, Nadel E, eds: Perspectives in Exercise and Sports Medicine, Vol 8. Exercise in Older Adults. Carmel, IN, Cooper Publishing, 1995, p 115-174.

38. McConaghy F: Thermoregulation. In Hodgson DR, Rose RJ, eds: The Athletic Horse: Principles and Practice of Equine Sports Medicine. Philadelphia, WB Saunders, 1994, p 181-191.

39. Geor RJ, McCutcheon LJ, Ecker Gayle L, et al: Thermal and cardiorespiratory responses of horses to submaximal exercise under hot and humid conditions. Equine Vet J Suppl 20:125, 1995.

40. Armstrong CG, Kenney WL: Effects of age and acclimation on responses to passive heat exposure. J Applied Physiol 75:2162, 1993.

41. Kenney WL: Body fluid and temperature regulation as a function of age. In Lamb DR, Gisolfi CV, Nadel E, eds: Perspectives in Exercise and Sports Medicine, Vol 8. Exercise in Older Adults. Carmel, IN, Cooper Publishing, 1995, p 305-351.

42. Kenney WL, Zappe DH: Effect of age on renal blood flow during exercise. Aging (Milano) 6:293, 1994.

43. Nieman DC: Immune function. In Lamb DR, Gisolfi CV, Nadel E, eds: Perspectives in Exercise and Sports Medicine, Vol 8. Exercise in Older Adults. Carmel, IN, Cooper Publishing, 1995, p 435-461.

44. Ho CW, Beard JL, Farrell PA, et al: Age, fitness, and regional blood flow during exercise in the heat. J Appl Physiol 82:1126, 1997.

45. Kearns CF, McKeever KH, Kumagai K, et al T: Fat-free mass is related to one mile race performance in elite Standardbred horses. Vet J 163:260, 2002.

46. Kearns CF, McKeever KH, John-Alder H, et al: Body composition and other predictors of maximal oxygen uptake. Equine Vet J Suppl 34:485, 2002.

47. Kearns CF, McKeever KH, Abe T: Overview of horse body composition and muscle architecture-implications for performance. Vet J 64:224, 2002.

48. Forbes GB, Reina JC: Adult lean body mass declines with age: some longitudinal observations. Metab Clin Exp 19:653, 1970.

49. Kohrt WM, Spina RJ, Ehsani AA, et al: Effects of age, adiposity, and fitness level on plasma catecholamine responses to standing and exercise. J Appl Physiol 75:1828, 1993.

50. Kohrt WM, Malley MT, Dalsky GP, et al: Body composition of healthy sedentary and trained, young and older men and women. Med Sci Sports Exerc 24:832, 1992.

51. Essen-Gustavsson B, Lindholm A: Muscle fibre characteristics of active and inactive Standardbred horses. Equine Vet J Suppl 17:434, 1985.

52. Gunn HM: Relative increase in areas of muscle fibre types in horses during growth. Equine Vet J Suppl 18:209, 1995.

53. Rivero JLL, Galisteo AM, Aguer E, et al: Skeletal muscle histochemistry in male and female Andalusian and Arabian horses of different ages. Res Vet Sci 54:160, 1993.

54. Roneus M, Lindholm A: Muscle characteristics in Thoroughbreds of different ages and sexes. Equine Vet J 23:207, 1991.

55. Snow DH, Billeter R, Jenny E: Myosin types in equine skeletal muscle fibres. Res Vet Sci 30:381, 1981.

56. Snow DH, Guy PS: Muscle fibre type composition of a number if limb muscles in different types of horses. Res Vet Sci 28:137, 1980.

57. van den Hoven R, Wensing TH, Breukink HJ, et al: Variation in fiber types in the triceps brachii, longissimus dorsi, gluteus medius, and biceps femoris of horses. Am J Vet Res 46:939, 1985.

58. Andersen JL, Terzis G, Kryger A: Increase in the degree of coexpression of myosin heavy chain isoforms in skeletal muscle fibers of the very old. Muscle Nerve 22:449, 1999.

59. Coggan AR, Abduljalil AM, Swanson SC, et al: Muscle metabolism during exercise in young and older trained and endurance trained men. J Appl Physiol 75:2125, 1993.

60. Coggan AR, Spina RJ, King DJ, et al: Histochemical and enzymatic characteristics of the gastrocnemius muscle of young and elderly men and women. J Gerontol 47:B71, 1992.

61. Frontera WR, Hughes VA, Fielding RA, et al: Aging of skeletal muscle: a 12-yr longitudinal study. J Appl Physiol 88:1321, 2000.

62. Cartee GD: Influence of age on skeletal muscle glucose transport and glycogen metabolism. Med Sci Sports Exerc 26:577, 1994.

63. Cartee GD, Farrar RP: Exercise training induces glycogen sparing during exercise by old rats. J Appl Physiol 64:259, 1988.

64. Tankersley CG, Smolander J, Kenney WL, et al: Sweating and skin blood flow during exercise: effects of age and maximal oxygen uptake. J Appl Physiol 71:236, 1991.

65. Lonnqvist F, Nyberg H, Wahrenberg H, et al: Catecholamine-induced lipolysis in adipose tissue of the elderly. J Clin Invest 85:1614, 1990.

66. Wade CE, Freund BJ, Claybaugh JR: Fluid and electrolyte homeostasis during and following exercise: hormonal and non-hormonal factors. In Claybaugh JR, Wade CE, eds: Hormonal Regulation of Fluid and Electrolytes. New York, Plenum, 1989, p 1-44.

67. Malinowski K, Shock EM, Roegner V, et al: Age and exercise training alter plasma β-endorphin, cortisol, and immune parameters in horses. J Animal Sci 80 (Suppl 1):156, 2003.

68. Mehl ML, Schott HC, Sarkar DK, et al: Effects of exercise intensity on plasma β-endorphin concentrations in horses. Am J Vet Res 61:969, 2000.

69. Sial S, Coggan AR, Carroll R, et al: Fat and carbohydrate metabolism during exercise in elderly and young subjects. Am J Physiol 271:E983, 1996.

70. Fiatarone MA, Morley JE, Bloom ET, et al: The effect of exercise on natural killer cell activity in young and old subjects. J Gerontol 44:M37, 1989.

71. Farquhar WB, Kenney WL: Age and renal prostaglandin inhibition during exercise and heat stress. J Appl Physiol 86:1936, 1999.

CHAPTER 9

Manual Therapy, Acupuncture, and Chinese Herbal Medicine in the Geriatric Equine

James D. Kenney,

William H. McCormick

Veterinary medicine has successfully managed to extend the lives of horses to the degree that our concerns now are with "quality of life" and performance issues in the geriatric animal. This extension of usefulness is a tribute to the effectiveness of the scientific method that is the basis of veterinary philosophy and to the dedicated clinicians who have persevered past the margins of medical orthodoxy.

Since antiquity, there has been a prejudice in favor of reason and against experiential knowledge. The longstanding dichotomy of medicine into science and art is a medical expression of this bias. However, knowledge, whether of medical science or the art of medicine, does not take care of sick persons or relieve their suffering; clinicians, who have integrated these kinds of knowledge, do.[1]

There are different ways to develop our diagnostic power. We may buy capital-intensive technology or we may develop our skills in palpation to the level of the hands-on, therapeutic modalities (i.e., acupuncture, manual therapy, massage, human chiropractics, and osteopathic medicine). As palpation is the primary focus of the hands-on therapies, it is learned in a more refined, comprehensive manner than the education we receive as veterinarians. An additional benefit of these hands-on therapies is that they are a means of sensory communication, of bridging the silence between you and your patient.[2]

To perform as the primary care practitioner, the veterinarian must acquire sufficient palpatory skills to assess upper body pain and function. Horse owners are subject to a plethora of complementary and alternative veterinary medicine from farriers, dentists, chiropractors, and other lay people. Having the capability to demonstrate the presence or absence of upper body pain rather than rejecting an unfamiliar therapy out of hand allows increased client rapport and demonstrates receptivity to clients' concerns and wishes, while placing veterinarians in the position of therapeutic quality control.

The Best Equine Geriatric Prescription

The best equine geriatric prescription is the same as it would be for you and me: proper diet and exercise. The only method proven to slow aging and extend the lifespan in mammals is caloric restriction of a nutrient-rich diet.[3] Exercise, as it is in elderly people, is extremely important in horses. Even though older horses have an age-altered endocrine response to exercise, they do have the capability to alter their body composition and improve aerobic capacity when exercised conditioned for 12 weeks.[4] Although aging may alter the control of cardiovascular function in the exercising horse, it does not produce the pronounced alterations that one would see in an exercising individual with a compromised cardiovascular system.[5] Many horses participate in athletic activities into their late teens and some do so beyond the age of 20 years; thus, the need exists to explore ways to adjust training programs for older horses.[6]

The geriatric animal requires an exacting approach. They are not simply older horses. They have needs stemming from aging physiology and age-related. The approach to the geriatric horse must be multidisciplinary and all-inclusive and must be driven by the goals of health maintenance and optimizing function. The aging process is far from being completely understood: "While aging and disease are distinctly different, the effects of the aging process on various organ systems are believed to reduce the organ's capacity to respond to increased demand. This has been called impaired homeostasis; it has significant clinical impact."[7]

Other theories of aging include weakened body defenses, hormonal and neuroendocrine failure, systemic inflammation, ischemia, and wear and tear.[3,7] Acupuncture and manual therapy may improve homeostasis, decrease wear and tear,[7,8] strengthen the body's defenses,[9] normalize hormonal and endocrine secretion,[10] decrease inflammation, and improve circulation.[11-14] A significant decrease in the prevalence of cell apoptosis occurred in the cerebral cortex on mice needled at true acupuncture points.[15] (Apoptosis has been implicated in the neurodegenerative pathophysiology of Alzheimer's, Parkinson's, and Huntington's diseases.[16])

Whether a horse develops some life-threatening affliction at an old age depends in part on its genetic constitution, in part on its lifelong exposure to environmental factors, and in part on the sheer luck of avoiding accidents. For disease that originates outside the body, it is relatively easy to identify the causative agents, such as pathogens and toxins, and do something about them. Most of the diseases of old age, however, result from the malfunctioning of the body itself, and their causes are rooted in the failure of defense and self-maintenance systems to function properly after a lifetime of hard work. Some problems are simply built into the system.

The horse's ability to perform the activities of daily living, gait disorders and instability, changes in postural control such as a decrease in proprioception and muscle tone, a slower righting reflex, degenerative joint disease, peripheral neuropathy, and muscle weakness all contribute to injuries and decreasing performance expectations.

Geriatric Issues

Aging studies in humans concur that musculoskeletal symptoms dominate the complaints of America's middle-aged and older adults for both men and women.[17] Pain is a common problem encountered among elderly people and is often underestimated, addressed inadequately, and undertreated.[18,19] Patient education and fitness walking can improve overall pain management and related functional limitations among elderly people with chronic musculoskeletal pain.[20] The management of chronic pain should be a priority in geriatric care, as it has tremendous potential to influence the physical function and quality of life of elderly people during their remaining years.[21] In one study, results indicate that 71% of the aged subjects had at least one pain complaint. Of subjects with pain, 34% described constant (continuous) pain and 66% described intermittent pain. Of 43 subjects with intermittent pain, 51% described pain on a daily basis. Major sources of pain included low back pain (40%), arthritis of appendicular joints (24 percent), previous fracture sites (14%), and neuropathies (11%).[22]

Osteoarthritis is a worldwide heterogeneous group of conditions that leads to joint symptoms, which are associated with defective integrity of articular cartilage, in addition to related changes in the underlying bone at the joint margins. The prevalence of the disease after the age of 65 years is about 60% in men and 70% in women. The cause of osteoarthritis is multifactorial, with the end result being mechanical joint failure and varying degrees of loss of joint function.[23]

An important iatrogenic problem is the failure to recognize special needs and weaknesses of geriatric animals. Unnecessary bed rest and immobility are common iatrogenic problems for the elderly human patient. Musculoskeletal activity is essential to maintain homeostatic mechanisms.[7] Weight loss in the geriatric horse may be related to inability to ambulate.[24] The human elderly also have a high frequency of adverse drug reactions (ADRs); studies show that the incidence of ADRs increases significantly with age. It has been reported that approximately 40% of hospitalized elderly patients develop ADRs. These observations are believed to occur because of a decrease in the therapeutic window with age. Both pharmacokinetic and pharmacodynamic changes occur that predispose the elderly to ADRs. Changes in body composition, altered hepatic function, and a decline in renal function all contribute to the pharmacokinetic alterations.[7] Adverse drug reactions are rare in horses but cause serious anxiety to patients, owners, and veterinarians when they occur and are frequently the reason for legal action.[25] Drug interactions are common in older people as they take more medications and have reduced ability to clear most analgesic and adjuvant medications; it is suggested that there exists a larger than usual role for nonpharmacological management strategies among these patients.[26,27]

Acupuncture and manual therapy are useful in the management of chronic pain, are safe, and decrease the need for medication.

Pain Is Common in the Geriatric Equine

Pain, especially in the locomotor system, is a curse humankind has always suffered.[28] The evolutionary purpose of pain is to warn of physical injury and to stimulate evasive action. On the one hand, injury often occurs without causing pain, for example on the sports field or more dramatically in battle, where traumatic limb amputation has occurred completely painlessly. On the other hand, chronic pain can and frequently does persist long after the original inflammation or injury has healed.[29] The difficulty in assessing pain is a serious handicap in ensuring the well-being of animals. This is important because chronic pain in animals may not have symptoms recognizable using prevailing veterinary protocol and thus often remains untreated.[30]

The geriatric equine may experience arthritis, degenerative joint disease, chronic lameness, bone deformity around joints, or inflexible joints due to chronic inflammation. Management includes scrupulous shoeing/trimming, proper bedding, and avoiding obesity and may include anti-inflammatory therapy. Phenylbutazone should be used judiciously in horses with osteoarthritis, because chronic administration may suppress proteoglycan synthesis and potentiate cartilage damage.[31] Intra-articular steroids have long been blamed for adverse effects such as "steroid arthropathy" in horses.[25] Osteoarthritis is a common indication for acupuncture and manual therapy. Treatment may make these animals comfortable and increase their level of physical activity. Acupuncture prescriptions for joint pain are discussed in great detail elsewhere.[32] Acupuncture points may be implanted as a means of decreasing or eliminating intra-articular injection.[33]

Back pain is common in the equine at any age and varies greatly in severity[34] and incidence (0.9%-94%) depending on the specialization or type of practice surveyed.[35] Thus, the geriatric equine may experience acute or chronic back pain with subsequent muscle spasm. Muscle spasm is a reflexive contraction mediated at the spinal cord level, presumably designed to protect and immobilize an injured part. Muscle spasm is a component of all acute injuries: as the reactive tissue of the musculoskeletal system, muscle responds to insult in the only way it can, by contracting. Persistent muscle spasm is a painful pathologic contraction resulting in limitation of motion and continued morbidity. Horses may recover spontaneously from back problems, irrespective of diagnosis and treatment or management regimen.[36] However, we must attend to those that have recurrent or persistent back pain. Long-term rest, in many cases, is neither feasible nor curative.[37] Pelvic asymmetry, often associated with poor performance,[38] is common in the geriatric equine. Functional assessment of the spine and pelvis is necessary to determine whether treatment is appropriate.

Complementary and adjunctive therapies are used in humans for low back pain more frequently than for any other indication. Expert opinions on the use of complementary and adjunctive therapies for low back pain indicate that for acute uncomplicated low back pain, most experts rated osteopathic and chiropractic medicine effective and for chronic uncomplicated low back pain, most experts considered acupuncture effective.[39] Use of acupuncture and manual therapy is valuable in managing pain in the geriatric horse.

Chronic forelimb lameness may be due to laminar corial hyperesthesia associated with cervicospinal pain and reduced spinal mobility.[40] Thoracolumbar spinal disease is often associated with lameness or limb gait abnormality (85 percent).[37] These lamenesses are characterized by a vague limb gait abnormality that eluded precise localization and inconsistently worsened with limb flexion. Careful limb palpation usually failed to help localize the site of pain and diagnostic regional anesthesia was similarly inconclusive. Absence of demonstrable pain did not exclude insidious spinal column disease, particularly kissing spines. Painful response to digital pressure on the tips of the dorsal spines or epaxial musculature was manifest in only half of these horses.

Chronic Pain: Mechanisms and Nociceptive Control

Mechanisms and nociceptive control of chronic pain are discussed in great detail elsewhere.[29] A stimulus is not regarded necessarily as painful. Rather, it indicates trauma and is therefore termed *nociceptive*. The nociceptive stimulus is processed or "modulated" on its passage through the central nervous system and may or may not result in the unpleasant experience that we recognize as pain. The process of preventing noxious stimuli from reaching consciousness is referred to as *nociceptive control*. Nociceptive stimuli activate small nerve fibers, including the unmyelinated C fibers and the myelinated Aδ fibers. Stimulation of the primitive C fibers produces pain with a profound quality (slow, deep, or chronic pain) and a strong emotional effect. C fibers may be inhibited by the action of larger myelinated fibers, including the Aδ and the Aβ groups, which developed later (in evolutionary terms) than C fibers.

C Fibers

Small, unmyelinated C fibers are the most numerous fibers in mammalian afferent nerves. Their threshold may be reduced in certain disease states and lead to.

Nerves respond to light pressure, which was previously subthreshold (allodynia). C fibers release the amino acids glutamate and aspartate as transmitters. The difference between acute and chronic pain, at least in part, has to do with the transmitters glutamate and aspartate. In acute pain, glutamate released by nociceptive impulses stimulates the α-amino-3-hydroxy-5-methyl-4-isoxalone propionic acid (AMPA) receptor, which responds to impulses on a strictly one-to-one basis. In chronic pain, repeated C-fiber stimulation leads to the release not only of the amino acids but also the peptides substance P, calcitonin gene-related peptide and neurokinin A. These rapidly activate a second receptor, known as N-methyl-d-aspartate (NMDA). The NMDA receptor does not respond on a one-to-one basis but produces a greatly amplified signal and the amplification can augment responses by 20-fold.

After being processed in the substantia gelatinosa cells in lamina II, the nociceptive signal activates the large transmission cells in lamina V. Transmission cells are fewer in number than the fibers in the dorsal root, so sensory information converges. This convergence occurs throughout the afferent system and offers important opportunities for influence, summation, and control of nociception. Nociceptive information then passes forwards, mainly to the intralaminar nuclei of the thalamus, which project diffusely throughout the cerebral cortex. Other fibers pass to the limbic system, including the cingulate gyrus, which is the seat of the emotional component of pain. Thus, noxious stimulation conveyed by the C-fiber system leads to a perception of pain that is poorly localized but has considerable emotional impact.

Aδ Fibers

Chronic pain can be the outcome of any (or a combination of) the following: (1) continuous stimulation of Aδ and C fibers from ongoing nociception (such as an unhealed fracture), or from ongoing inflammation (rheumatoid arthritis, for instance); (2) psychogenic factors (which are outside the present discussion); and (3) functional disturbances in the nervous system, when there may be supersensitivity in the pain sensory system but no actual excitation of nociceptors from extrinsic sources.[29]

Radiculopathic (and neuropathic) pain belongs to category 3; it typically occurs in the absence of ongoing tissue injury, nociception, or inflammation. It is secondary to a functional disturbance in the nervous system (radiculopathy) and is always, therefore, accompanied by signs of neuropathy, which resolve after successful treatment. Other features of neuropathic pain include (1) delay in onset after precipitating injury (supersensitivity takes at least 5 days to develop); (2) unpleasant sensations such as dysesthesias, or deep, aching pain; (3) pain felt in a region of sensory deficit; and (4) paroxysmal, brief, shooting or stabbing pain. Mild stimuli can be very painful (allodynia). Significantly, additional pain may be produced mechanically by muscle shortening.[41]

Frontier Diagnosis: Emerging Methods of Pain Assessment

Palpation provides sensory information that the brain interprets as manifestations of or changes in temperature, texture, surface humidity, elasticity, turgor, tissue tension, thickness, shape, irritability, and motion. We must learn to observe through our fingers in order to heighten our ability to perceive and differentiate from among these aspects listed. With training and practice, palpatory skills allow us to detect extremely subtle changes in the body. Tissue movements as small as 1 μm are perceptible to the trained individual.[42] Osteopathic medicine describes pathologic tissue changes using the term *somatic dysfunction*: "Impaired or altered function of related components of the somatic (body framework) system: skeletal, arthrodial, and myofascial structures, and related vascular, lymphatic, and neural elements."[43]

Motion palpation skills must be developed over time. In the beginning, it is natural to feel overwhelmed and distracted by the mass of palpatory data available, until a filtering process is developed that reduces the data to relevant and clinically significant findings. Common palpation errors are a lack of concentration, too much pressure, and excess movement by the examiner's hands and fingers during the palpatory examination. The learning curve for developing motion palpation skills is similar to developing joint flexion techniques in that it takes a number of horses to develop the tactile sense to recognize what is normal. One does spend the rest of his or her career refining technique. It is a natural progression from joint flexion techniques to assessing the lateral bending, flexion/extension, and rotation of individual spinal segments in the context of facet angle and other anatomic specifics.

Musculoskeletal examination for somatic dysfunction has been discussed in great detail in the human osteopathic literature.[44] What will be presented here will be a simple, subjective, effective examination of joint motion in the spine and pelvis of the horse See Appendix 9B: "A guide to motion palpation of the equine spine and pelvis for the veterinarian". Education of the: motor components of motion palpation is largely a subjective, experiential process. Gatterman suggests that the following steps be taken to improve the reliability of palpatory procedures: Standardization of test procedures, repetition of test findings, corrobora-tion of test findings, identification of suitable patient subpopulations, and re-evaluation of specificity assumption.[45]

Some pain provocation studies have shown poor reliability, and the unreliable nature of motion palpation has been discussed at length.[45,46] However, when using a combination of pain provocation and motion palpation, the reliability appears to increase.[47] A study that demonstrated 100% agreement for manual diagnosis compared with a diagnostic joint block manual diagnosis was based on the assessment of three clinical features: pain, quality of motion, and range of motion/end feel. This manual examination had a κ score of 1 for detecting the painful zygapophysial joint associated with the patient's cervicogenic headache as confirmed by intra-articular joint block.[48]

Human osteopathy includes extensive training in palpatory diagnosis. Diagnostic criteria for the human osteopathic evaluation of somatic dysfunction that are available through palpation comprise the mnemonic TART (Box 9-1).[44]

Motion Palpation

In order to understand motion palpation, one must examine each articulation with a focus on the specific characteristics of each articulation. It is important to develop consistency in standardization of examination. Of particular note is the horse's position, the veterinarian's position in relation to the horse, the specific area in which the veterinarian touches the horse and what part of the veterinarian's anatomy contacts the horse. The horse as well as the veterinarian must be stable. Static palpation findings indicate present anatomic relationships. Motion palpation findings are a description of altered joint end-feel, restricted joint motion, or asymmetric motion of a joint in one, two, or three planes of movement (e.g., flexion or extension, left or right lateral bending, left or right axial rotation).

One must proceed with caution because horses with painful articulations in the spine or pelvis may be defensive and react violently when examined. As noted by Kevin Haussler, DVM, PhD, DC, manual therapy is not a "cure-all" for every back problem and is not suggested for treatment of fractures, infections, neoplasia, metabolic disorders, or nonmechanically related joint disorders. Acute episodes of sprains or strains, degenerative joint disease, or impinged spinous processes are also relative contraindications for chiropractic adjusting. All neurologic diseases should be fully worked up to assess the potential risks or benefits of chiropractic treatment. Serious diseases requiring immediate medical or

surgical care need to be ruled out and treated by conventional veterinary medicine before routine manual therapy is begun. Nevertheless, manual therapy may contribute to the rehabilitation of most post-surgical cases or severe medical conditions by helping in the restoration of normal musculoskeletal function. Manual therapy cannot reverse severe degenerative processes or overt pathologic lesions. Manual therapy works optimally in the early clinical stages of disease versus end-stage disease, at which stage reparative processes have been exhausted. This is why manual therapy and other complementary and alternative modalities often fail to produce their fully desired therapeutic effects when used as a last resort.[35]

Box 9-1

Diagnostic Criteria for the Human Osteopathic Evaluation of Somatic Dysfunction: TART

T: Tissue texture abnormalities. This is palpatory assessment of quality of tissues, usually paraspinal. Tissue changes accompany somatic dysfunction. Tissue texture change is evaluated in layers, from superficial or skin to deep, such as deep muscle. Tissue texture changes are described as acute or chronic.

A: Asymmetry in tonicity, turgor, color, temperature, and static and motion palpation.

R: Restriction of motion. Active motion testing involves instructing the patient to move, with the physician observing and recording range of motion. Passive motion testing involves the physician slowly introducing motion (with the patient inactive or passive). Taking the joint to the endpoint of motion in both directions, or in all directions if multiple planes of motion are being assessed, assesses the quantity of motion. Quality of motion is assessed by palpation; that is, the physician introduces motion and assesses compliance or resistance to the motion being introduced.

T: Tenderness (in the dysfunctional location). Tenderness is said to be present when the physician applies a stimulus, usually palpatory pressure, and the patient reports discomfort, flinches, has a facial change, or otherwise indicates discomfort. The test is objective in that the physician applies a measured force to the patient. Patient response involves a degree of subjectivity, depending on the individual's sensitivity or threshold for pain. Tenderness differs from pain. Pain is a totally subjective cerebral (cortical) perception of nociceptive input reported by the patient in the absence of palpatory stimulus.

Manual Therapy

Between 60% and 80% of the human population suffers low back pain during their lives.[35] Many affected individuals turn to manual therapy for their own pain problems, often with effective and consistent results.[49] Some clients prefer manual therapy (such as chiropractic) to medication or surgery for their animals as well. Human research shows that manual therapy can provide as much relief as conventional treatment but with less or no medications.[50] Training in veterinary manual therapy provides veterinarians the opportunity to gain further expertise in evaluating joint and spine disorders. It equips veterinarians with treatment options for effectively diagnosing and treating musculoskeletal dysfunction in pain conditions, performance problems, and gait abnormalities. Early intervention may prevent irreversible pathologic structural changes from occurring in the ensuing months or years. Clients would likely prefer to have their animals treated by a veterinarian, but it is difficult to find veterinary professionals trained in this modality.

Equine Manual Therapy: Manual therapy provides important diagnostic and therapeutic approaches that are not currently available in veterinary medicine.[35] Most of what we know about equine manual therapy has been borrowed from human chiropractic techniques, theories, and research and adapted to our animal patients. Therapeutic trials of chiropractic adjustments are often used, since we currently have limited knowledge about the effects of manual therapy in animals. Manual therapy addresses mechanically related disorders of the musculoskeletal and nervous systems and provides a conservative means of treatment for horses with spinal problems. Chiropractic techniques involve a controlled force applied to a specific anatomical region or osseous structure to produce a desired therapeutic response (i.e., restore joint motion and reduce pain). The applied treatment influences both mechanoreceptor and nociceptor function via mechanical and biological mechanisms.[51]

Recent equine manual therapy research has demonstrated that forces applied to instrumented vertebral segments do induce substantial vertebral motion, usually beyond the normal range of segmental motion that occurs during locomotion.[52] Segmental vertebral motion characteristics induced during manual therapy treatment in horses are similar to those reported in humans.[53] The induced vertebral motion supports current theories on the effects of chiropractic manipulations on joint physiology. Future studies need to evaluate the long-term mechanical and neurophysiologic effects of manual therapy techniques in horses. Compared to a control group, a series of chiropractic treatments produced a measurable increase in pain pressure thresholds in 10 of 10 vertebral locations treated. However, only 5 of 10 of these vertebral locations had a statistically significant increase in values.[54] Girth pain may respond to manual therapy.[55] Knowledge of normal segmental vertebral motion and response to manual therapies will further our future understanding of the pathophysiology, clinical diagnosis, and treatment of spinal problems in horses. Manual therapy adjustments are usually done without any sedation or other medications but may occasionally be done under anesthesia if indicated.[56]

Joint Motion Equals Joint Health: Chiropractors, osteopaths, medical doctors, and physical therapists describe joint complex dysfunction in the literature. All agree that reduced mobility promotes pathologic changes in the structures that make up the joint complex. Pain, inflammation, and stiffness are common manifestations. Restoring mobility is often a primary objective of care. Muscles often develop weakness or tightness in typical imbalance patterns that promote faulty movement patterns. In addition, muscles play a role in stabilizing the spinal column and muscle weakness may predispose the spine to injury.[57]

Joint motion has been equated to joint health: a joint that loses its ability to move properly also loses its ability to nourish itself and maintain tissue integrity and therefore begins to degenerate.[58] When researchers wish to reproduce arthritis in experimental animals, the most common procedure is to immobilize the joints.[59-62] Restoration of movement can decrease the rate of degeneration or even restore the joint to its normal structure and function.[63-66]

The mechanisms underling the benefits of spinal manipulation are not well understood. It has been suggested that the effect of a chiropractic treatment is not due to correction of a subluxation; rather, it stimulates mechanoreceptors and causes reflex relaxation.[67] When motor neuron pool excitability is measured directly by central corticospinal activation with transcranial magnetic stimulation techniques, a transient but significant facilitation occurs as a consequence of spinal manipulation.[68] Spinal manipulation in humans provided a repeatable and systematic electromyographic response that extended beyond the immediate area of force application. In symptomatic patients, local muscle hypertonicity was largely abolished immediately after the spinal manipulation induced electromyographic response, supporting the idea that spinal manipulation reduces hyperactivation of muscles in areas of back pain.[69]

In a study to determine response of muscle proprioceptors to spinal manipulative-like loads in the anesthetized cat and to measure whether muscle spindles and Golgi tendon organs in paraspinal muscles respond to a mechanical load whose force-time profile is similar to that of a spinal manipulation, the data suggest that the high-velocity, short-duration load delivered during the impulse of a spinal manipulation can stimulate muscle spindles and Golgi tendon organs more than the preload. The physiologically relevant portion of the manipulation may relate to its ability to increase as well as decrease the discharge of muscle proprioceptors. In addition, the preload, even in the absence of the impulse, can change the discharge of paraspinal muscle spindles.[70]

Efficacy of Manual Therapy: There are more than 30 randomized controlled clinical trials in humans studying the effectiveness of spinal manipulation in the relief of spinal pain, the majority of which have looked at acute low back pain.[71] These studies have been subjected to a number of meta-analyses that have consistently demonstrated a beneficial effect of manipulation on the duration and severity of low back pain. Manipulation has been compared to most nonsurgical treatment modalities including placebo, ultrasound, traction, exercise, bed rest, analgesics, and corsets. The meta-analyses performed by Anderson et al.[49] led to the conclusion that the average patient receiving spinal manipulation is better off than 54% to 85% of the patients receiving the comparison treatment. There are 11 studies on the effectiveness of manipulation on chronic low back pain. Each of these studies reported short-term positive results in one or more parameters of pain or disability.[71] For cervical manipulation, the systematic literature review indicated efficacy for neck pain and for patients with muscle-tension-type headache.[72] In patients with chronic spinal pain syndromes, spinal manipulation, if not contraindicated, results in greater improvement than acupuncture and medicine.[73]

Spinal manipulation of the cervical spine increases active range of motion.[74] Mechanical force spinal manipulation increases trunk muscle strength assessed by electromyography.[75] It can be shown that back pain and muscle spasm are elicited or reduced in different positions.[76] This may explain the beneficial effects of spinal manipulation as it demonstrates that mechanoreceptors some distance from the affected facet joint are sensitive to facet motion.

The nocireaction caused by a somatic joint dysfunction proceeds predominantly via the dorsal ramus of the spinal nerve that supplies the back muscles. This is electromyographically demonstrated by continued spontaneous activity in the respective segmental muscle. If the afferent information from the restricted joint is blocked with local anesthetic injection, the spontaneous activity disappears. The same result can be achieved with injection into the corresponding segmental muscle with a delay of 4 minutes. Manipulation (thrust techniques)

results in the immediate disappearance of spontaneous activity.[77]

Knee-joint pathologies, such as anterior knee pain, are associated with strength deficits and reduced activation of the knee extensors, which is referred to as *muscle inhibition*. Muscle inhibition is thought to prevent full functional recovery, and treatment modalities that help to reduce or eliminate muscle inhibition appear necessary for successful rehabilitation. Clinical observations suggest that anterior knee pain is typically associated with sacroiliac joint dysfunction. In a randomized controlled trial, it was demonstrated that conservative lower back treatment (i.e., spinal manipulation of the sacroiliac joint) reduces inhibition in knee-extensor muscles.[78]

Another human study indicates that the mortise separation adjustment is superior to detuned ultrasound therapy in the management of subacute and chronic grade I and grade II inversion ankle sprains.[79]

A recent well-designed study published by a physical therapist with a master's degree in orthopedic manual therapy provides strong evidence that spinal manipulation in conjunction with stabilization exercises can provide better 2- and 3-month outcomes than the same stabilization exercise program alone for acute low back pain patients. It is the first relative efficacy trial that clearly demonstrates better results for a rehabilitation program that combines spinal manipulation with exercise rather than just the same exercise program by itself. Not only are the results better with the combined treatment plan; the outcomes are dramatically better.[80] Spinal manipulation also appears to be cost-effective.

In a randomized, controlled trial (n = 21) comparing three treatment groups (thoracic adjustment, placebo adjustment, and no treatment), the thoracic adjustment group had significant short-term reductions in both systolic and diastolic blood pressure.[81] Spinal manipulation in humans is effective in relieving infantile colic compared to treatment with the drug dimethicone.[82] Spinal manipulation may impact most efficiently on the complex process of proprioception and dizziness of cervical origin when compared to acupuncture, nonsteroidal anti-inflammatory drugs (NSAIDs), or no therapy.[83] Another study demonstrates a significant improvement in cognitive function, as measured by an improved reaction time to a mental rotation task, after upper cervical adjustments.[84]

Spinal manipulative therapy may improve athletic performance without a history of pain. Asymptomatic patients demonstrated improved performance in agility, balance, speed reaction time, kinesthetic perception, and power and increased biomechanical efficiency and proprioception with chiropractic treatment.[85] In measuring right-to-left weight distribution using dual scales, 12 weeks of chiropractic care improved weight distribution symmetry 3.7 pounds versus 12.8 pounds.[86] Using force plates to measure symmetry of force distribution during walking, chiropractic treatment improved symmetry to normal force profiles.[87]

Safety of Manual Therapy: Spinal manipulative therapy in humans is relatively safe. For both cervical manipulation and manipulation for low-back pain, the literature reports low levels of complications. For cervical manipulation, the estimated risk for serious complications is 6.39 per 10 million manipulations. For lumbar manipulation, the estimate is 1 serious complication per 100 million manipulations. The risk from manipulation is low and compares favorably to other forms of therapy for the same conditions (e.g., 15.6 complications per 1000 cervical spine surgeries, 3.2 per 1000 subjects for NSAIDs).[72] There are no clinical or case-control studies that show spinal manipulative therapy is unsafe for the treatment of low back pain. The literature suggests that chiropractic manipulation is safer than medical management of low back pain.[88]

In 1996, Dabbs and Lauretti reviewed the literature from 1966 to 1994 to assess the evidence that cervical manipulation is an effective treatment for mechanical pain and to evaluate the risk of serious injury or death resulting from cervical manipulation in addition and to assess the risks and effectiveness of NSAIDs, which are often used as the conventional first-line treatment for similar musculoskeletal conditions. They found that although there are a small number of well-performed trials of cervical manipulation for neck pain, they were unable to locate even a single randomized, controlled trial examining NSAID use specifically for neck pain. As for comparative safety, the best available evidence indicates that NSAID use poses a significantly greater risk of serious complications and death than the use of cervical manipulation for comparable conditions.[89]

Acupuncture

Acupuncture may be defined as the stimulation of specific predetermined points on the body to achieve a therapeutic or homeostatic effect. Acupuncture has been a diverse tradition with many voices and styles, both in historical and modern periods. It is generally believed to have originated in China, has an extensive body of literature that began around 200 BCE,[29] and is an aspect of Traditional Chinese Medicine (TCM). Around 650 BCE, Bai-le wrote *Bai-le's Canon of Veterinary Medicine*, one of the first veterinary textbooks.[90] It was primarily on acupuncture and moxibustion and emphasized equine medicine.

One helpful aspect of Traditional Chinese Acupuncture (TCA) is that no matter what clinical situation arises, there is a treatment associated with it. Acupuncture originally developed in a virtually technology-free

culture and depended on naked sense observations to gather data about patient problems. The traditionally based acupuncture diagnosis makes no effort to objectively describe disease; rather, it seeks to classify various signs and symptoms according to traditional notions of health, eventually categorizing these as a "pattern," which in turn always has a prescribed treatment associated with it.[29]

The metaphysics that emphasizes the perception of patterns is basic to Chinese thinking. It results in part from Taoism, which altogether lacks the idea of a creator, and whose concern is insight into the web of phenomena, not the weaver. For the Chinese, that web has no weaver, no creator; in the West, the final concern is always the creator or cause and the phenomenon is merely its reflection. The Western mind seeks to discover and encounter what is beyond, behind, or the cause of phenomena. In the Chinese view, the truth of things is imminent; in the Western, truth is transcendent. Knowledge, within the Chinese framework, consists in the accurate perception of the inner movement of the web of phenomena. The desire for knowledge is the desire to understand the interrelationships or patterns within that web and to become attuned to the unfolding dynamic.[91]

It is important to develop an understanding of what perspective the Chinese intended and not react to our own mistranslations or misconceptions of TCM. For example, to characterize *Qi* as energy is to invoke a worldview the Chinese never had, in which matter and energy are different things. To call *Qi* energy or life force is probably as erroneous as it is to call it matter.[91] The Chinese character for *Qi* is composed of the vapor radical enclosing the radical for rice or grain. It is said to be a picture of fumes wafting up from a batch of fermenting rice. *Qi* is therefore a smell or gas, and, by extension, something that moves yet cannot be seen and is detected only by the effects it has on other things.[92]

What then, would be the contemporary equivalent of *Qi*? Perhaps the concept most central to all of science is energy. The combination of energy and matter makes up the universe: matter is substance, and energy is the mover of substance. The idea of matter is easy to grasp. Matter is the stuff that we can see, smell, and feel. It has mass and occupies space. Energy, on the other hand, is abstract. We cannot see, smell, or feel most forms of energy. Although energy is familiar to us, it is difficult to define, because it is not only a thing but also a process, as if it were both a noun and a verb. Persons, places, and things have energy, but we usually observe energy only when it is happening—only when it is being transformed. It comes to us in the form of electromagnetic waves from the sun and we feel it as thermal energy; it is captured by plants and binds molecules of matter together; it is in the food we eat, and we receive it by digestion. Even matter itself is condensed bottled-up energy, as set forth in Einstein's famous formula, $E = mc^2$.[93]

Chinese thought does not distinguish between matter and energy, but we can perhaps think of *Qi* as matter on the verge of becoming energy, or energy at the point of materializing. But the concept is far beyond this simple attempt to bridge the chasm of a Western dichotomy. In a single syllable, the word *Qi* proclaims one of the deepest root intuitions of Chinese civilizations.[91] In any case, *Qi* is perceived functionally, by what it does.

In *The Web That Has No Weaver*, Ted Kaptchuk addresses the question of whether Chinese medicine is an art or a science. If science is the relatively recent intellectual and technological development in the West, then Chinese medicine is not scientific. It is a pre-scientific tradition that has survived into the modern age and remains another way of doing things. Chinese medicine does resemble science in that it is grounded in conscientious observation of phenomena, guided by rational, logically consistent, and communicable thought process. It has a body of knowledge with standards of measurement that allow systematic description, diagnosis, and treatment of illness. Its measurements are not the linear, fixed yardsticks of weight, number, time, and volume but rather flexible images of the phenomenal world. Because it deals with situationally dependent images, Chinese medicine allows and demands a recognition and assessment of quality and context.[91]

Acupuncture Points

The concept of the acupuncture point may be better understood by examining Chinese point nomenclature, which cannot be disassociated with the pervasive philosophical and metaphysical worldview of Taoism and Confucianism, veneration for custom and history, a propensity to observe and correlate the phenomena of nature, and a long medical tradition of apprenticeship and secret teaching.

Xuè is the character used in Chinese to represent the acupuncture points. Its translation is cave, den, hole, underground dwelling, or to bore a hole. The top part of the character represents a roof. The bottom portion means "to divide." Therefore, the meaning of the character is derived from the idea of a space that is obtained by the removal of rocks and dirt.[92] This concept of a hole that one must search for is lacking if one uses the Western meaning of *point*: an intersection of two lines or a spot on a map.

"The names of the points are not merely nominal; each has a profound meaning."[92] In China, the acupuncture points are somatotopically organized on the body. If you know the name of the acupuncture point, then you know where the point is located. If you know

where the point is located, then you know the function of the point. The Western system of acupuncture nomenclature is convenient, logical, and easy to learn. Points are numbered, grouped according to function, and arranged in a linear fashion (meridians).

Stimulation of acupuncture points has many and various physiologic effects on all systems throughout the body. No one mechanism can explain all the physiologic effects observed. The traditional Chinese medical theories have explained these effects based on empirical observations and descriptions of naturally occurring phenomena. Essentially, acupuncture stimulates various sensory receptors, which stimulates sensory afferent nerves that transmit the signal through the central nervous system to the hypothalamic/pituitary system. Various neurotransmitters and neurohormones are then released and have their subsequent effects throughout the body.

Palpation of Acupuncture Points: It is important to have an idea of where to begin looking for the acupuncture point that needs treating. If, in a treatment formula, a specific acupuncture point is listed, this generally means going to the standard anatomical location for that point and then palpating around it to find the reactive point, which may be indicated by the presence of pressure pain or a small knot or indentation.[94]

It has been suggested that reactive points are far more effective than textbook points for chronic pain management and that acupuncture points refer to general potential sites in the myofascial territory that are predisposed to dysfunction concomitantly.[95] Acupuncture images called *meridians* are but early maps of myofascial pain and dysfunction made by acupuncturists thousands of years ago without the benefit of dissection and autopsy.[95] Matsumoto and Birch have also made a highly articulate case made for viewing acupuncture as a myofascial, connective tissue therapy.[96]

Tender points can be described as *a shi* points (Chinese) or *kori* (Japanese). An *a shi* point, as described in Chinese acupuncture, is any point where, upon palpation, the patient expresses pain and discomfort in response to pressure. In Japanese acupuncture, *kori* is a general term used to describe areas of bodily stiffness and constriction with discomfort. *Kori* is defined as tight myofascial constriction, which the practitioner can definitely feel as a constriction beneath probing fingers, which may or may not elicit discomfort when pressed. Some Japanese texts describe more than a dozen different shapes and textures for *kori*, all of which constitute different types of myofascial constriction. When *kori* are present in the muscles and fascia, they block that area and thus the four circulatory systems of the body are impeded: lymphatic drainage, venous transport, arterial circulation, and nervous conduction. When these systems are blocked, not only will there be pain and discomfort, but the internal regulatory and immune functions will also be compromised.[95]

Human acupuncturists use certain visual clues that can indicate that a point needs treatment. These include signs of swelling, tight underlying musculature, and depressions in the skin or musculature. Upon touching the point, there might be very subtle signs, primarily at the skin level, such as sponginess of the skin, dryness or roughness of the skin, stickiness of the point, or a palpable "hole." As a little pressure is applied to the point, there is some resistance, hardness, a knot, a very subtle response of the tissues that can feel like a nonsymmetric compression of the tissues rather than a smooth compression of the tissues, or a feeling that almost appears to be avoidance.[94]

Another method of determining the appropriateness of point selection is to select a point that was reactive before needle application and palpate it again to see whether the reaction at the point is different. If the reaction is dramatically reduced, this is an indication of the accuracy of the location and the appropriateness of the technique used on the point. The other obvious way of assessing the accuracy of point location is to see how the patient's symptoms change after needle application. In cases of pain or restricted range of motion, this is easily determined.[94]

Equine acupuncturists have described the acupuncture points as firm, yielding to pressure, tightening under pressure, warm, cold, and so on. A reactive point may trigger a muscle spasm or an evasive or aggressive reaction. Some horses will feel so much pain when pressure is applied to a point that they will bite or kick. Generally, a reaction to light pressure indicates a more acute condition, and response to deep pressure indicates a long-standing condition.[97]

By objectifying and confirming the existence of conditions of extreme subtlety, palpation serves us as the major methodology when symptomatic data may be "normal" or extremely difficult to evaluate. If palpation is able to cue us to the existence of pre-disease tendencies or states that have some probability of developing into specific pathologies, it thereby achieves a unique place in the diagnostic tool chest. However, pressure-induced pain is a sign of imbalance that may not have progressed to the point of manifestation on the symptomatic level. They may indicate tendencies that precede some more specific pathologic state. Thus, treating distal acupuncture points to eliminate the pain found on palpation, or treating the reactive acupuncture points themselves, may change these subtle influences.

Reactive Acupuncture Points: Reactive acupuncture points and sensitivity at Pailleux's points of tension[2] may indicate the appropriate treatment to alleviate pain. Equine acupuncturists have emphasized careful palpation of the musculature as a screening test to ascertain areas of abnormal sensitivity. Abnormally sensitive

acupuncture points may refer to intra-articular pathology.[98-100] The combination of reactive points may assist your diagnosis and aid you in localizing the cause of the problem. Acupuncture diagnosis is an excellent adjunct to your equine lameness examination. Diagnostic acupuncture should be used with other modalities, including nerve blocks, flexion tests, ultrasonography, radiology, and nuclear scintigraphy to achieve the best diagnosis and the best possible treatment.

Acupuncture points project a quality that reflects the state of the body. This is why palpation is so important. Not only does it help us find the acupuncture points we want to treat, but these acupuncture points project certain qualities relative to the nature of the problems we seek to cure: pressure pain, tension, tightness, swelling, indentation, thickness and suppleness of the skin, and temperature variation. Through palpation we are able simultaneously to gain diagnostic information and find the acupuncture points. Based on the patterns of reactivity found and the records of many years of research and practice, we are able to interpret this information and to further understand the body.[96]

Acupuncture: A Heuristic Device

Birch and Kaptchuk propose that the TCA diagnosis may be a heuristic device for selecting treatment, or a stepping-stone in the therapeutic process, but does not necessarily describe an objective entity as biomedicine attempts to do.[29] The focus of TCA is always on what treatment should be administered. This focus is particularly helpful with the aged equine patient, as clinical signs are a hodgepodge (which may or may not be significant) and client complaints are vague. One may, subsequently, use TCA as a starting point to provide symptomatic relief until diagnostics or the course of the clinical syndrome becomes apparent.

If one is not well versed in traditional Chinese notions of health, one could replace TCA concepts and practice a contemporary version that is better attuned to familiar neuroanatomic principles. Examination, diagnosis, and treatment, as well as progress of therapy, are all determined according to physical signs of peripheral neuropathy.* This system, referred to as intramuscular stimulation (IMS) to distinguish it from other forms of needling, is based on the Radiculopathy Model proposed by C. Chan Gunn and is used at many pain centers throughout the world.[41]

Other ways to view acupuncture are the neuroanatomic approach, which offers tangible, scientifically based expla-

---

*Peripheral neuropathy is a disease that causes disordered function in the peripheral nerve characterized by supersensitivity that can generate spontaneous electrical impulses triggering false pain signals or provoking involuntary muscle activity.

nations of the effects of needle stimulation, or the segmental approach, which traces the symptoms that are found in the dermatome, myotome, sclerotome, and viscerotome and translates them into acupuncture therapy.[29]

Radiculopathy Model

Gunn's Radiculopathy Model[8] of acupuncture proposes that the many and various conditions amenable to needle therapy, including chronic pain, are essentially epiphenomena (or signs and symptoms) of abnormal physiology in the peripheral nervous system that occur with radiculopathy. These various conditions (including any accompanying pain) improve when normal function is restored. The needle is a simple yet unique tool, able to access the peripheral nervous system to restore normal function. In other words, although the needle in acupuncture helps many conditions, they are but different facets of a single underlying condition: radiculopathy. Needle therapy does not treat individual diseases. Rather, it aims to restore homeostasis to the entire patient. It helps many conditions by a single expedient: restoring normal function to the peripheral nervous system.

Any circumstance that impedes the flow of motor impulses for a period of time can rob the effector organ of its excitatory input and can cause disuse supersensitivity in that organ and in associated spinal reflexes. The importance of disuse supersensitivity cannot be overemphasized. When a nerve malfunctions, the structures it supplies become supersensitive and will behave abnormally. These structures overreact to many forms of input, not only chemical but physical inputs including stretch and pressure. Disuse supersensitivity is basic and universal, yet not at all well known or credited.

It is not unusual for the flow of nerve impulses to be obstructed. Peripheral neuropathy, which is often accompanied by partial denervation, is not exceptional in adults. There are innumerable causes of peripheral nerve damage, such as trauma, inflammation, and infection. They may be from metabolic, degenerative, toxic, or other conditions. The nerve's response to any agent, however, is always the same: dysfunction of the nerve. Spondylosis is probably the most common cause of peripheral neuropathy. The spinal nerve root, because of its vulnerable position, is notably prone to injury from pressure, stretch, angulation, and friction. Because spondylosis follows wear and tear, radiculopathy is typically seen in middle-aged individuals.

Radiculopathic (and neuropathic) pain is characterized by functional disturbances in the nervous system, when there may be supersensitivity in the pain sensory system, but no actual excitation of nociceptors from extrinsic sources; it typically occurs in the absence of ongoing tissue injury, nociception, or inflammation. Neuropathy can cause muscle contracture, with concurrent muscle short-

ening. These constant companions of musculoskeletal pain can be palpated as ropy bands in muscle. Muscle shortening can cause further pain through mechanical pull. Physical force generated by a shortened muscle can give rise to many painful conditions (Box 9-2).

The key to treating all radiculopathic conditions is releasing the shortened paraspinal muscles. This is where the acupuncture needle plays its unsurpassed role.

Gunn believes that the needle is more than a therapeutic tool; it is a diagnostic tool as well.[41] It transmits feedback on the nature and consistency of the tissues it is penetrating. When it penetrates normal muscle, the needle meets with little hindrance; when it penetrates a contracture, there is firm resistance and the needle is grasped; and when it enters fibrotic tissue, there is a grating sensation (like cutting through a pear). Guided by the needle-grasp (De *Qi*), an examiner is able to identify the distressed segment quickly, and with greater accuracy than with x-rays, scans, or magnetic resonance imaging.

Neuroanatomic Acupuncture

Neuroanatomical acupuncture adds an intriguing new dimension to acupuncture by correlating traditionally described points and channels with neurologic pathways and influences. In so doing, neuroanatomic acupuncture offers tangible, scientifically based explanations of the effects of needle stimulation. A neuroanatomic approach to pain involves rebalancing neural regulation to an area in

---

Box 9-2

Physical Force Generated by a Shortened Muscle Can Give Rise to Many Painful Conditions

Shortening gives rise to tension in tendons and their attachments—when protracted, tension can cause such syndromes as epicondylitis, tendonitis, tenosynovitis, or chondromalacia patellae. When muscles acting on a joint shorten, they limit the joint's range.

Chronic restriction of joint range, misalignment, and increased pressure on articular surfaces can eventually lead to degenerative arthritis or osteoarthritis.

Pressure on a nerve can produce an entrapment syndrome. Shortening in the pronator teres or pronator quadratus, for example, can give rise to symptoms of a carpal tunnel syndrome.

The most critical of all the muscles that can shorten and press on, or pull on, supersensitive structures to cause pain, are the paraspinal muscles that act across an intervertebral disc space. They draw adjacent vertebrae together, compress the disc, and narrow the intervertebral foraminae compressing or irritating the nerve root.

order to optimize endogenous pain control systems, reduce inflammation, and resolve somatic dysfunction. This technique involves selecting points that relate to one or all of the three following levels of nerve input: spinal nerves, peripheral nerves, and autonomic input. The spinal nerves addressed are those that give rise to the innervation of the painful region. Points along the peripheral nerve are chosen that relate to the sensorimotor input to the area. It is important, also, to consider the autonomic (i.e., sympathetic) contributions to the region, both at the local site related to the vasculature and at the spinal segmental levels from which the autonomic innervation arises, because dysfunctional pain patterns become further perpetuated by heightened and unresolved sympathetic tone.[101]

Segmental Acupuncture

Segmental acupuncture is the technique of needling an area innervated by the same spinal segment as the disordered structure under treatment. It has been practiced since the earliest use of acupuncture therapies, though not by name or design. The use of "local" points and *a shi* points will almost inevitably involve treatment of the correct level in segmental terms. "Distant" points are less likely to fall within the same segment. However, there are a number of examples of classical points that do, such as *San Yin Jiao* (SP6), which is in the S2 myotome, for uterine problems.[29] A segmental diagnosis traces the symptoms that are found in the dermatome, myotome, sclerotome, and viscerotome and translates them into acupuncture therapy. For example, superficial shoulder pain (dermatome) can point to a disturbed C4; a trigger point in the deltoid muscle (myotome) with referred pain patterns to the upper arm can have a relationship with a segmental disturbance in C5/C6; an epicondylitis lateralis humeri (sclerotome) can point to a disturbance in C6; and stomach complaints (viscerotome) can be associated with a disturbance in T6.[41]

Mechanisms of Acupuncture

Acupuncture stimulates Aδ or group III small myelinated primary afferents in skin and muscle and produces a segmental and heterosegmental effect. In the segmental mechanism, acupuncture stimulates the larger myelinated Aδ fibers, which stimulate the inhibitory enkephalinergic stalked cells in the outer part of lamina II (substantia gelatinosa) of the spinal gray matter, on which the unmyelinated C fibers (pain fibers) end.

Heterosegmental acupuncture involves a generalized neurohormonal mechanism: release of β-endorphin and met-enkephalin. Extensive work has been done to demonstrate that stimulation of certain acupuncture points will induce the release of endogenous opioids and hence provide analgesia. There are 17 different lines

of experimental evidence that have independently supported this fact.[102] There are two descending neuronal mechanisms, the serotonergic and the adrenergic.[41]

Acupuncture reacts in local, regional (spinal cord), and general (brain) levels. Therefore, placing one or more needles on a particular point or area of the body activates neural pathways on three different levels, provoking local, regional, and general reactions. The local reaction is a multifactorial phenomenon. The electric injury potential due to the needle, the presence and synthesis of opioid peptides at the place of the injury, the substance P, and histamine-like substances bradykinin, serotonin, proteolytic enzymes all around the needle occurred during every needling therapy. The regional reaction concerns the activation of a larger area (two or three dermatomes) through reflex arches. The general reaction mainly activates the brain central mechanism of internal homeostasis and releases central neurotransmitters.[103] Researchers have suggested that noxious stimuli, when applied to any part of the body, can produce analgesic effects at distant sites (diffuse noxious inhibitory control). This response is thought to markedly modify the C-fiber response and is thought to be a key mechanism in acupuncture analgesia.[104]

Acupuncture also affects the levels of nitric oxide in plasma. This may explain acupuncture's rapid and complex action of interconnecting various systems and organ complexes, as nitric oxide is an important determinant of basal vascular tone. Nitric oxide is involved in a number of interneuronal functions, including long-term potentiation, memory synapse formation and plasticity, intracellular signal transmission, release of neurotransmitters, modulation of sensory and motor pathways, regulation of local cerebral circulation and cerebral blood flow, neuroendocrine regulation, feeding, and sexual behavior.[105]

Efficacy of Acupuncture

The level of scientific proof of the efficacy of human acupuncture has improved dramatically. Clinical researchers have devised a variety of protocols to test acupuncture efficacy according to generally accepted standards for randomized controlled trials.[106] Recently reported by Reuters Health (January 30, 2002) are the preliminary results of a large acupuncture study. The study, involving some 40,000 patients, is the largest acupuncture study ever undertaken. Of the patients in the study, almost 90% claimed that acupuncture treatments had resulted in relief from pain. Of those patients, around half suffered from back pain, some 26% from headaches, and 10% from knee or hip arthrosis. Of the patients who experienced relief from the treatments, some 51 percent did so within 2 weeks, usually after four treatments. Some 2% of patients needed more than 10 treatments before feeling relief. Severe side effects, such as local infection, occurred "very seldom," at a rate of "much less than 1%." The average age of study participants was around 58 years.

The largest scientific randomized controlled acupuncture study in the world, with 250,000 patients and approximately 10,000 established physician, demonstrated that acupuncture works reliably and durably with headache, chronic neck pain (neck spinal column syndrome), and hay fever. The results of the study are to determine whether acupuncture is included in the regular service catalog of the health insurance companies. Although the first results are ready now, the research will continue until 500,000 participants are reached. The study will end in October of 2008.[107]

According to a National Institute of Health[108] consensus panel of scientists, researchers, and practitioners who convened in November 1997, clinical studies have shown that acupuncture is an effective treatment for nausea caused by surgical anesthesia and cancer chemotherapy: 27 of 29 clinical trials, involving nearly 2000 patients, favored acupuncture.[106] Acupuncture is effective in alleviating pain during or after dental operations.[109] When compared with real acupuncture, placebo (sham) acupuncture was associated with more adverse effects directly related to tooth excision procedure. The panel also found that acupuncture is useful by itself or combined with conventional therapies to treat addiction, headaches, menstrual cramps, tennis elbow, fibromyalgia, myofascial pain, osteoarthritis, lower back pain, carpal tunnel syndrome, and asthma and to assist in stroke rehabilitation.

The existing evidence supports the value of acupuncture for the treatment of idiopathic headaches.[110] Acupuncture has demonstrated usefulness in treatment of radiation-induced xerostomia,[111-119] treatment of chemotherapy-induced leukocytopenia,[120] and urinary incontinence caused by detrusor hyperreflexia in patients with chronic spinal cord injuries.[121] Acupuncture possesses therapeutic effects for age-related problems, such as Parkinson's disease, by improving the clinical symptoms and signs, delaying the disease's progression, allowing a decrease in the dosage of antiparkinsonian drug, and providing expectant treatment of the complications and symptoms induced by the drug side-effects.[122,123] Acupuncture treatment was superior in immediate therapeutic effect on senile vascular dementia when compared with drug treatment. The statistical data showed that the total effective rate in the treatment group (80.6%) was significantly higher than in the control group (25%).[124]

Acupuncture has proven useful in human obstetrics.[106] There are controlled clinical trials on the use of acupuncture on breech presentation, pain relief during labor, and the duration and preparation for labor. One particular study (Romer et al.) in the duration of labor is particularly impressive. It has a large sample size (n = 878), good methodology, and very good assessments, and the results demonstrate significant benefits from acupuncture treatment versus standard care or sham acupuncture. Acupuncture increases the chance of pregnancy for women undergoing in vitro fertilization.[125] In a study on acupuncture and moxibustion therapy for female urethral syndrome, the short-term effective rate in the acupuncture and moxibustion group was 90.6% and the long-term effective rate was 80.4%, whereas the short-term effective rate of the control group was 26.9% ($P < .01$). The maximal uroflow rate increased by an average of 4.6 mL/sec after acupuncture and moxibustion treatment ($P < .001$) and the mean uroflow rate increased by an average of 3.1 mL/sec ($P < .001$); in contrast, no changes were found in the control group ($P > .05$). Sixty-nine cases from the acupuncture and moxibustion group and 39 from the control group were subjected before and after treatment to determinations of the maximal bladder pressure, maximal abdominal pressure, bladder-neck pressure, and maximal urethral closure pressure during urination. All these indexes were decreased remarkably in the acupuncture and moxibustion group, and no changes were observed in the control group.[126]

Existing data support the effect of acupuncture on the physiology of the gastrointestinal tract, including acid secretion, motility, neurohormonal changes, and changes in sensory thresholds. Much of the neuroanatomic pathway of these effects has been identified in animal models. Prospective randomized controlled trials have also shown the efficacy of acupuncture for analgesia for endoscopic procedures, including colonoscopy and upper endoscopy. Acupuncture has also been used for a variety of other conditions including postoperative ileus, achalasia, peptic ulcer disease, functional bowel diseases (including irritable bowel syndrome and non-ulcer dyspepsia), diarrhea, constipation, inflammatory bowel disease, expulsion of gallstones and biliary ascariasis, and pain associated with pancreatitis.[127] Acupuncture may enhance the regularity of gastric myoelectrical activity in diabetic patients.[128]

Low back pain may be effectively managed with acupuncture. A large, methodologically rigorous trial assessed two questions: can acupuncture contribute as an adjunctive therapy to conservative management of low back pain and is real acupuncture superior to sham acupuncture? This trial was a three-arm parallel group design involving 186 patients with pain of greater than 6 weeks' duration. Patients in both acupuncture groups were blinded, and the outcomes assessor for all three groups was also blinded. The primary outcome was 50% pain reduction at 3 months after the end of treatment. The results are as follows:

- Real acupuncture: 76.6%
- Sham acupuncture: 29.3%
- Conservative orthopedic therapy: 13.9%

For low back pain patients with pain lasting more than 5 years, the relative probability of experiencing 50% or greater pain reduction was 10 times higher with real acupuncture than with sham acupuncture.[106]

Acupuncture is useful in the treatment of osteoarthritis. Comparing real versus sham acupuncture (n = 97), real acupuncture significantly outperformed sham acupuncture for pain relief at 3 months after the end of treatment ($P < .05$). Comparing acupuncture as an adjunct to standard medical care versus standard medical care alone, showed significantly more improvement in the acupuncture group ($P < .05$) in both pain and functional indices.[106]

In acupuncture treatment of fibromyalgia, a high-quality randomized controlled trial (scoring a perfect quality score) demonstrated that real acupuncture is more effective than sham acupuncture in relieving pain, increasing pain thresholds, and improving global ratings.[106] Somatic sympathetic vasomotor changes may be documented by medical thermographic imaging during acupuncture analgesia.[129]

Asthma patients benefit from acupuncture treatment given in addition to conventional therapy.[130] TCM-based acupuncture therapy showed significant immune-modulating effects: CD3+ and CD4+ lymphocytes increased significantly, interleukin-6 and interleukin-10 decreased, interleukin-8 rose significantly, in vitro lymphocyte proliferation rate increased significantly, and eosinophils decreased. Acupuncture treatment of people with asthma resulted in decreased airway resistance.[131,132] Acupuncture is an effective and safe alternative treatment for the management of seasonal allergic rhinitis.[133]

Increasingly, acupuncture is complementing conventional therapies. Doctors may combine acupuncture and drugs to control surgery-related pain in their patients.[134] By providing both acupuncture and certain conventional anesthetic drugs, doctors have found it possible to achieve a state of complete pain relief for some patients. They also have found that using acupuncture lowers the need for conventional pain-killing drugs and thus reduces the risk of side effects.[135,136]

Bidirectional Effects of Acupuncture

Acupuncture facilitates the physiologic reflexes in response to changes in internal or external environment. Thus, acupuncture can lower high blood pressure in hypertensive subjects, elevate low blood pressure in hypotensive subjects, and promote urinary sodium excretion during hyperosmotic challenge, for example.[137] Blood pressure and heart rate in strains of rats bred to be either congenitally hypotensive or hypertensive were "normalized" by acupuncture. Similar normalizing effects of acupuncture have been described in rats made hypotensive by withdrawing blood and in dogs made hypertensive by intravenous infusion of epinephrine.[106]

Safety of Acupuncture

Acupuncture may be much safer than the alternative conventional treatment. Recently, Lazarou et al. showed that drugs are between the fourth and sixth leading cause for deaths in the United States and in 1994 accounted for approximately 2.22 million serious ADRs[†] and approximately 106,000 fatal ADRs.[138] So it is hardly surprising that there is unprecedented interest in non-drug treatment worldwide. Acupuncture is not without potential side effects, but as Edzard Ernst points out, "The side effects of acupuncture are dimensions less than those of drugs."[29] Previous surveys indicate that there is a significant but low risk of serious side effects of acupuncture from 1:10,000 to 1:100,000.[29] A comprehensive review of the complementary and alternative therapies database and MEDLINE database (1966-1993) with extensive cross-referencing concluded that there were 216 reported instances of serious complications worldwide over a 20-year period.[41] Recent reports published with a total of 32,000,[139] 34,000,[140] and 65,482[141] treatments indicated that none of the adverse events were life threatening and all the adverse events had ceased within 2 weeks. In comparison, it has been estimated that 1 in 1200 human patients will die from gastroduodenal complications when treated with NSAIDs for 2 months[142] and that people who often take acetaminophen or NSAIDs have an increased risk of end-stage renal disease.[143] The serious adverse affects of acupuncture treatment reported in the literature may easily be prevented by straightforward precautions.[29]

Application of State of the Art Technology to Acupuncture

Use of state of the art medical technology to assess the low-tech, millennia-old practice of acupuncture has yielded interesting results. Functional magnetic resonance imaging has demonstrated activity in the visual lobes of the brain during needling of distal acupuncture points on the leg and foot that Eastern medicine selects for treating eye problems.[106] Conceptual relationships between the brain, organs, and acupuncture points can be examined by functional magnetic resonance imaging. These relationships suggest functional interactions between acupuncture points and the cortical areas related to disease treatment by each acupuncture point. To test the hypothesis that sensory-related acupuncture points have brain cortical correspondence, functional magnetic resonance imaging signals were sought in the visual cortex after needling of GB37 (used to treat eye-related diseases such as itchiness or pain in the eyes, cataracts, night blindness, and optic atrophy) and BL67

[†]Serious ADRs were defined as those that required hospitalization, were permanently disabling, or resulted in death.

(conditions of head and sense organs, headache, neck pain, ophthalmalgia.) The careful and systematic examination of the hundreds of currently known acupuncture points and the mapping of corresponding cortical activation may well reveal evidence of homeostatic regulatory mechanisms not yet understood by Western physiology and medicine. Such research will also contribute significantly to creating more accurate and reliable treatment for the millions of patients who may benefit from acupuncture.[144]

Clinical Applications of Acupuncture

Currently, much acupuncture practice in horses is based on limited evidence, such as small-scale research, case studies, and clinical experience. In a mature science, this would be undesirable, but acupuncture is in the early stages of development as a science, and many of its practices depend on relatively informal knowledge. To encourage the spread of potentially valuable ideas, practitioners must be willing to share their clinical experience. High-quality research is essential to the long-term development of evidence-based practice, but it is crucial at the present stage of acupuncture that we do not become too concerned with perfect research methodology at the expense of good ideas. This particularly applies to tests of statistical significance. If we accept only information that has demonstrated statistical significance, we risk the dismissal of qualitative research and other information that may be extremely valuable but that has not yet been fully investigated. Statistical significance is not the only way to judge clinical importance. Decisions on what should be submitted and accepted for clinical practice should be based on potential clinical relevance as well as statistical analysis.

Current equine acupuncture studies show potential usefulness in treatment of pain,[145-150] lameness,[145,152-155] head shaking,[155] chronic diarrhea,[156] allergic dermatitis,[157] equine ataxia,[158] chronic laminitis,[97,159-161] and chronic navicular disease.[97] When electroacupuncture was used in the treatment of chronic lameness, 7 of 10 animals with chronic laminitis improved clinically, and 6 of 10 with navicular disease improved, but there were no significant differences between treatment and control groups.[162] Acupuncture has been used to treat rectal prolapse in a mare,[163] traumatic facial hemiplegia,[164] radial nerve paralysis,[97] and severe stringhalt,[97] as an adjunct in the treatment of a horse with tetanus,[165] as management of lumbar and croup myopathy associated with distal tarsitis,[166] and in the diagnosis and treatment of equine immune-mediated myofascial syndrome.[167] Acupuncture has been used to decrease the number of joints injected in the sports horses by implanting acupuncture points[33] or used to treat chronic back pain,[168-172] including chronic back pain that presents as a fibromyalgia syndrome.[173] Moxibustion can

prevent the incidence and attenuates the developement of collagen-induced arthritis in mice.[174]

Acupuncture is used as treatment for infertility in mares,[175-177] including those who fail to cycle normally[97] or who experience urine pooling or uterine fluid,[97] decreased libido in stallions,[97] post-foaling bladder paralysis,[97] and other animal reproductive disorders.[178,179] Aquapuncture is a simple and effective method to treat repeat breeders in dairy herds.[180] EA and moxibustion may be convenient, safe, and economic therapeutic alternatives available to surgical procedures on abomasal displacement in dairy cattle.[181] Moxibustion could be used as the alternative to PGF2 alpha and antibiotics for treating delayed uterine involution in cows.[182]

The effects of acupuncture have been studied on gastrointestinal motility and blood concentration of endocrine substances in horses.[183] Electroacupuncture and butorphanol (0.1 mg/kg, IV) may provide useful rectal analgesia in horses.[184] Acupuncture may produce significant visceral analgesia with minimal cardiovascular and respiratory changes.[185] Administration of EA was more effective than acupuncture for activating the spinal cord to release beta-endorphins into the CSF of horses. Acupuncture and EA provided cutaneous analgesia in horses without adverse cardiovascular and respiratory effects.[148] Bilateral EA at Guan-yuan-shu was ineffective in reducing signs of discomfort induced by small intestinal distention.[186] Electroacupuncture has been used for treatment of intestinal impaction of the horse.[187] Acupuncture is useful for chronic diarrhea in foals[97] and is effective in controlling induced E. coli diarrhea at its early stage in pigs.[188,189] Acupuncture is used as a diagnostic aid and adjuvant therapy for ulcerative gastritis in the horse.

Acupuncture is used for analgesia in equine surgery,[191-195] sheep,[196] and cattle.[197,198] There are several papers that measure the release of β-endorphin and cortisol during equine acupuncture.[186,199,200] Electroacupuncture elevates blood cortisol levels in naive horses, whereas sham treatment has no effect.[201] There are papers that discuss the use of acupuncture in general practice,[202] review acupuncture's effect on the body's defense systems,[203] in addition to prolonged[204] and uncommon effects.[205] There are papers that discuss clinical trials of acupuncture in the horse,[206] the analgesic and immunologic effects of acupuncture in domestic animals,[207] and its neuroimmunomodulatory effects in mice.[208] There are case studies covering a period of time from 3 months to 10 years, which suggest that acupuncture treatment of "extreme" COPD is suitable in countering allergic regulatory disorders.[209] A single acupuncture treatment during an attack of heaves causes no more improvement in lung function than does handling the horse.[210]

Acupuncture may be suitable as a postoperative rehabilitation treatment for animals with fractures. Sheep treated with acupuncture, after mid-diaphyseal transverse fractures of the femur were created, regained functional activity in the affected limb and showed a significant decrease in total leukocyte and neutrophil counts compared with untreated controls.[211] Electroacupuncture enhanced the myocardial protection of hypothermia on myocardial ischemic and reperfusion injury in pigs.[212] A clinical randomized trial of treatment of Wobbler syndrome in dogs, with EA—and in a few cases, surgical intervention—compared to orthodox medical and surgical intervention, demonstrated an 85 percent vs. 20 percent success rate. The number of treatments required to achieve full recovery depended on the severity of the case: Grade I: 18.5 ± 2.5; Grade II: 25 ± 5.4; Grade III: 34 ± 6.7 (r = 0.962). Electroacupuncture treatments were given every other day, delivering 150 to 300 mVolts at 125 Hz (equivalent to approximately 20 microAmps) in 10 acupuncture points per treatment. No adverse effects were observed with acupuncture.[213]

Equine acupuncturists have emphasized careful palpation of the musculature as a screening test to ascertain areas of abnormal sensitivity. Abnormally sensitive acupuncture points may refer to intra-articular pathology.[98-100] Thermal imaging can provide objective, measurable evidence of the ability of acupuncture to restore normal homeostasis in the autonomic regulation of vasomotor tone.[214] Results of the meridian test in case horses were associated with sensitivity reactions similar to those detected by physical and neurological examinations; however, an unequivocal association with EHV-1 or EHV-4 infection was not detected.[215] Acupuncture is not effective in diagnosing equine protozoal myelitis.[216]

Controversy exists in the current state of understanding of TCM and application of acupuncture to modern medicine.[217-219] Evidence-based traditional Chinese medicine is attainable.[220]

Treatment of the Geriatric Equine with Myofascial Therapies

Acupuncture therapy and manual therapy need not treat individual diseases. Rather, the clinician helps many conditions by a single expedient: restoring normal function to the peripheral nervous system. It is said in Chinese medicine: *Yi bing tong zhi, Tong bing yi zhi* ("One disease, different treatments; different diseases, one treatment").[221] Acupuncture and manual therapy address impaired function and restore homeostasis to the entire patient, which may correct many of the myriad of tribulations experienced by the geriatric equine.

After completion of standard dental, physical, and lameness examinations, it is then appropriate to assess upper body pain and function. Palpating the acupuncture points and performing motion palpation achieves this and suggests the probable value of treatment. Once an assessment is made, the clinician performs the various manipulations indicated by motion palpation findings. At this point, acupuncture point palpation should be performed again, as points reactive due to local muscle spasm may no longer be reactive. Points that continue to be reactive are assessed to ascertain a therapeutic pattern that may involve aspects of visceral somatic reflex or may suggest joints that require acupuncture or physical therapy. Appropriate acupuncture treatment may then be instituted. On occasion, a horse presents with such severe muscle spasm that manipulation is problematic. It is advisable in these cases to acupuncture local points, such as needling the *Huatuo Jiaji* points (located in the juxtavertebral muscles of the spine), thereby decreasing muscle spasm and providing relief of myofascial pain before performing manual therapy. Treatment at *Huatuo Jiaji* points may be superior in analgesic effect and clinical total effective rate to that by conventional acupuncture.[222] It is considered that the mechanism of treatment at *Huatuo Jiaji* points is related to the trunk of posterior ramus of the spinal nerve where the points are located. It is important to reassess the reactivity of the acupuncture points after manual therapy is performed because reactivity may change with treatment.

With experience, the clinician is able to differentiate between primary pathology and pain that may be compensatory in nature and act accordingly. Treatment of the upper body using acupuncture and/or manual therapy in many cases resolves chronic pain and improves ambulation even in the severely arthritic horse. Use of these modalities is desirable, as they represent conservative therapy with a low risk of adverse circumstances in the hands of the experienced practitioner. NSAIDs and/or joint injection are potentially hazardous and rarely efficacious in the long run in the aged equine.

Chronic parasite damage, reduced activity, and reduced intestinal motility may predispose some senior horses to experience digestive disorders, including chronic colic. Acupuncture may improve gastrointestinal motility and blood concentration of endocrine substances.[223] Manual therapy may be helpful by provoking somatovisceral reflexes.

Treatment of the Geriatric Equine with Traditional Chinese Medicine

Use of modern TCM in the geriatric patient is worthwhile, as there are inherent differences from the Western medical approach. The promotion of longevity has been an important concern in Chinese civilization for at least a few millennia. The First Emperor, Hwang Di, is said to have poisoned himself with mercury-based longevity tonics in the 2nd century BCE. At a later date, the fourth of the Manchu Emperors of the Qing Dynasty, Qian Long, who reigned 60 years from 1736 to 1796, had three basic recommendations: (1) a regular life-style, (2) *Qi Gong* exercises, and (3) the use of herbs and foods to restore one's *Qi*.[224] The statements of this political figure emphasize the importance of avoiding sex, drugs, and rock and roll; engaging in physical exercise; and, most importantly, supporting the source *Qi* by medicinals. It is fundamental to the Chinese world view that cultivation of the life forces, *Qi*, blood, *Yin* and *Yang*, should be pursued to enhance and prolong one's life.

The Eastern examination is the key to the management of the equine geriatric patient with herbs and acupuncture. The basis of the TCM examination is pattern differentiation. This principle as stated in Chinese is "*bien jheng lun jhi*," or in translation, "treatment is based on the pattern."[225] The *si jhun*, or four examinations of looking, asking, palpating, and listening/smelling, outline the procedure for determining patterns. A patient's pattern is defined by the sum total of the signs, symptoms, tongue, and pulse as determined by the *si jhun*.[225] The results of the four examinations are interpreted in light of the 10 sanctioned theories of TCM in China today.

How does the Eastern pattern-based therapy differ from the Western disease-based approach? The Western practitioner arrives at a diagnosis by heavy dependence on the use of objective imaging technologies and laboratory tests. The strict TCM examiner must rely on the traditional patterns demonstrated by the patient using the *si jhun* without technical support. In the hypothetical case of arthritic disease, one might expect the following patterns, to name only a few: *Blood Stasis* or fixed pain, *Qi Stagnation* or moving, referred muscle pain, *Liver Depression* or anger perhaps expressed in stereotypical behavior, *Heart Qi Vacuity* or anxiety, with a probable underlying *Vacuity* of the *Spleen, Lung, or Kidney*. The total of the patterns is a description of the presentation of the disease in TCM. Any disease can manifest with a number of different patterns. Furthermore, therapy will be defined by the pattern because each pattern must be addressed in the subsequent therapeutic principles used in treatment. In other words, the pattern of blood stasis (fixed pain) requires the use of a TCM therapy that will quicken the blood and resolve stasis; for liver depression, *Qi* stagnation will require coursing the liver and rectifying the *Qi*, and so on. The stated functions of each acupoint or herbal medicinal will be used to determine which acupoints or medicinals to select. The proper use of the descriptive methodology of TCM forces the practitioner to depict each individual in terms of patterns that will then be used to direct therapy. Whether acupuncture, herbs, or both are used will depend on the practitioner's skill in the individual modalities. At a fundamental level, the stated function of any one acupuncture technique can be theoretically duplicated by the proper herbal formula and visa versa. The specifics of the pattern will dictate the use of one modality over another. For instance, if nausea were a symptom, an acupuncture technique would be preferred over unpalatable herbs. On the other hand, if supplementation were required over a long time, herbs would be preferred to repeated supplementation by acupuncture stimulation. One must evaluate the use of therapy by the resultant effect on the described pattern or patterns. However, any therapy, be it Western or Eastern, can also be evaluated in terms of its effect on the pattern.

The TCM description of *shuai lao* or "detriment due to aging" depends on some of the terms in the following text. Health in TCM is defined as a balance or harmony of the difficult to define concepts of *Qi*, blood, *Yin*, and *Yang*. Yan De-Xin stated the relationship as follows: "Although there are many forms of change from birth through growth, youth, old age, and disease to death, yet in the final analysis, these are all inseparable from changes in *Qi* and blood. If *Qi* and blood lose their harmony and the vessels and network vessels become static and obstructed, then phlegm turbidity will be engendered internally and may lead to a chain of pathologic changes, such as heat, cold, vacuity, and repletion in the viscera and bowels."[226] *Qi* is the motivating force behind all thought, transformation, and action in TCM. O'Connor and Bensky describe *Qi* as "a tendency, a movement, something on the order of energy," but on the other hand "matter without form," and "an example of the absence of the matter/energy dichotomy in Chinese medicine."[227] Diseased *Qi* stems from hereditary factors, lifestyle excess, chronic enduring disease, and aging. The chief symptoms of *Qi* vacuity (deficiency) are fatigue, depression, poor appetite, abdominal distention, loose stools, and digestive upsets as well as the TCM signs of a pale, fat tongue and a vacuous, floating, forceless pulse.

Qi and blood exist as a *Yin/Yang* pair. That is to say, *Qi* and blood represent opposite qualities but are necessarily coexistent in the same individual. "In addition to being a substance, blood is also regarded as a force, a level of activity in the body which is involved with the sensitivity of the sense organs . . . and the major function of blood is to carry nourishment and moisture to all parts of the body."[228] Blood can be damaged by hemorrhage, lack of nutrition, defective nutrition, and the TCM concept of blood stasis. Blood vacuity/deficiency results in dry skin, loss of hair, pale mucous membranes and tongue, and a fine pulse. Because blood is dependent on *Qi* for blood formation from air and food and for the power to circulate within the channels, *Qi* is said to govern blood. On the other hand, the strength of *Qi* depends on the nutrition and moisture of blood, which is referred to as the "Mother of *Qi*." Thus, *Qi* and blood have an archetypal *Yin/Yang* relationship in which, in vivo, both are always present. One does not exist without the other, and a balanced and harmonious juxtaposition is the healthiest relationship. It should follow that in a case of clinical vacuity, one might preferentially supplement one but that the other might need therapeutic benefit as well. As a rule, *Qi* vacuity will precede blood vacuity; therefore, fatigue is a common clinical finding. However blood vacuity will further be characterized by pale mucous membranes and dryness, as for example in dry mucous membranes of the eyes, intestines, or lungs.

Yin and *Yang* are descriptions of the ultimate source of blood and *Qi*. Therapeutic medicinals classified as *Yin* supplements are more nourishing and fluid engendering than blood supplements and are thus used on occasion of more profound vacuity. *Yang* is the presence of *Qi* in such quantity that there is associated warmth; therefore, a *Yang* vacuity is associated with signs of cold, such as cold back, cold extremities, or loss of libido.

The essence, or *Jing*, "is that which is responsible for growth, development and reproduction and determines the strength of the constitution."[229] In TCM, an individual is born with a certain amount and quality of prenatal or preheaven *Jing*. The postnatal or post-heaven *Jing* is derived from daily excess *Jing*, which has been produced from food but not immediately consumed. The prenatal and postnatal *Jing* combine within the concept of the Chinese *kidney* and are held in reserve to be converted to *Yin* or *Yang* as the need arises. The aging individual can no longer as efficiently produce postnatal *Jing*; therefore, when *Yang Qi* is needed, the stores of prenatal *Jing* will be converted. Ultimately, the inherited prenatal *Jing* will be exhausted. "We are only as old as the essence we have consumed."[230]

The TCM concept of kidney organ function governs the ears, bones, teeth, genitalia, reproductive capacity, and mental clarity. Consequently, aging results in loss of hearing, brittle bones, lost teeth, and diminished reproduction and thought processes. Furthermore, there is in TCM an order of diminishment of *Qi* (*Yang*) and blood (*Yin*) over time. "By 40 [human] years of age, the healthy *Yin Qi* is automatically reduced by half, since the process of life itself is the consumption and transportation of *Yin* substance by *Yang Qi*."[224] *Yin* vacuity begins in middle age, especially with a decline in body warmth.[224] Skin becomes dry and wrinkled and hair turns white because of *Yin* blood failure to nourish skin and hair. *Yang*, which is rooted in *Yin*, will ultimately become affected by a loss of *Yin* substance. Loss of energy, cold extremities, and increase in frequency of urination are all attributes of *Yang* vacuity.

The preceding description of TCM statements of doctrine would mean little if they did not lead to beneficial action in the development of therapeutic action stated as acupuncture or herbal medicinal formulas. "Unbalance of *Yin* and *Yang* is the underlying cause of all disease, therefore health arises from a balance of *Qi*, blood, *Yin* and *Yang*, [when] *Qi* and blood will be maximally produced."[228]

Inappropriate supplementation may lead to imbalance or exacerbation of an existing imbalance. With respect to the aging equine patient, the primary assumption is that the underling pattern is one of vacuity. There may be overlying patterns of repletion/excess, such as pain or infectious disease, which must be addressed in the short term. However, ultimately the root pattern of vacuity requires supplementation. If there is *Qi* vacuity, then *Qi* supplements are indicated. If there is blood vacuity, then blood supplements will nourish the blood. However, a TCM pattern of *Yin* vacuity, if supplemented with *Yang* supplements, will become more pronounced. There is little risk of prolonged *Yin* supplements in the aged patient so long as loose stools or diarrhea are not a part of the pattern. Other possible untoward results would be expected if splecn vacuity were to be treated with bitter or cold medicinals or blood-quickening agents, which have an attacking nature. Likewise, exterior releasing medicinals will over time injure the source *Qi*. The established, ultimate goal of TCM therapy is to maximize *Qi* and *Jing*-essence production, minimize the consumption of the same, and protect the health of the TCM concept of the spleen and kidney.[224]

To state a goal of supplementation requires a starting point. The Shanghai Encyclopedia of Chinese Medicinals cites 5762 medicinals that could have a therapeutic role in medical formulas.[229] Given that most formulas are composed of four to 10, or more, medicinals, the potential for combinations and permutations is astronomical. However, some semblance of control can be established by the use of classic supplementing formulas. The choice of the proper formula will be based on the four TCM examinations. Furthermore, the practitioner will be required to modify most formulas based on his or her knowledge of individual medicinals or acupoints.

Si Jun Zi Tang, or The Four Gentleman Decoction, is a classic formula of the Tai Ping period to boost the *Qi* and fortify the Chinese concept of the spleen, or digestion (Table 9-1).

This formula is rarely used alone, because most patients will have multiple patterns that require therapy and not simply spleen vacuity. Among the modifications one might make would be the addition of Citri

TABLE 9-1

Si Jun Zi Tang[230]

Radix Ginseng	Ren Shen	3-9 g
Rhizoma Atractylodes Macrocephali	Bai Zhu	6-9 g
Sclerotium Poriae Cocos	Fu Ling	6-9 g
Radix Glycyrrhizae Uralensis	Jhi Gan Cao	3-6 g

Reticulatae (*Chen Pi*) and Rhizoma Pinelliae Ternatae (*Ban Xia*) or *Er Chen Tang* for the presence of copious white phlegm. For Stomach Heat Pattern (gastric ulcers) one could add some or all of the following: Radix Scutellaria Baicalensis (*Hwang Qin*), Rhizome Coptidis Chinensis (*Hwang Lian*), Pueraria Lobatae (*Ge Gen*), Gypsum Fibrosum (*Shi Gao*), and Tuber Ophiopogonis Japonici (*Mai Men Dong*).

Another supplementing formula close to *Si Jhun Zi Tang* and attributed to the Jin-Yuan Dynasty Master Li Dong-yuan (1180-1251 CE) is *Bu Zhong Yi Qi Tang* or Supplement the Center and Boost the *Qi* Decoction (Table 9-2).

Like *Si Jhun Zi Tang*, *Bu Zhong Yi Qi Tang* supplements the *Qi* (*Huang Qi, Ren Shen, Gan Cao*) with mild supplementation of the blood (*Dang Gui*) and clears pathogenic heat (*Sheng Ma* and *Chai Hu*) without specific heat-clearing medicinals. This latter quality is an advantage in horses because most heat-clearing medicinals are quite bitter and decrease palatability. Beyond spleen/stomach vacuity, this formula is most appropriate in enduring diarrhea and prolapsed conditions of the rectum or uterus due to vacuity detriment or the TCM pattern of *Central Qi Downward Fall*. Fatigue and undiagnosed chronic diarrhea are commonly seen in geriatric horses. *Bu Zhong Yi Qi Tang* is a useful base formula for a number of chronic functional diseases such as chronic glomerulonephritis and hemorrhagic disorders. For prolonged diarrhea, add Fructus Terminalis Chebulae (*He Zi*), Semen Myristicae Fragrantis (*Rou Dou Kou*), Fructus Schizandra Chinensis (*Wu Wei Zi*), and Fructus Pruni Mume (*Wu Mei*).[233] For abdominal distension, add Fructus Immaturus Citri Aurantii (*Zhi Shi*), Cortex Magnoliae Officianalis (*Huo Po*), Radix Auklandia Lappae (*Mu Xiang*), and Fructus Amomi (*Sha Ren*).[233] For constipation, add Radix and Rhizoma Rhei (*Da Huang*), Honey (*Mi Tang*), and sesame oil (*Xiang You*).[233] *Bu Zhong Yi Qi Tang* is a good example of the use of the five principles of *Li Dong-yuan* in formula preparation. The principles are to (1) supplement the spleen with sweet and warming medicinals, (2) regulate upbearing and downbearing with acrid and *Qi* rectifying medicinals, (3) clear heat with bitter and cold medicinals as necessary, (4) address other concerns, and (5) prioritize.[234]

Shi quan Da Bu Tang (Ten Complete Great Supplementing Decoction) was first codified in the Song Dynasty (960-1280 CE). It is another major and important variation on the base formula of *Si Zhun Zi Tang*. The most important application of *Shi quan Da Bu Tang* is debilitation after surgery, chronic or acute illness, and post parturition.

The vacuity detriment addressed by this formula falls under three patterns in TCM:

"1. Insufficient *Qi* and blood, heart-spleen dual vacuity,
2. Spleen-kidney dual vacuity, former heaven–latter heaven lack of nourishment, and
3. Liver-kidney dual vacuity, aging and bodily weakness."[235]

The formula consists of the addition of one formula and two medicinals to the base formula. *Si Wu Tang* (Four Materials Decoction) consists of Radix Angelica Sinensis (*Dang Gui*), cooked Rehmannia (*Shu Di Huang*), Rhizoma Ligustici Wallichii (*Chuan Xiong*), and Radix Albus Paeonia Lactiflora (*Bai Shao*). The indications for *Si Wu Tang* alone are anemia of numerous causes, postpartum weakness, and constipation. For severe anemia or blood loss, *Si Wu Tang* should at least be added to *Si Jhun Zi Tang* to boost the *Qi*, a necessary antecedent to supplementing the blood in TCM. With poor appetite and chronic diarrhea, neither *Shu Di* nor *Dang Gui* should be used. Lastly, Cortex Cinnamomi (*Rou Gui*) and Radix Astragali Membranacei (*Huang Qi*) warm the center and kidney and supplement the *Qi*. The final formula results in supplementation of spleen and kidney and *Yin* and *Yang* (Table 9-3).

TABLE 9-2
Bu Zhong Yi Qi Tang[231]

Radix Astragali Membranacei	Huang *Qi*	12-24 g
Radix Ginseng	Ren Shen	9-12 g
Rhizoma Atractylodis Macrocephali	Bai Zhu	9-12 g
Radix Glycyrrhizae Uralensis	Zhi Gan Cao	3-6 g
Pericarpium Citri Reticulatae	Chen Pi	6-9 g
Rhizoma Cimicifugae	Sheng Ma	3-6 g
Radix Bupleuri	Chai Hu	3-9 g

TABLE 9-3
Shi Quan Da Bu Tang[230]

Radix Panacis Ginseng	Ren Shen	6-9 g
Rhizoma Atractylodes Macrocephali	Bai Zhu	9-12 g
Sclerotium Poriae Cocos	Fu Ling	12-15 g
Radix Glycyrrhizae	Jhi Gan Cao	3-6 g
Radix Rehmannia Glutinosae	Shu Di Huang	15-18 g
Radix Paeonia Lactiflorae	Bai Shao	12-15 g
Radix Angelicae Sinensis	Dang Gui	12-15 g
Radix Ligustici Wallichii	Chuan Xiong	6-9 g
Cortex Cinnamomi Cassiae	Rou Guai	6-9 g
Radix Astragali Membranacei	Huang *Qi*	15-18 g

Box 9-3

Herbal Formulas

Shi Quan Da Bu Fang of Golden Needle Wang Li-ting (1894)

Zhang Men (LIV 13) supplements the five viscera with the effect of Ren Shen

Zu San Li (St 36) fortifies spleen, disperses food, and upbears the clear with the effect of *Bai Zhu*.

Nei Guan (PC 6) quickens the blood, fortifies spleen, and disinhibits damp with the effect of Fu Ling.

Jhong Wan (CV 12) governs the five viscera and six bowels with the effect of Gan Cao.

San Yin Jiao (SP 6) nourishes the blood with the effect of Dang Gui.

Qu Chi (LI 11) dispels Wind and Wind Stroke with the effect of Chuan Xiong.

Tai Chong (LIV 3) stops abdominal pain and quickens the blood as does Bai Shao.

Guan Yuan (CV 4) dispels blood stasis and engenders new blood as does Shu Di Huang.

He Gu (LI 4) rules the Defensive *Qi* and frees the flow of channel and network vessels as does Huang Qi.

Yang Ling Quan (GB 34) soothes the sinews, supplements the center and boosts the *Qi* as does Rou Gui.

Box 9-4

Patterns Associated with Cushing's Syndrome

1. Yin Vacuity with ascendant Liver Yang Hyperactivity Pattern
2. Yin Vacuity Fire Effulgence Pattern
3. Ascendant Liver Yang Hyperactivity with Phlegm Fire Pattern
4. Yin Vacuity with Heat Toxins Pattern
5. Spleen Qi Vacuity with Phlegm Damp Pattern
6. Spleen-Kidney Yang Vacuity Pattern
7. Yin and Yang Dual Vacuity Pattern

Unlike most herbal formulas, *Shi Quan Da Bu Tang* has been rigorously tested using Western methods. The effects are thought to be due to the immune modulating effects of several different pectic polysaccharides. "It significantly enhanced antibody responses to SRBC (Komatsu, 1986), phagocytosis (Maruyama, 1988), and mitogenic activities against splenic B cells in mice (Takemoto et al. 1989). Peripheral blood cell counts in patients treated concomitantly with JTT (*Shi Quan Da Bu Tang*) orally and the antineoplastic drug mitomycin C were higher in patients treated with the antineoplastic drug alone (Nabeya and Ri, 1983)."[236] *Si Quan Da Bu Tang* has a direct acupuncture analogue in the acupuncture formula *Shi Quan Da Bu Fang* of Golden Needle Wang Li-ting (1894) (Box 9-3).[235]

Yin and *Yang* supplementation is appropriate in cases of enduring and less responsive *Qi* and blood vacuities. In Western medicine, the term *Cushing's syndrome* is used to describe the signs exhibited by patients who have been exposed to high levels of endogenous and exogenous cortisol. In the horse, the clinical signs may include fatigue, polyuria, polydipsia, obesity, fluid retention, muscle wasting, hirsutism, and dorsal periorbital fat pads. In the geriatric equine, the TCM origin of

Cushing's syndrome would be aging, iatrogenesis, prolonged disease, vacuity of prenatal *Jing*-essence, or damage of the seven affects (emotions). Injudicious use of the exterior releasing medication, corticosteroid, will damage *Yang Qi* by out-thrusting *Qi* to the surface of the body as well as depleting *Yin* fluids. Ultimately, the source of the out-thrust *Yang Qi* will be kidney essence-*Jing*. Flaws and Sionneau list the patterns associated with Cushing's syndrome (Box 9-4).[237] Basically, these patterns fall into two categories: (1) Spleen *Qi* and kidney *Yang* vacuity and (2) *Yin* vacuity with effulgent fire. A pattern of pathologic dampness can occur with any of these patterns as a result of fluid accumulation.

The basic formula most appropriate for use with the pattern of *Yin* vacuity would be *Liu Wei Di Huang Wan* or Rehmannia 6. Created in the Song Dynasty (960-1279 CE), the formula treats kidney *Yin* and liver blood vacuity (Table 9-4).

By the addition of Radix Lateralis Aconiti Carmichaeli Preparata (*Fu Zi*) and Ramulus Cinnamomi Cassiae (*Gui Jhi*), *Liu Wei Di Wan Huang* is easily converted into a formula that supplements both *Yin* and *Yang*: *Jin Gui Shen Qi Wan* (Golden Cabinet Kidney Pills), to which the first recorded reference is during the Late Han Dynasty, approximately 200 BCE. Prepared Rehmannia serves to supplement kidney *Yin*, whereas Diascorea and Cornis supplement the spleen

TABLE 9-4

Liu Wei Di Huang Wan[230]

Radix Rehmannia Glutinosa	Shu Di Huang	240 g
Fructus Corni Officianalis	Shan JuYu	120 g
Radix Diascorea Oppositae	Shan Yao	120 g
Sclerotium Poriae Cocos	Fu Ling	90 g
Cortex Moutan Radicis	Mu Dan Pi	90 g
Rhizoma Alismatis Orientalis	Ze Xie	90 g

TABLE 9-5

Rehmannia 14[238]

Radix Rehmannia Glutinosa	Sheng Di Huang	80 g
Radix Diascorea Oppositae	Shan Yao	40 g
Radix Paeonia Lactiflora	Bai Shao	30 g
Radix Astragali Membranacei	Huang *Qi*	45 g
Radix Anemarrhenae Aspheloidis	Zhi Mu	30 g
Cortex Phellodendri	Huang Bai	30 g
Fructus Schisandrae Chinensis	Wu Wei Zi	45 g
Tuber Ophiopogonis Japonica	Mai Men Dong	45 g
Sclerotium Poria Cocos	Fu Ling	30 g
Rhizoma Alismatis Orientalis	Ze Xie	30 g
Ramulua Cinnamomi Cassiae	Gui Jhi	30 g
Radix Lateralis Aoniti Carmichaeli	Fu Zi	30 g
Fructus Corni Officianalis	Shan Zhu Yu	40 g
Cortex Moutan Radicis	Mu Dan Pi	30 g

and liver *Yin,* respectively. The formula can actually be used with these three ingredients alone if dampness need not be drained. Otherwise, Alisma and Poria clear pathogenic *Dampness* and Moutan quickens the blood while clearing liver heat. Cinnamon and Aconite, when added to from *Jin Gui Shen Qi Wan* warm and supplement both kidney *Yin* and *Yang,* as well as Astragali to supplement the spleen. A further modification is found in the formula Rehmannia 14 (Table 9-5), in which kidney *Yin, Yang,* and *Jing* are supplemented along with strong heat clearing.

The modern Chinese physician and geriatric specialist Yan De-Xin placed a special emphasis on blood-quickening agents such Cortex Moutan Radicis (Mu Dan Pi), which is used in the preceding formula. Other agents that Master Yan preferred were Salvia Milthorrhizae (*Dan Shen*), Radix Pseudogensing (*San Qi*), and Radix Paeonia Rubrus (*Chi Shao*). He believed that although the classic manifestations of aging were related to the kidney, the function of kidney was compromised by blood stasis. In this case, blood stasis might refer to microcirculatory disturbances as well as to fixed pain. Microcirculatory disturbances would be a result of blood vacuity leading to the inability of the blood to circulate vigorously, itself a cause of blood vacuity in TCM. "In clinical practice, if one simply employs supplementary formulas in their treatment of diseases; the more one supplements the patient, the more stagnant they become. And the more stagnant they become, the more vacuous they become. However, if we adapt the methods of quickening the blood and transforming stasis, we may get unexpectedly good therapeutic results. This also proves the credibility of the view point that static blood is the origin of senility."[232]

With respect to Rehmannia 14, two further modifications are particularly important in the aged patient. In the case of loose stool or diarrhea and a need for blood supplementation, then Rehmannia could be removed and substituted with the ruling ingredients in the formula Er Zhi Wan, the Two Ultimates. They are Fructus Ligustri Lucidi (*Nu Zhen Zi*) and Herba Ecliptae Prostratae (*Han Lian Cao*).[230] Neither medicinal is slimy nor will they damage the spleen, that is, cause diarrhea. In breeding animals with kidney *Yang* vacuity, one should add *Er Xian Tang,* or the Two Immortals, which consist of Rhizoma Curculiginis Orchioidis (*Xian Mao*) and Hera Epimedii (*Yin Yang Huo*).[230]

Chronic allergic lung disease in TCM is the result of an invasion of wind toxin combined with deep phlegm in the presence of a preexisting lung and kidney vacuity. The lung dominates respiration and is in the physical position as the "florid canopy" of the Zang Fu organs. However, the kidney, in the lowest position must "grasp the *Qi*" from the lungs. Allergic lung disease can be divided into acute attack and remission phases.[237] The following formula from Xie's Veterinary Herbal Handbook addresses the acute phase but not the remission phase (Table 9-6). The treatment principles are to supplement kidney *Qi* and lung *Qi* vacuity, nourish lung *Yin,* and stop asthma and cough.

TABLE 9-6

Allergic Lung Disease Formula[238]

Gecko	Ge Jie	3-6 g
Radix Panacis Ginseng	Ren Shen	3-10 g
Radix Platycodi Grandiflori	Jie Geng	3-10 g
Bulbus Lilii	Bai He	10-30 g
Lumbricus	Di Long	6-15 g
Bulbus Fritillaria Cirrhosae	Chuan Bei Mu	3-10 g
Bulbus Fritillaria Thunbergii	Zhe Bei Mu	3-10 g
Fructus Schisandrae Chinensis	Wu Wei Zi	3-10 g
Tuber Ophiopogon Japonica	Mai Men Dong	10-15 g

Box 9-5

Goals of Remission Therapy

1. Course the Liver and rectify the *Qi.*
2. Fortify the Spleen and boost the *Qi.*
3. Transform Phlegm and eliminate Damp.
4. Clear Heat if appropriate.
5. Nourish and enrich *Yin* if a *Yin* Vacuity.
6. Warm and invigorate *Yang* if a *Yang* Vacuity.
7. Quicken the Blood and transform Blood Stasis if present.

In this formula, Ginseng and Gecko supplement lung and kidney *Qi*, Platycodon, Fritillaria, and Lilly transform phlegm, Schisandra and Ophiopogon nourish lung *Yin*, and lastly Gecko and Lumbricus stop cough. Insect medicinals such as Periostricum Cicadae (*Chuan Tui*), Lumbricus (*Di Long*), and Buthus Martensis (*Quan Xie*) are best used for the wheezing and panting phase but not for remission.[233] In the remission phase, the probable disharmony between liver and spleen with subsequent phlegm and damp engenderment must be addressed as well as the lung-kidney vacuity.[233] The goal of remission therapy is listed in Box 9-5.

Further medicinals that could be used in Xie's formula during the remission phase would be Cortex Magnoliae Officianalis (*Huo Po*), Semen Pruni Armeniacae (*Xing Ren*), and Semen Ginkgonis Bilboae (*Bai Guo*).

There is a logical TCM thought process and progression of action used in the treatment of the geriatric patient. The aging patient is assumed to sustain progressively greater loss of *Yin* as time goes on. Ultimately, *Yang* will be lost as well, but initially *Qi* and blood will be weakened. Although the kidney, as the source of *Jing*-essence, is thought to be central to the process of detriment due to aging, spleen function is a root of equal importance for many important practitioners, such as Wang Li-ting and Li Dong-yuan. Furthermore, Yan De-xin has found blood stasis to be a root cause for the loss of kidney function. All of the above theories can be accommodated by use of classic supplementing formulas, such as *Liu Wei Di Hwang Wan* and *Bu Jhong Yi Qi Tang*. However, to make the appropriate modifications, be they acupunctural or herbal, the practitioner must have an intimate knowledge of the individual medicinals and be skilled in the application of the four examinations.

Conclusion

If the veterinary profession is to continue as a primary care model, we must acquire a better understanding of current modes of treatment of various disorders affecting the musculoskeletal system that are used by different health care providers. By applying these different theories that have been used successfully to treat various disorders, we may find ways of improving our capabilities in addressing difficult-to-treat patients and managing animals that are suffering.

Although the veterinarian's role is to offer advice and professional guidance based on existing evidence, it is ultimately the client who decides on treatment. Evidence-based medicine is defined as "the integration of best research evidence combined with clinical expertise and patient values."[240] The test of a system of medicine should be adequacy in the face of suffering. It has been suggested that modern medicine fails this test: *"The moral compulsion of their responsibilities exposes physicians to the peril of unavoidable uncertainty and overwhelming subjectivity created by serious illness and suffering. It can only be through education and method that these dangers are converted into therapeutic power. It follows that medicine needs a systematic and disciplined approach to the knowledge that arises from the clinician's experience rather than artificial divisions of medical knowledge into science and art. The timeless goal of the relief of suffering remains the challenge to change and the enduring test of medicine's success."*[1]

Respect, love, compassion, wisdom, care, and directed intention to heal are the other essential components of good medicine. They cost nothing but our time and energies and are renewable resources. Both Western and Eastern medical systems have their strengths and weaknesses. Neither is a perfect system, but the integration of the best from both systems would be the basis of a better and more sustainable medicine than either system can offer alone.[239]

REFERENCES

1. Cassell EJ: The Nature of Suffering and the Goals of Medicine. New York, Oxford University Press, 1991.
2. Denoix JM, Pailloux JP: Physical Therapy and Massage for the Horse, 2nd ed. North Pomfret, VT, Trafalgar Square Publishing, 2001.
3. Ricklefs RE, Finch CE: Aging: A Natural History. New York, Scientific American Library HPHLP, 1995, p 58.
4. McKeever KH, Malinowski K, et al: Effects of aging and twelve weeks of training on aerobic performance and plasma β-endorphin and cortisol concentrations in horses. Presented at the Equine Research Update, October 20, 2001, Cook College-Rutgers University, New Jersey.
5. McKeever KH, Malinowski K: Endocrine response to exercise in young and old horses. Equine Vet J Suppl 30:561, 1999.
6. McKeever KH, Malinowski K: Exercise capacity in young and old mares. AJVR 58:1468, 1997.
7. Cavalieri TA: Geriatrics. In Ward RC, editor: Foundations for Osteopathic Medicine. Baltimore, Lippincott Williams & Wilkins, 1997.
8. Gunn CC: Treatment of Chronic Pain: Intramuscular Stimulation for Myofascial Pain of Radiculopathic Origin, 2nd ed. London, Churchill Livingstone, 1996.
9. Chen J, Chen M, Zhao B, et al: Effects of acupuncture on the immunological functions in hepatitis B virus carriers. J Tradit Chin Med 19:268, 1999.
10. Zhu D, Ma Q, Li C, Wang L: Effect of stimulation of shenshu point on the aging process of genital system in aged female rats and the role of monoamine neurotransmitters. J Tradit Chin Med 20:59, 2000.
11. Litscher G, Wang L, Yang NH, Schwarz G: Ultrasound-monitored effects of acupuncture on brain and eye. Neurol Res 21:373, 1999.
12. Shi R, Ji G, Zhao L, Wang S, et al: Effects of electroacupuncture and twirling reinforcing-reducing manipulations on volume of microcirculatory blood flow in cerebral pia mater. J Tradit Chin Med 18:220, 1998.
13. Thomas D, Collins S, Strauss S: Somatic sympathetic vasomotor changes documented by medical thermographic imaging during acupuncture analgesia. Clin Rheumatol 11:55, 1992.
14. Litscher G, Wang L, Huber E, et al: Changed skin blood perfusion in the fingertip following acupuncture needle introduction as evaluated by laser Doppler perfusion imaging. Lasers Med Sci 17:19, 2002.

15. Xuemin S, Shu W, Qingzhong L, et al: Brain atrophy and ageing: Research on the effect of acupuncture on neuronal apoptosis in cortical tissue. Am J Acupuncture 26:251, 1998.
16. Carson DA, Riberio JM: Apoptosis and disease. Lancet 15:1251, 1993.
17. Verbrugge L: Gender, aging and health. In Markides K, editor: Aging and Health: Perspectives on Gender, Race Ethnicity, and Class. Newbury Park, CA, Sage, 1989, pp 23-78.
18. Ferrell BA. Pain management. Clin Geriatr Med 16:853, 2000.
19. Landi F, Onder G, Cesari M, et al: Pain management in frail, community-living elderly patients. Arch Intern Med 161:2721, 2001.
20. Ferrell BA, Josephson KR, Pollan AM, et al: A randomized trial of walking versus physical methods for chronic pain management. Aging (Milano) 9:99, 1997.
21. Ferrell BA, Ferrell BR: Principles of pain management in older people. Compr Ther 17:53, 1991.
22. Ferrell BA, Ferrell BR, Osterweil D: Pain in the nursing home. J Am Geriatr Soc 38:409, 1990
23. Chikanza I, Fernandes L: Novel strategies for the treatment of osteoarthritis. Expert Opin Investig Drugs 9:1499, 2000.
24. Steffanus D: Help horses, owners cope with geriatric lameness: Age plays a dramatic role in how or if this condition can be treated. Vet. Practice News 14:9, 2002.
25. Dowling PM: Adverse drug reactions in horses. Clin Techn Equine Pract 1:58, 2002.
26. Helme RD: Chronic pain management in older people. Eur J Pain 5(Suppl A):31, 2001.
27. Miaskowski C: The impact of age on a patient's perception of pain and ways it can be managed. Pain Manag Nurs 1(3 Suppl 1):2, 2000.
28. Lewit K: Manipulative Therapy in Rehabilitation of the Locomotor System, 3rd ed. Oxford, England, Butterworth-Heinemann, 1999, p 3.
29. Ernst E, White A: Acupuncture: A Scientific Appraisal. Oxford, Butterworth-Heinemann, 1999.
30. Anil SS, Anil L, Deen J: Challenges of pain assessment in domestic animals. JAMA 220:3, 2002.
31. Beluche LA, Bertone AL, et al: Effects of oral administration of phenylbutazone to horses on in vitro articular cartilage metabolism. AJVR 62:1916, 2001.
32. Fleming P: Acupuncture for musculoskeletal and neurologic conditions in horses. In Schoen AM, editor: Veterinary Acupuncture: Ancient Art to Modern Medicine, 2nd ed. St. Louis, Mosby, 2001.
33. McCormick WH: The use of implants in the treatment of gall bladder and bladder channel imbalance in the horses: A review of 114 cases. In the Proceedings of the Sixteenth Annual International Congress on Veterinary Acupuncture, 1990, Noordwijk, Holland.
34. Haussler KK, Stover SM: Stress fractures of the vertebral lamina and pelvis in Thoroughbred racehorses. Equine Vet J 30:374, 1998.
35. Haussler KK: Chiropractic evaluation and management: Back problems. Vet Clin North Am Equine Pract 15:195, 1999.
36. Jeffcot LB: Back problems in the horse: A look at past, present and future progress. Equine Vet J 11:129, 1979.
37. Steckel RR, Kraus-Hansen AE, Fackleman GE, et al: Scintographic diagnosis of thoracolumbar spinal disease in horses: A review of 50 cases. Proc Am Assoc Equine Pract 37:583, 1991.
38. Dalin G, Magnusson LE, Thafvelin BC: Retrospective study of hindquarter asymmetry in Standardbred Trotters and its correlation with performance. Equine Vet J 17:292, 1985.
39. Ernst E: Experts' opinions on complementary/alternative therapies for low back pain. JMPT 22:87, 1999.
40. Ahern TJ: Laminar corial hyperaesthesia in chronic forelimb lameness. JEVS 15:460, 1995.
41. Filshie J, White A: Medical Acupuncture: A Western Scientific Approach. London, Churchill Livingstone, 1998, p 139-145.
42. Greenman PE: Principles of Manual Medicine, 2nd ed. Baltimore, Williams & Wilkins, 1997, p 473-477.
43. Kappler RE: Palpatory skills. In Ward RC, editor: Foundations for Osteopathic Medicine. Baltimore, Lippincott Williams & Wilkins, 1997, p 475.
44. Kuchera WA, Jones JM III, Kappler RE, et al: Musculoskeletal examination for somatic dysfunction. In Ward RC, editor: Foundations for Osteopathic Medicine. Baltimore, Lippincott Williams & Wilkins, 1997, p 489.
45. Gatterman MI: Foundations of Chiropractic. St. Louis, Mosby-Year Book, 1995, p 63.
46. Troyanovich SJ: Motion palpation: It's time to accept the evidence. JMPT 21:568, 1998.
47. Jull G, Zito G, Trott P, et al: Inter-examiner reliability to detect painful upper cervical joint dysfunction. Aust Physiother 43:125, 1997.
48. Jull G, Bogduk N, Marsland A: The accuracy of manual diagnosis for cervical zygapophysial joint pain syndromes. Med J Aust 148:233, 1988.
49. Anderson R, Meeker WC, Wirick BE, et al: A meta-analysis of clinical trials of spinal manipulation. JMPT 15:181, 1992.
50. Gunnar BJ: A comparison of osteopathic spinal manipulation with standard care for patients with low back pain. N Engl J Med 342:1426, 1999.
51. Leach RA: The Chiropractic Theories: Principles and Clinical Applications, 3rd ed. Baltimore, William & Wilkins, 1994.
52. Haussler KK, Bertram JEA, Gellman K: In-vivo segmental kinematics of the thoracolumbar spinal region in horses and effects of chiropractic manipulations. Proc AAEP 45:327, 1999.
53. Gál JM, Herzog W, Kawchuk GN, et al: Movements of vertebrae during manipulative thrusts to unembalmed human cadavers. JMPT 20:30, 1997.
54. Haussler KK, Erb HN: Pressure algometry: Objective assessment of back pain and effects of chiropractic treatment. AAEP Proceedings 49:66-70, 2003.
55. Bidstrup IS: That "girthy" horse is suffering pain, not just behaving badly. Girth Pain Syndrome, March 2003. Available at: http//www.chirovet.com.au/girthyhorse.pdf.
56. Ahern TJ: Cervical vertebral mobilization under anesthetic (CVMUA): A physical therapy for treatment of cervico-spinal pain and stiffness. JEVS 14:540, 1994.
57. Seaman D: Joint complex dysfunction, a novel term to replace subluxation/subluxation complex: etiologic and treatment considerations. JMPT 20:634, 1997.
58. Gottlieb MS: Conservative management of spinal osteoarthritis with glucosamine sulfate and chiropractic treatment. JMPT 20:400, 1997.
59. Peacock EE: Some biomechanical and biophysical aspects of joint stiffness: Role of collagen synthesis as opposed to altered molecular bonding. Ann Surg 16:1, 1966.
60. Moskowitz R: Experimental models of degenerative joint disease. Semin Arthritis Rheum 2:95, 1972.
61. Langenskoid A, et al: Osteoarthritis of the knee in the rabbit produced by immobilization. Acta Orthop Scand 50:1, 1979.
62. Videman T: Experimental osteoarthritis in the rabbit. Acta Orthop Scand 53:339, 1982.
63. Jayson M: Intra-articular pressure. Clin Rheum Dis 7:149, 1981.
64. Valias AC, et al: Physical activity and its influence on the repair process of medial collateral ligaments. Connect Tissue Res 9:25, 1981.
65. Videman T: Connective tissue and immobilization. Clin Orthop 221:26, 1987.
66. Salter R, et al: The biological effect of continuous passive motion on the healing of full-thickness defects on articular cartilage. J Bone Joint Surg Am 62:1232, 1980.
67. Cassidy JD: The immediate effect of manipulation versus mobilization on pain and range of motion in the cervical spine: A randomized controlled trial. JMPT 15:570, 1992.
68. Dishman JD, Ball KA, Burke J: Central motor excitability changes after spinal manipulation: A transcranial magnetic stimulation study. JMPT 25:1, 2002.
69. Herzog W, et al: Electromyographic responses of back & limb muscles associated with spinal manipulative therapy. Spine 24:146, 1999.
70. Pickar JG, Wheeler JD: Response of muscle proprioceptors to spinal manipulative-like loads in the anesthetized cat. JMPT 24:2, 2001.
71. Haldeman S: Chiropractic: Clinical Practice and State of the Science. Presented at the Complementary & Integrative Medicine Conference, Harvard Medical School, Boston, MA, 2001.

72. Coulter ID: Efficacy and risks of chiropractic manipulation: What does the evidence suggest? Int Med 1:61, 1998.

73. Giles LG, Müller, R: Chronic spinal pain syndromes: A clinical pilot trial comparing acupuncture, a nonsteroidal anti-inflammatory drug, and spinal manipulation. JMPT 22:376, 1999.

74. Whittingham W, Nilsson N: Active range of motion in the cervical spine increases after spinal manipulation (toggle recoil). JMPT 24:552, 2001.

75. Keller TS, Colloca CJ: Mechanical force spinal manipulation increases trunk muscle strength assessed by electromyography: A comparative clinical trial. JMPT 23:585, 2000.

76. Pickar JG, et al: Responses of mechanosensitive afferents to manipulation of the lumbar facet in the cat. Spine 20:2379, 1995.

77. Thabe H: Electromyography as tool to document diagnostic findings and therapeutic results associated with somatic dysfunction in the upper cervical spinal joints and sacroiliac joints. Manual Med 2:53, 1986.

78. Suter E, McMorland G, Herzog W, et al: Conservative lower back treatment reduces inhibition in knee-extensor muscles: A randomized controlled trial. JMPT 23:76, 2000.

79. Pellow JE, Brantingham HW: The efficacy of adjusting the ankle in the treatment of subacute and chronic grade I and grade II ankle inversion sprains. JMPT 24:17, 2001.

80. Morton J: Manipulation in the treatment of acute low back pain. J Manual Manip Ther 7:182, 1999.

81. Yates RG, et al: Effects of chiropractic treatment on blood pressure and anxiety: A randomized, controlled trial. JMPT 11:484, 1988.

82. Wiberg JMM, Nordsteen J, Nilsson N: The short-term effect of spinal manipulation in the treatment of infantile colic: A randomized controlled clinical trial with a blinded observer. JMPT 22:517, 1999.

83. Heikkila H, Johansson M, Wenngren BI: Effects of acupuncture, cervical manipulation and NSAID therapy on dizziness and impaired head repositioning of suspected cervical origin: A pilot study. Man Ther 5:151, 2000.

84. Kelly DD, Murphy BA, Backhouse DP: Use of mental rotation reaction-time paradigm to measure the effects of upper cervical adjustments on cortical processing: A pilot study. JMPT 23:246, 2000.

85. Lauro A, Mouch B: Chiropractic effects on athletic ability. Chiro Res Clin Invest 6:84, 1991.

86. Seemann W: Bilateral weight differential and functional short leg: An analysis of pre and post data after reduction of an atlas subluxation. Chiro Res J 2:33, 1993.

87. Herzog W, et al: Effects of different treatment modalities on gait symmetry and clinical measures for sacroioiliac joint patients. JMPT 14:104, 1991.

88. Manga P, Angus D, Papadopoulos C, et al: The Effectiveness and Cost-Effectiveness of Chiropractic Management of Low-Back Pain. Ontario, Canada, The Ontario Ministry of Health, 1993.

89. Dabbs V, Lauretti WJ: A risk assessment of cervical manipulation vs. NSAIDs for the treatment of neck pain. JMPT 19:220, 1996.

90. Jaggar DH, Robinson NG: History of veterinary acupuncture. In Schoen AM, editor: Veterinary Acupuncture: Ancient Art to Modern Medicine, 2nd ed. St. Louis, Mosby, 2001, p 3-18.

91. Kaptchuk T: The Web That Has No Weaver: Understanding Chinese Medicine. Lincolnwood, IL, Contemporary Books, 2000, p 15

92. Ellis A, Wiseman N, Boss K: Grasping the Wind: An exploration into the meaning of Chinese acupuncture point names. Brookline, MA, Paradigm Publications, 1989.

93. Hewitt PG: Conceptual Physics, 8th ed. Reading, MA, Addison Wesley Longman, 1998, p 100.

94. Birch S, Ida J: Japanese Acupuncture: A Clinical Guide. Brookline, MA Paradigm Publications, 1998.

95. Seem M: A New American Acupuncture: American Osteopathy. Boulder, CO, Blue Poppy Press, 1993.

96. Matsumoto K, Birch S: Hara Diagnosis: Reflections on the Sea. Brookline, MA, Paradigm Publications, 1988.

97. Rathgeber R: Understanding Equine Acupuncture. Lexington, KY, The Blood Horse, 2001.

98. McCormick WH: Traditional Chinese channel diagnosis, myofascial pain syndrome and metacarpophalangeal joint trauma in the horse. JEVS 16:562, 1996.

99. McCormick WH: Oriental channel diagnosis in foot lameness of the equine forelimb. Proc AAEP 43:330, 1997.

100. McCormick WH: The Origins of Acupuncture Channel Imbalance in Pain of the Equine Hindlimb. Presented at the Annual International Congress on Veterinary Acupuncture, Lexington, Kentucky, 1998.

101. Robinson NG: Neuroanatomic Acupuncture Approaches to Pain. Course notes from Colorado State University Veterinary Medical Acupuncture Training Program, Fort Collins, CO, 2001.

102. Stux G, Pomeranz B: Basics of Acupuncture, 4th ed. New York, Springer-Verlag, 1998.

103. Karavis MK: Neuroscience, Neurophysiology and Acupuncture. ICMART '96, VII's World Congress. Copenhagen, May 9-12, 1996.

104. Konttinen YT: Peripheral and spinal neural mechanism in arthritis, with particular reference to treatment of inflammation and pain. Arthritis Rheum 37:965, 1994.

105. Xuemin S, Ping L, Shu W, et al: Nobel Prize opens possibilities for exploring acupuncture mechanisms and dementia: The effects of needling on nitric oxide levels in plasma and myocardium. Am J Acupuncture 26:255, 1998.

106. Stux G, Hammerschlag R: Clinical Acupuncture: Scientific Basis. New York, Springer-Verlag, 2001.

107. Acupuncture study available at: http://www.medizin.auskunft.de/artikel/aktuell/28_01_04_akupunkturstudie.php&p.

108. National Institutes of Health. Available at: http://nccam.nih.gov/nccam/fcp/factsheets/acupuncture

109. Ernst E, Pittler MH: The effectiveness of acupuncture in treating acute dental pain: A systematic review. Br Dent J 184:443, 1998.

110. Melchart D, Linde K, Fischer P, et al: Acupuncture for idiopathic headache (Cochrane Review). In The Cochrane Library, Issue 1. Oxford, Update Software, 2002.

111. Blom M, Dawidson I, Angmar-Mansson B: The effect of acupuncture on salivary flow rates in patients with xerostomia. Oral Surg Oral Med Oral Pathol 73:293, 1992.

112. Blom M, Dawidson I, Angmar-Mansson B: Acupuncture treatment of xerostomia caused by irradiation of the head and neck region: Case reports. J Oral Rehabil 20:491, 1993.

113. Blom M, Dawidson I, Fernberg JO, et al: Acupuncture treatment of patients with radiation-induced xerostomia. Eur J Cancer B Oral Oncol 32B:182, 1996.

114. Blom M, Kopp S, Lundeberg T: Prognostic value of the pilocarpine test to identify patients who may obtain long-term relief from xerostomia by acupuncture treatment. Arch Otolaryngol Head Neck Surg 125:561, 1999.

115. Dawidson I, Angmar-Mansson B, Blom M, et al: Sensory stimulation (acupuncture) increases the release of calcitonin gene-related peptide in the saliva of xerostomia sufferers Neuropeptides 33:244, 1999.

116. Dawidson I, Angmar-Mansson B, Blom M, et al: Sensory stimulation (acupuncture) increases the release of vasoactive intestinal polypeptide in the saliva of xerostomia sufferers Neuropeptides 32:543, 1998.

117. Rydholm M, Strang P: Acupuncture for patients in hospital-based home care suffering from xerostomia. J Palliat Care 15:20, 1999.

118. Blom M, Lundeberg T: Long-term follow-up of patients treated with acupuncture for xerostomia and the influence of additional treatment Oral Dis 6:15, 2000.

119. Johnstone PA, Peng YP, May BC, et al: Acupuncture for pilocarpine-resistant xerostomia following radiotherapy for head and neck malignancies. Int J Radiat Oncol Biol Phys 50:353, 2001.

120. Chen HL, Huang XM: Treatment of chemotherapy-induced leukocytopenia with acupuncture and moxibustion. Zhong XiYi Jie He Za Zhi 11:350, 1991.

121. Honjo H: Acupuncture on clinical symptoms and urodynamic measurements in spinal-cord-injured patients with detrusor hyperreflexia. Urol Int 65:190, 2000.

122. Zhuang X, Wang L: Acupuncture treatment of Parkinson's disease: A report of 29 cases. J Tradit Chin Med 20:265, 2000.

123. Wang L, He C, Liu Y, Zhu L: Effect of acupuncture on the auditory evoked brain stem potential in Parkinson's disease. J Tradit Chin Med 22:15, 2002.

124. Gao H, Yan L, Liu B, et al: Clinical study on treatment of senile vascular dementia by acupuncture. J Tradit Chin Med 21:103, 2001.

125. Pins and needles: Can acupuncture help promote pregnancy? ABC-NEWS.com, April 16, 2002.

126. Zheng H, Wang S, Shang J, et al: Study on acupuncture and moxibustion therapy for female urethral syndrome. J Tradit Chin Med 18:122, 1998.

127. Diehl DL: Acupuncture for gastrointestinal and hepatobiliary disorders. J Altern Complement Med 5:27, 1999.

128. Chang CS, Ko CW, Wu CY, et al: Effect of electrical stimulation on acupuncture points in diabetic patients with gastric dysrhythmia: A pilot study. Digestion 64:184, 2001.

129. Thomas D, Collins S, Strauss S: Somatic sympathetic vasomotor changes documented by medical thermographic imaging during acupuncture analgesia. Clin Rheumatol 11:55, 1992.

130. Joos S, Schott C, Zou H, et al: Immunomodulatory effects of acupuncture in the treatment of allergic asthma: A randomized controlled study. J Alt Comp Med 6:519, 2000.

131. Nolte D: Acupuncture in bronchial asthma: Body-plethysmographic measurements of acute bronchospasmolytic effects. Comp Med East West 5:265, 1977.

132. Tashkin DP, Bresler DE, Kroening RJ, et al: Comparison of real and simulated acupuncture and isoproteronal in methacholine-induced asthma. Allergy 39:379, 1977.

133. Xue CC, English R, Zhang JJ, et al: Effect of acupuncture in the treatment of seasonal allergic rhinitis: A randomized controlled clinical trial. Am J Chin Med 30:1, 2002.

134. Robinson NG: Acupuncture-assisted anesthesia reduces patient pain. Veterinary Practice News July:36, 2002.

135. Wang HH, Chang YH, Liu DM, et al: A clinical study on physiological response in electroacupuncture analgesia and meperidine analgesia for colonoscopy. Am J Chin Med 25:13, 1997.

136. Wang RR, Tronnier V: Effect of acupuncture on pain management in patients before and after lumbar disc protrusion surgery: A randomized control study. Am J Chin Med 28:25, 2000.

137. Yao T: Acupuncture and somatic nerve stimulation: Mechanism underlying effects on cardiovascular and renal activities. Scand J Rehabil Med Suppl 29:7, 1993.

138. Lazarou J, Pomeranz BR, Corey PN: Incidence of adverse drug reactions in hospitalized patients: A meta-analysis of prospective studies. JAMA 279:1200, 1998.

139. White A, Hayhoe S, Hart A, et al: Adverse events following acupuncture: Prospective survey of 32,000 consultations with doctors and physiotherapists. BMJ 323:485, 2001.

140. MacPherson H, Thomas K, Walters S, et al: The York acupuncture safety study: Prospective survey of 34,000 treatments by traditional acupuncturists. BMJ 323:486, 2001.

141. Yamashita H, Tsukayama H, Tanno Y, et al: Adverse events in acupuncture and moxibustion treatment: A six-year survey at a national clinic in Japan. J Altern Complement Med 5:229, 1999.

142. Tramer MR, Moore RA, Reynolds DJ, et al: Quantitative estimation of rare adverse events which follows a biological progression: A new model applied to chronic NSAID use. Pain 85:169, 2000.

143. Penreger TV, Whelton PK, Klag MJ: Risk of kidney failure associated with use of acetaminophen, aspirin, and nonsteroidal anti-inflammatory drugs. N Engl J Med 331:1675, 1994.

144. Cho ZN, Wong EK, Fallon J: Neuro-Acupuncture: Scientific Evidence of Acupuncture Revealed. Los Angeles, Q-Puncture, 2001.

145. Xie H, Ott EA, Harkins JD, et al: Influence of Electroacupuncture Stimulation on Pain Threshold and Neuroendocrine Responses in Horse. In Sustainable Medicine for Animals, the Proceedings of the 24th Annual International Congress on Veterinary Acupuncture, August 12-15, 1998, Chitou, Taiwan, Republic of China.

146. Hackett GE, Spitzfaden DM, May KJ, et al: Acupuncture versus phenylbutazone. JEVS 19:326, 1999.

147. Hackett GE, Spitzfaden DM, May KJ, et al: Acupuncture: Is it effective for alleviating pain in the horse? Proc AAEP 43:333, 1997.

148. Skarda R, et al: Cutaneous Analgesic, Hemodynamic and Respiratory Effects, and Beta-Endorphin Concentration in Lumbar Spinal Fluid After Bilateral Percutaneous Electrical Stimulation of Acupuncture points BL18, 23, 25, and 28 in Healthy Mares. In the Proceedings IVAS 2000 World Congress, Vienna, Austria, p 118-121.

149. Bossut DF: Production of cutaneous analgesia by electro-acupuncture in horses: Variations dependent on sex of subject and locus of stimulation. AJVR 45:620, 1984.

150. Yamaguchi T, Kastumi A, Igarahi K, et al: Effect of Moxaneedle Therapy on Chronic Back Pain and Hip Pain in Race Horses. In the Proceedings of the Twenty-Fourth Annual International Congress on Veterinary Acupuncture Taiwan, Republic of China, 1998, p 129-131.

151. Jin-Zhong Y: Studies on the treatment of lameness in horses by acupuncture. Sci Agricul Sinica 5:90, 1981.

152. Rogers PAM, Cain MJ, Kent E, et al: Physiotherapy, homeopathy, and acupuncture in the treatment and prevention of lameness and the maintenance of peak fitness in horses. International Journal of Veterinary Acupuncture 2:14, 1991.

153. Xie H: Influence of acupuncture on experimental lameness in horses. Proceedings AAEP 47:347, 2001.

154. Xie H: Treating equine lameness with acupuncture. Compendium 23:838, 2001.

155. Bidstrup IS: Equine headshaking: a case study. Available at: http://users.med.auth.gr/~karanik/english/articles/headshake.html

156. Bobis S: Chronic diarrhoea in a Thoroughbred filly. Int J Vet Acupuncture 3:17, 1992.

157. Cochran SL: Acupuncture therapy for the treatment of allergic dermatitis in a horse. Int J Vet Acupuncture 4:21, 1993.

158. Hoogenraad RR: Equine ataxia. Int J Vet Acupuncture 6:1, 1995.

159. Klide AM: Acupuncture for the Treatment of Chronic Laminitis in the Horse. In the Proceedings of the Sixteenth Annual International Congress on Veterinary Acupuncture, Noordwijk, Holland, 1990.

160. Landholm JE, Mills LI: Use of acupuncture in treatment of laminitis in a horse. VMSAC 76:405, 1981.

161. Chen YY, Marshall D, et al: Alternate adjunct therapy can enhance coffin bone (P3) stabilization after laminitis and rotation. Meridian 4:4, 2002.

162. Steiss JE, White NA, Bowen JM: Electroacupuncture in the treatment of chronic lameness in horses and ponies: A controlled clinical trial. Can J Vet Res 53:239-243, 1989.

163. Puertas D: Acupuncture treatment of rectal prolapse in a mare: A clinical case. Available at http://users.med.auth.gr/~karanik/english/articles/rect.html

164. Schmitz WG: Transcutaneous electroacupuncture used in left traumatic facial hemiplegia on one mare. Int J Vet Acupuncture 7:4, 1996.

165. White SS, Christie MP: Acupuncture used as an adjunct in the treatment of a horse with tetanus. Austr Vet J 62:25, 1985.

166. Mitchell RD: Acupuncture Management of Lumbar and Croup Myopathy Associated with Distal Tarsitis in the Horse: A Case Report. Presented at the Lameness in the Show Hunter/Jumper, Equine Practitioners' Workshop, Ohio State University, January, 1990.

167. Schoen AM: Equine Immune-Mediated Myofascial Syndrome: Acupuncture Diagnosis and Treatment. In the Proceedings of the Twenty-Fourth Annual International Congress on Veterinary Acupuncture, Taiwan, Republic of China, 1998, p 1157-1163.

168. Klide AM, Martin BB Jr: Methods of stimulating acupuncture points for treatment of chronic back pain in horses. JAVMA 195:1375, 1989.

169. Martin BB Jr, Klide AM: Acupuncture for the treatment of chronic back pain in horses. In Schoen AM, editior: Veterinary Acupuncture: Ancient Art to Modern Medicine, 2nd ed. St. Louis, Mosby, 2001, p 467-473.

170. Merriam JG: Acupuncture in the treatment of back and hindleg pain in sport horses. Proc AAEP 43:325, 1997.

171. Uwe P: The Role of Laser Acupuncture in Equine Back Problems. In the Proceedings of the Twenty-Sixth Annual International Congress on Veterinary Acupuncture, Vienna, Austria, 2000, p 144-147.

172. Xie H, Asquith RL, Kivipelto J, et al: A review of the use of acupuncture for treatment of equine back pain. JEVS 16:285, 1996.

173. Ridgway K: Acupuncture as a treatment modality for back problems. Vet Clin North Am Equine Pract 15:211-221, 1999.

174. Fang JQ, Aoki E, Seto A, et al: Influence of moxibustion on collagen-induced arthritis in mice. In Vivo 12:421-426, 1998.

175. Hao LC: Electropuncture therapy trial for treating infertility in mares. Theriogenology 28:301, 1997.

176. Xie H: Infertility in the mare: an alterative approach. In the Proceedings of the Twenty-Third Annual International Congress on Veterinary Acupuncture, 1997, p 114-122.

177. Muxeneder R: Treatment of ovarian dysfunction in mares by acupuncture and biological remedies as an alternative to hormone therapy. Praktische Tierarzt 72:88, 1991.

178. Lin JH, Chen WW, Wu LS: Acupuncture Treatments for Animal Reproductive Disorders Available at http://users.med.auth.gr/~karanik/english/articles/lin99rep.html

179. Lin JH, Liu SH, Chan WW, et al: Effects of electroacupuncture and gonadotropin-releasing hormone treatments on hormonal changes in anoestrous sows. Am J Chin Med 16:117-126, 1988.

180. Lin JH, Wu LS, Wu YL, et al: Aquapuncture therapy of repeat breeding in dairy cattle. Am J Chin Med 30:397-404, 2002.

181. Jang KH, Lee JM, Nam TC: Electroacupunture and moxibustion for correction of abomasal displacement in dairy cattle. J Vet Sci 4:93-95, 2003.

182. Korematsu K, Takagi E, Kawabe T, et al: Therapeutic effects of moxibustion on delayed uterine involution in postpartum dairy cows. J Vet Med Sci 55:613-616, 1993.

183. Kim BS: The effects of electroacupuncture on gastrointestinal motility and blood concentration of endocrine substances in horses. In Schoen AM, editor: Veterinary Acupuncture: Ancient Art to Modern Medicine, 2nd ed. St. Louis, Mosby, 2001, p 57.

184. Skarda RT, Muir WW 3rd: Comparison of electroacupuncture and butorphanol on respiratory and cardiovascular effects and rectal pain threshold after controlled rectal distention in mares. AJVR 64:137-144, 2003.

185. Skarda RT, Muir WW: Visceral Analgesis, Respiratory and Cardiovascular Effects of Electroacupuncture and Butorphanol in Mares: A Comparative study Using Controlled Rectal Distension. In Proceedings of the 28th international Congress on Veterinary Acupuncture, 2002, Kawaii, Hawaii.

186. Merritt AM, Xie H, Lester GD, et al: Evaluation of a method to experimentally induce colic in horses and the effects of acupuncture applied at the Guan-yuan-shu (similar to BL-21) acupoint. AJVR 63:1006-1011, 2002.

187. Feng KR: A method of electro-acupuncture treatment for equine intestinal impaction. Am J Chin Med 9:174-180, 1981.

188. Park ES, Jo S, Seong JK, et al: Effect of acupuncture in the treatment of young pigs with induced Escherichia coli diarrhea. J Vet Sci 4:125-128, 2003.

189. Hwang YC, Jenkins EM: Effect of acupuncture on young pigs with induced enteropalthogenic Escherichia coli diarrhea. Am J Vet Res 49:1641-1643, 1988.

190. Mitchell RD: Acupuncture as a diagnostic aid and adjuvant therapy for ulcerative gastritis in the horse. Int J Vet Acupuncture 4:18, 1999.

191. Hussain SS: Techniques of acupuncture analgesia for equine surgery. Centaur Mylapore 12:8, 1995.

192. Hwang YC, Held H: Some experimental observations on acupuncture analgesia in the pony. Anat Histol Embryol 6:88, 1997.

193. Klide AM, Gaynor JS: Acupuncture for Surgical Analgesia and Postoperative Analgesia. In Schoen AM, editor: Veterinary Acupuncture: Ancient Art to Modern Medicine, 2nd ed. St. Louis, Mosby, 2001, p 295-302.

194. Klide AM: Acupuncture produced surgical analgesia. Prob Vet Med 4:200, 1992.

195. Rogers PAM, White SS, Ottaway CW: Stimulation of the acupuncture points in relation to therapy of analgesia and clinical disorders in animals. Vet Ann 17:258, 1976.

196. Bossut DF, Stromberg MW, Malven PV: Electroacupuncture-induced analgesia in sheep: Measurement of cutaneous pain thresholds and plasma concentrations of prolactin and beta-endorphin immunoreactivity. Am J Vet Res 47:669-676, 1986.

197. Kim DH, Cho SH, Song KH, et al: Electroacupuncture analgesia for surgery in cattle. Am J Chin Med 32:131-140, 2004.

198. White SS, Bolton JR, Fraser DM: Use of electroacupuncture as an analgesic for laparotomies in two dairy cows. Aust Vet J 62:52-54, 1985.

199. Bossut DFB, Leshin LS, Stromberg MW, et al: Plasma cortisol and beta-endorphin in horses subjected to electro-acupuncture for cutaneous analgesia. Peptides 4:501, 1983.

200. Luna SPL, Taylor PM: Effect of electroacupuncture on endogenous opioids, AVP, ACTH, cortisol and catecholamine concentrations measured in the cerebrospinal fluid (CSF), peripheral and pituitary effluent plasma of ponies. In the Proceedings of the Twenty-Fourth Annual International Congress on Veterinary Acupuncture Taiwan, Republic of China, 1998, p 172-174.

201. Cheng R, Mckibbin L, Roy B, ct al: Electroacupuncture elevates blood cortisol levels in naive horses; sham treatment has no effect. Int J Neurosci 10:95-97, 1980.

202. Chan WW, Chen KY, Liu H, et al: Acupuncture for general veterinary practice. J Vet Med Sci 63:1057-1062, 2001.

203. Lin JH, Rogers PAM: Acupuncture effects on the body's defense systems: A veterinary review. Vet Bull 50:8, 1980.

204. Klide AM: An hypothesis for the prolonged effect of acupuncture. Acupuncture Electrother Res Int J 14:141, 1989.

205. Hwang YC: Pilomotor Reaction of Equine Bladder Channel Points Following Acupuncture Treatment. In the Proceedings of the Twenty-Fourth Annual International Congress on Veterinary Acupuncture Taiwan, Republic of China, 1998, p 106-109.

206. Gideon L: Acupuncture: Clinical trials in the horse. JAVMA 170:220, 1977.

207. Mittleman E, Gaynor, JS: A brief overview of the analgesic and immunologic effects of acupuncture in domestic animals. JAMA 217:8, 2000.

208. Lundeberg T, Eriksson SV, Theodorsson E: Neuroimmunomodulatory effects of acupuncture in mice. Neurosci Lett 128:161-164, 1991.

209. Uwe P: Laser acupuncture on horses with COPD. Proceedings of the Twenty-Sixth Annual International Congress on Veterinary Acupuncture, Vienna, Austria, 2000, p. 144-147.

210. Wilson DV, Lankenau C, Berney CE, et al: The effects of a single acupuncture treatment in horses with severe recurrent airway obstruction. Equine Vet J 36:489-494, 2004.

211. Bakhtiari J, Zama MMS: Acupuncture Therapy in Postoperative Rehabilitation of Sheep with Fracture of Femur. In Sustainable Medicine for Animals, the Proceedings of the 24th Annual International Congress on Veterinary Acupuncture, August 12-15, 1998, Chitou, Taiwan, Republic of China.

212. Wang XR, Xiao J, Sun DJ: Myocardial protective effects of electroacupuncture and hypothermia on porcine heart after ischemia/reperfusion. Acupunct Electrother Res 28:193-200, 2003.

213. Sumano H, Bermudez E, Obregon K: Treatment of Wobbler syndrome in dogs with electro-AP. Dtsch Tierarztl Wochenschr 107:231-235, 2000.

214. Von Schweinitz DG: Thermographic evidence for the effectiveness of acupuncture in equine neuromuscular disease. Acupuncture Med J Br Med Acupuncture Soc 16:14, 1998.

215. Chvala S, Nowotny N, Kotzab E, et al: Use of the meridian test for the detection of equine herpesvirus type 1 infection in horses with decreased performance. JAVMA 225: 554-559, 2004.

216. Fenger CK, Granstrom DE, Langemeier JL, et al: Equine protozoal myelitis: Acupuncture diagnosis. Proc AAEP 43:327, 1997.

217. Ramey DW: Do Acupuncture points and meridians actually exist? Compendium 22:1132, 2000.

218. Ramey DW, Imrie RH, Buell PD: Veterinary acupuncture and traditional Chinese medicine: Facts and fallacies. Compendium 23:188, 2001.

219. Ramey DW, Buell PD: Acupuncture and "traditional Chinese medicine" in the horse. Equine Vet Education/AE/August 2004, 275-282.

220. Critchley JA, Zhang Y, Suthisisang CC, et al: Alternative therapies and medical science: Designing clinical trials of alternative/complementary medicines. Is evidence-based traditional Chinese medicine attainable? J Clin Pharmacol 40:462, May.

221. Flaws B: Sticking to the Point: A Rational Methodology for the Step by Step Formulation and Administration of a TCM Acupuncture Treatment. Boulder, CO, Blue Poppy Press, 1990, p 8.

222. Wang S, Lai X, Lao J: The third lumbar transverse process syndrome treated by electroacupuncture at huatuojiaji points. J Tradit Chin Med 19:190, 1999.

223. Kim BS: The effects of electroacupuncture on gastrointestinal motility and blood concentration of endocrine substances in horses. Doctoral thesis, Seoul National University, 1997. Veterinary acupuncture: Ancient art to modern medicine, Schoen AM, editor, 2nd ed. St. Louis, Mosby, p. 57.

224. Flaws B: Imperial Secrets of Health and Longevity. Boulder, CO, Blue Poppy Press, 1994.

225. Flaws B: The Secret of Chinese Pulse Diagnosis. Boulder, CO, Blue Poppy Press, 1995.

226. Yan De-Xin: Ageing and Blood Stasis, trans. by Tang Guo-shun and B. Flaws. Boulder, CO, Blue Poppy Press, 1995.

227. O'Connor J, Bensky D: Acupuncture, A Comprehensive Text. Seattle, WA, Eastland Press, 1981.

228. Wiseman N, Feng Y: A Practical Dictionary of Chinese Medicine, 2nd ed. Brookline, MA, Paradigm Publications, 1998.

229. The Encyclopedia of Chinese Medicinals. Shanghai, Shanghai Science and Technology Press, 1991.

230. Bensky D, Barolet R: Formulas and Strategies. Seattle, WA, Eastland Press, 1990.

231. Li D-Y, Pi WL: Treatise on the Spleen and Stomach, trans. by Yang S-Z, Li J-Y. Boulder, CO, Blue Poppy Press, 1993.

232. Yan D-X: Ageing and blood stasis. Boulder, CO, Flaws Blue Poppy Press, 1995, p. 34.

233. Flaws B: Seventy Essential TCM Formulas. Boulder, CO, Blue Poppy Press, 1991.

234. Flaws B: A Certificate Program in Chinese Medical Herbology: Course 5. Boulder, CO, Blue Poppy Press, 1999.

235. Wang LT: Golden Needle, trans. Yu H-C, Han F-R. Boulder, CO, Blue Poppy Press, 1997.

236. Wu LS, Lin JH, Rogers PAM: Pharmacological Effects of Chinese Medicinal Formulas. In the Proceedings of the Twenty-Third Annual International Congress on Veterinary Acupuncture, St. Sauveur, Quebec, Canada, 1997, p 32.

237. Flaws B, Sionneau P: The Treatment of Modern Western Medical Diseases with Chinese Medicine. Boulder, CO, Blue Poppy Press, 2001.

238. Xie H, Xiaolin D, Mani D: Chinese Veterinary Herbal Handbook. Reddick, FL, Chi Institute of Chinese Medicine, 2000.

239. Sackett D: Evidence-Based Medicine. London, Livingstone Churchill, 2001.

240. Lin JH, Wu LS, Rogers PAM: Sustainable Medicine for Veterinarians in the New Millennium. In the Proceedings of the 24th Annual International Congress on Veterinary Acupuncture, August 12-15, 1998, Chitou, Taiwan, Republic of China.

241. Haussler K: Course notes: 2001 Manual Therapy Course, Colorado State University, Fort Collins, CO.

Extensive Continuing Education Programs Are Recommended

Specific therapeutic techniques are beyond the scope of this chapter, and it is recommended that extensive continuing education programs be undertaken before a veterinarian is considered competent to perform manual therapy or acupuncture. (These therapies are most successful when used in conjunction with careful physical and lameness examinations.)

Postgraduate education in manual therapy is offered by the following institutions:

Colorado State University College of Veterinary Medicine
(Narda Robinson, DO, DVM, DABMA)
105 Equine Center, Fort Collins, CO 80523-1679

American Veterinarians and Chiropractors Association
623 Main St, Hillsdale, IL 61275

The Healing Oasis Wellness Center
2555 Wisconsin St., Sturtevant, WI 53177-1825

Veterinary Acupuncture Training Programs are offered by the following institutions:

Chi Institute for Traditional Chinese Medicine

(Huisheng Xie, DVM, PhD)
9708 W. Hwy. 318, Reddick, FL 32686

Colorado State University College of Veterinary Medicine
(Narda Robinson, DO, DVM, DABMA),
105 Equine Center, Fort Collins, CO 80523-1679

International Veterinary Acupuncture Society
P. O. Box 1478, Longmont, CO 80502

Tufts University School of Veterinary Medicine—Acupuncture
Office of Continuing Education
200 Westboro Road, North Grafton, MA 01536

A Guide to Motion Palpation of the Equine Spine and Pelvis for the Veterinarian[241]

To understand motion palpation, one must examine each articulation with a focus on the specific characteristics of each articulation. It is important to develop consistency in standardization of examination. Of particular note is the horse's position, the veterinarian's position in relation to the horse, the specific area in which the veterinarian touches the horse and what part of the veterinarian's anatomy contacts the horse. In general, the veterinarian contacts the horse with his or her hands. Areas of the hand that are commonly used for contact are the pisiform (accessory carpal), the thenar pad (the muscle over the first metacarpal of the thumb), and the calcaneal area (between the pisiform and thenar contacts). The horse as well as the veterinarian must be stable. Static palpation findings indicate present anatomic relationships. Motion palpation findings are a description of altered joint end-feel, restricted joint motion, or asymmetric motion of a joint in one, two, or three planes of movement (e.g., flexion or extension, left or right lateral bending, left or right axial rotation).

Occipitoatlantal Articulation (Occiput-C1)

Normal Joint Biomechanics

Articular processes support both vertebral stability and mobility due to the interlocking articular surfaces. The occiput-C1-C2 articulations are not considered typical vertebral articulations, since the synovial articular surfaces are modified and specialized, and the intervertebral disks are absent. The occiput-C1 articulation supports vertical motion in the median plane (i.e., shaking the head in a "yes" motion).

Restriction of Flexion

Upon palpation of the anatomic relationships, the veterinarian finds symmetrical space between the caudal ramus of the mandible and the cranial wing of the atlas. Pain is localized to the poll region and hypertonicity of the poll muscles (e.g., rectus capitis dorsalis) bilaterally. Upon motion palpation, the veterinarian finds restriction in flexion of the occiput-C1 articulation. The horse is not able to flex at the poll (especially with certain dressage movements). The horse's position is standing with head and neck extended and relaxed. The veterinarian's position is standing directly in front of the horse on either side of the restricted joint motion, facing caudally. The veterinarian contacts the horse bilaterally at the ventrocaudal aspect of the wing of C1 with both hands, bilateral fingertip contact. The veterinarian stabilizes the horse by resting the dorsal aspect of the horse's muzzle under veterinarian's axilla. The veterinarian motions the atlas caudal to cranial, to induce increased flexion of the occiput-C1 articulation. Caution: the horse may toss his head, striking the veterinarian in the face.

Restriction of Extension

Upon palpation of the anatomic relationships, the veterinarian finds a symmetrical space between the caudal ramus of the mandible and the cranial wing of the atlas.

Upon motion palpation, the veterinarian finds restriction in extension of the occiput-C1 articulation. The horse's position is standing, with head and neck extended and relaxed. The veterinarian stands directly in front of the horse, on either side of the restriction, facing caudally, in a broad-based stance. The veterinarian contacts the horse bilaterally at the dorsal aspect of the wing of C1 with loosely crossed finger contact. The veterinarian stabilizes the horse by resting the ventral aspect of the mandible on his or her shoulder. The veterinarian motions C1 dorsal to ventral and slightly caudal to cranial, to induce increased extension of the occiput-C1 articulation. Caution: the horse may unexpectedly rear up and strike with front feet. Caution: loosely cross fingers so that if the horse suddenly raises head and neck, your will not be lifted off the ground and lose your footing.

Restriction in Ipsilateral Lateral Bending of the Occiput Cranial

Upon palpation of the anatomic relationships, the veterinarian finds an ipsilaterally widened (asymmetrical) space between the caudal ramus of the mandible and the cranial wing of the atlas. Pain is localized to poll muscles, and there may be hypertonicity of the poll muscles either unilaterally or bilaterally. Upon motion palpation, the veterinarian finds restriction in ipsilateral lateral bending of the occiput-C1 articulation. If the occiput is relatively cranial on one side, the occiput on the opposite side will appear to be caudally restricted or displaced. Motion palpation will help to determine which side is restricted. The horse's position is standing, with head and neck extended and relaxed. The veterinarian's position is standing next to the patient's head, ipsilateral to the side of restriction, facing toward the patient's head. The veterinarian contacts the horse at the lateral aspect of the occiput, ventral and caudal to the base of the ear, ipsilateral to the affected articulation with his or her caudal hand, with pisiform or thenar contact. The veterinarian stabilizes the horse by holding the lateral aspect of the muzzle and nasal bones using the cranial hand, with palmar contact. The veterinarian motions lateral to medial and cranial to caudal, to induce increased lateral bending of the occiput-C1 articulation. Follow the angle of the occipital condyle from cranial to caudal.

Restriction in Ipsilateral Lateral Bending of the Atlas Caudal

Upon palpation of the anatomic relationships, the veterinarian finds an ipsilaterally widened (asymmetrical) space between the caudal ramus of the mandible and the

cranial wing of the atlas. Upon motion palpation, the veterinarian finds restriction in ipsilateral lateral bending of the occiput-C1 articulation. The horse's position is standing, with head and neck extended and relaxed. The veterinarian's position is standing to side of the patient, ipsilateral to the side of restriction, facing toward the patient's head. The veterinarian contacts the horse at the ventrocaudal aspect of the wing of C1, ipsilateral to the affected articulation with the caudal hand, with pisiform contact. The veterinarian stabilizes the horse by the halter on the ipsilateral side of restriction using the cranial hand on the halter. After bringing the head and neck into slight lateral bending on the ipsilateral side of veterinarian's position, the veterinarian motions caudal to cranial and slightly lateral to medial, to induce increased lateral bending of the occiput-C1 articulation.

Restriction in Contralateral Lateral Bending of the Occiput-C1 Articulation Occiput Caudal

Upon palpation of the anatomic relationships, the veterinarian finds an ipsilaterally narrowed (asymmetrical) space between the caudal ramus of the mandible and the cranial wing of the atlas. Upon motion palpation, the veterinarian finds restriction in contralateral lateral bending of the occiput-C1 articulation. The horse's position is standing, with head and neck extended and relaxed. The veterinarian's position is standing next to the patient's head, contralateral to the side of restriction, facing toward the patient's head. The veterinarian contacts the horse at the lateral aspect of the occiput, ventral and caudal to the base of the ear, contralateral to the affected articulation with the caudal hand, with pisiform or thenar contacts. The veterinarian stabilizes the horse by lateral aspect of the muzzle and nasal bones using the cranial hand, with palmar contact to stabilize the horse. The veterinarian motions lateral to medial and cranial to caudal to induce increased lateral bending of the occiput-C1 articulation. Follow the angle of the occipital condyle from cranial to caudal.

Restriction in Contralateral Lateral Bending of the Occiput-C1 Articulation Atlas Cranial

Upon palpation of the anatomic relationships, the veterinarian finds an ipsilaterally narrowed (asymmetrical) space between the caudal ramus of the mandible and the cranial wing of the atlas. Upon motion palpation, the veterinarian finds restriction in contralateral lateral bending of the occiput-C1 articulation. The horse's position is standing, with head and neck extended and relaxed. The veterinarian's position is standing directly in front of the patient's head, ipsilateral to the side of restriction, facing caudally. The veterinarian contacts the horse at the craniodorsal aspect of the wing of C1, ipsilateral to the affected articulation with the caudal hand, with thenar contact. The veterinarian stabilizes the horse by the halter on the ipsilateral side of restriction using the cranial hand on the halter to stabilize the horse and brings the head and neck into slight lateral bending on the ipsilateral side of veterinarian's position.

Atlantoaxial Articulation (C1/C2)

Normal joint biomechanics: Axial rotation in the cervical region occurs primarily at the Cl/C2 articulation in the transverse plane (i.e., shaking the head in a "no" motion).

Atlas Restricted Motion Occurs Dorsal to Ventral or Ventral to Dorsal

Upon palpation of the anatomic relationships, the veterinarian finds the dorsal landmarks of the wing of the atlas are not horizontally level (i.e., the wing of the atlas is higher on side of restriction). Pain is localized to poll muscles and there is hypertonicity of the poll muscles either unilaterally or bilaterally. Upon motion palpation, the veterinarian finds restriction in dorsal to ventral rotation of the atlas. The horse's position is standing. The veterinarian's position is standing directly in front of patient, contralateral to the side of restriction, facing caudally. The veterinarian contacts the horse at the dorsal aspect of the wing of C1, ipsilateral to the affected articulation with webbed fingers or with ipsilateral thenar contact over the dorsal wing of the atlas. The veterinarian stabilizes the horse by resting the ventral aspect of the patient's mandible on the veterinarian's shoulder on the contralateral side of restriction to stabilize the horse. The veterinarian motions dorsal to ventral to induce increased rotation of the C1/C2 motion segment. Caution: patient may unexpectedly rear up and strike with front feet. Caution: loosely cross fingers so that if patient suddenly raises head and neck, you will not be lifted off the ground and lose your footing.

Middle and Lower Cervical Region (C2 to C7)

Normal Joint Biomechanics

Articular processes support both vertebral stability and mobility due to the interlocking articular surfaces. The cervical vertebrae have relatively large articular facets compared to the vertebrae in other vertebral regions. The articular facet orientation of the caudal C2 to T2 vertebrae, relative to the lateral aspect of the neck, lie at about 45 degrees to the long axis of the neck. The C2-T2 articular facet orientations support relatively large ranges of flexion extension and coupled motion of combined rotation and lateral bending.

C2 to C5, Restriction in Flexion

The horse is not able to lower head and neck. It eats or drinks from ground with a scissor stance (foal posture). Upon motion palpation, the veterinarian finds restriction in flexion of the C2 to C5 vertebrae. The horse's position is standing. The veterinarian's position is standing directly in front of the patient, ipsilateral to the side of restriction, facing caudally. The veterinarian contacts the horse at the ventral aspect of the transverse process, ipsilateral to the affected cervical motion segment with the caudal hand, with thenar contact. The veterinarian stabilizes the horse by holding the halter on the ipsilateral side of contact using the cranial hand on the halter and brings the head and neck into slight lateral bending on the ipsilateral side of the veterinarian's position. The veterinarian motions ventral to dorsal and cranial to caudal and medial to lateral through the cervical facet plane to induce increased flexion of the C2 to C5 motion segments.

C2 to C4, Restriction in Extension

The horse is not able to raise the head and neck normally and holds the head in horizontal position. Gait and performance may be affected. Upon motion palpation, the veterinarian finds restriction in extension of the C2 to C4 vertebrae. The horse's position is standing. The veterinarian's position is standing directly in front of the patient, to either side of restriction, facing caudally in a broad-based stance. The veterinarian contacts the horse at the bilateral, dorsal aspect of the crest and nuchal ligament over the affected cervical motion segment with a loosely crossed webbed finger contact and brings the head and neck into extension to induce joint tension at the articulation. The veterinarian stabilizes the horse by placing the ventral aspect of the mandible on the veterinarian's shoulder using either shoulder. The veterinarian motions dorsal to ventral and caudal to cranial to induce increased extension of the C2 to C4 motion segments. Caution: patient may unexpectedly rear up and strike with front feet.

C2 to C6, Restriction in Lateral Bending

Horses exhibit a reduced ability to do lateral bending, typically worse on one side than the other. Upon palpation of the anatomic relationships, the veterinarian finds prominent transverse processes on either side of restriction due to local muscle atrophy of the cervical muscles or prominent articular processes on either side of restriction due to proliferation associated with osteoarthritis. Pain and hypertonicity is localized to the multifidus, intertransversarii, omotransvarsarius, or brachiocephalic muscles ipsilateral to the side of restriction. Motion palpation findings: Primary restriction in lateral bending of the C2 to C6 vertebrae, secondary axial rotation restriction due to coupled motion. The horse's position is standing; head and neck should be lowered to horizontal if possible to open the articular processes. Cervical extension induces joint interlocking (i.e., close packed position) of the articular processes and limits the effectiveness of manual treatment. The veterinarian's position is standing next to the patient's neck, ipsilateral to the side of restriction, facing cranially and laterally (veterinarian's trunk at 45 degrees to the long axis of the patient). The veterinarian contacts the horse at the dorsolateral aspect of the transverse process or articular process, ipsilateral to the affected cervical motion segment over the joint facet capsule with his caudal hand, with pisiform contact. The veterinarian stabilizes the horse by holding the halter on the ipsilateral side of restriction using his cranial hand on the cheek piece of the halter and bringing the head and neck into ipsilateral lateral bending. The joint is brought to tension by bending the neck to the ipsilateral side of restriction to induce joint tension at the restricted articulation. Caution: the halter on the opposite side may slide up into the patient's eye. Careful manipulation of the halter and head is required to prevent ocular injuries. The veterinarian motions dorsal to ventral and caudal to cranial and lateral to medial, through the cervical facet plane, approximately 45 degrees (tangential) to the horizontal plane to induce increased lateral bending and rotation of the C2 to C6 motion segments.

C6/C7, Restriction in Lateral Bending

Motion palpation findings: Primary restriction in lateral bending of the C6/C7 vertebrae, secondary axial rotation due to coupled motion. The horse's position is standing. The veterinarian's position is standing next to the base of the patient's neck, ipsilateral to the side of restriction, facing caudally and medially. The veterinarian contacts the horse at the dorsolateral aspect of the articular process or lamina pedicle junction, ipsilateral to the affected cervical motion segment. The veterinarian contacts the horse with the caudal hand, with closed fist contact. An assistant lifts and holds the ipsilateral forelimb in flexion as retraction of the forelimb caudally opens the access to the C6 to T1 motion segments. The veterinarian uses the cranial hand on the lateral halter on the ipsilateral side of restriction to stabilize the horse and brings the head and neck into ipsilateral lateral bending. The veterinarian motions lateral to medial and dorsal to ventral, to induce increased lateral bending and rotation of the C6-C7 motion segment.

Cranial and Middle Thoracic Region (T3 to T16)

Articular facets are coronal from T1 to T16. The veterinarian cannot readily access T1-T2 motion segments due to deep location, medial to the scapula.

T11 to T16 (not routinely T3 to T10), Restriction in Extension, Dorsal Spinous Process Contact

The horse exhibits kyphotic posture—that is, the trunk is held in flexion. Upon palpation of the anatomic relationships, the veterinarian finds dorsally prominent dorsal spinous process. Upon motion palpation, the veterinarian finds restriction in extension of the T11 to T16 vertebrae. The horse's position is standing. The veterinarian's position is standing on a stable elevated surface, next to the horse's trunk, on either side of the restriction. The veterinarian contacts the horse at the dorsal aspect of the spinous process, dorsal to the affected thoracic motion segment with his caudal hand, calcaneal contact. The stabilization of the horse is inherent in the motion segment. The veterinarian uses the cranial hand, with supported wrist contact, to contact the horse. The veterinarian motions dorsal to ventral, to induce increased extension of the T11 to T16 motion segments. Follow the inclination of the spinous processes: T3 to T11 are angled approximately 70 degrees caudally; T12 to T15 are angled approximately 80 degrees caudally; T16 is the anticlinal vertebra.

T11 to T16 (not routinely T3 to T10), Restriction in Flexion, Dorsal Spinous Process Contact

Upon palpation of the anatomic relationships, the veterinarian finds a ventrally prominent (dip) in the dorsal spinous process. Upon motion palpation, the veterinarian finds restriction in flexion of the T11 to T16 vertebrae. The horse's position is standing. The veterinarian's position is standing on a stable elevated surface, next to the horse's trunk, on either side of the restriction, facing toward the horse. The veterinarian contacts the horse at the dorsal aspect of the spinous process, dorsal to the affected thoracolumbar motion segment with the caudal hand, with calcaneal contact. The veterinarian motions dorsal to ventral, to induce increased flexion of the T11 to T16 motion segments. Consider spinous process inclination: T3 to T11 are angled approximately 70 degrees caudally; T12 to T15 are angled approximately 80 degrees caudally; T16 is the anticlinal vertebra; T17 to L6 are angled approximately 80 to 90 degrees cranially.

T3 to T11, Restriction in Rotation, Dorsal Spinous Process

Upon palpation of the anatomic relationships, the veterinarian finds muscle sensitivity on either side of withers. Check scapular height and dorsal scapular muscle symmetry. Pain and hypertonicity of the spinalis muscle is common and there may be sensitivity at the dorsolateral aspect of the dorsal spinous processes. Chronicity will affect the entire wither region bilaterally. Chronicity may be due to improper mounting and lameness in the forelimb. Symptoms include cinchy or girthy with saddle placement, decreased cervical extension, decreased forelimb extension, anhydrosis, and poor lead changes. Upon motion palpation, the veterinarian finds restriction in rotation of the T3 to T11 vertebrae. The horse's position is standing. The veterinarian's position is standing next to the horse's withers, ipsilateral to the side of restriction, facing toward the horse in a fencer's stance. The veterinarian contacts the horse at the dorsolateral apex of the spinous process, ipsilateral to the affected thoracic motion segment with the cranial hand with fingers directed caudally so that the fifth metacarpus is parallel to the angle of the dorsal spinous process (i.e., inclined caudally). Spinous process inclination of T3-T11 are angled approximately 70 degrees caudally. The stabilization of the horse is inherent in the motion segment. The veterinarian motions lateral to induce increased rotation of the motion segment.

T12 to T16, Restriction in Lateral Bending

Symptoms include cinchy, cold-backed, difficulty in lateral movement, difficult extension at trot, transition problems form a walk to canter, Standardbreds are on one shaft, and bearing in or out. Upon motion palpation, the veterinarian finds primary restriction in lateral bending of the T12-T16 vertebrae and secondary axial rotation restriction due to coupled motion. The horse's position is standing. The veterinarian's position is standing on a stable elevated surface, next to the horse's trunk, ipsilateral to the side of restriction, facing toward the horse in a fencer's stance. The veterinarian contacts the horse at the dorsolateral apex of the spinous process, ipsilateral to the affected thoracic motion segment with either cranial or caudal hand,

pisiform contact. The stabilization of the horse is inherent in the motion segment. The veterinarian motions dorsal to ventral and lateral to medial, to induce increased lateral bending of the T12 to T16 motion segments. Along the angle of the facet plane: T12-T15 are angled approximately 80 degrees caudally; T16 is the anticlinal vertebra.

Rib 10 to Rib 18, Dorsal Contact

Symptoms include cinchy, breathing problems, fatiguing easily, poor inspiration, kicking at belly while grooming, bending problems, and ears back when the saddle is brought out or when groomed. Upon palpation of the anatomic relationships, the veterinarian finds a palpable dorsal rib compared to the adjacent ribs. Pain is localized along the rib. There may be bilateral pain. Often there is hypertonicity of the iliocostalis muscle. Upon motion palpation, the veterinarian finds restriction in ventral movement of ribs 10 through 18. The horse's position is standing. The veterinarian's position is standing on a stable elevated surface, next to the horse's trunk, ipsilateral to the side of restriction, facing toward the horse. The veterinarian contacts the horse at the dorsal arch or dorsal aspect of the neck of the rib, ipsilateral to the affected rib with the cranial hand, with pisiform contact. The stabilization of the horse is inherent in the costotransverse and costovertebral articulations. The veterinarian motions dorsal to ventral and cranial to caudal to induce increased ventral motion of ribs 10 through 18.

T17 to L6, Restriction in Extension, Dorsal Spinous Process Contact

The horse exhibits kyphotic posture (roached back)—that is, the trunk is held in flexion. Upon palpation of the anatomic relationships, the veterinarian finds dorsally prominent dorsal spinous process. Upon motion palpation, the veterinarian finds restriction in extension of the T17 to L6 vertebrae. The horse's position is standing. The veterinarian's position is standing on a stable elevated surface, next to the horse's trunk, on either side of the restriction, facing toward the horse. The veterinarian contacts the horse at the dorsal aspect of the spinous process, ipsilateral to the affected thoracolumbar motion segment with the cranial hand, with calcaneal contact. The stabilization of the horse is inherent in the motion segment. The veterinarian motions dorsal to ventral, to induce increased extension of the T17 to L6 motion segment. Follow the inclination of the spinous processes: T16 is the anticlinal vertebra; T17 to L6 are angled approximately 80 degrees to 90 degrees cranially. The spinous processes are divergent at the lumbosacral joint.

T17 to L6, Restriction in Lateral Bending, Spinous Process Contact

Symptoms include rear leg lameness, back pain on extension, decreased lateral bending, resistance to leg aids, hunter's bump, grunting at canter, toe drag, abnormal shoe wear, poor attitude, difficulty in balancing over back legs, interfering, hock problems, difficulty in rounding, hiking rear leg, cold back, bucking, limited back motion, exploding over jumps, refusing jumps, not lying down, and loss of power from behind. Upon motion palpation, the veterinarian finds primary restriction in lateral bending of the T17 to L6 vertebrae and secondary axial rotation restriction due to coupled motion. The horse's position is standing. The veterinarian's position is standing on a stable elevated surface, next to the horse's trunk, ipsilateral to the side of restriction, facing toward the horse. The veterinarian contacts the horse at the lateral aspect of the apex of the spinous process, ipsilateral to the affected thoracolumbar motion segment with the cranial hand while the caudal hand holds the sacral apex. The stabilization of the horse is inherent in the motion segment. The veterinarian motions lateral to medial and dorsal to ventral, to induce increased lateral bending and rotation of the T17 to L6 motion segment.

The Sacroiliac Joint

Upon motion palpation, the veterinarian finds restriction in extension of the pelvis unilaterally. The veterinarian's position is standing on a stable elevated surface, next to the horse's pelvis, on the contralateral side of restriction, facing toward the horse, in a fencer's stance. The veterinarian contacts the horse at the dorsal aspect of the tuber sacrale, ipsilateral to the affected tuber sacrale with the caudal hand, with pisiform or thenar contacts. The stabilization of the horse is inherent in the motion segment. The veterinarian motions dorsal to ventral, medial to lateral, and caudal to cranial through the sacroiliac joint plane (45 degrees to the horizontal plane) to induce increased extension of the sacroiliac joint.

Restriction in Extension, Tuber Coxae Contact

Upon motion palpation, the veterinarian finds restriction in extension of the pelvis unilaterally. The horse's position is standing square. The veterinarian's position is standing on a stable elevated surface, next to the horse's pelvis, on the ipsilateral side of restriction, facing toward the horse, in a fencer's stance, arm dropped, and facing cranially. The veterinarian contacts the horse at the dorsal aspect of the tuber coxa, ipsilateral to the affected tuber coxa with the caudal hand, with pisiform contact. The stabilization of the horse is inherent in the pelvis and sacroiliac joint ligaments. The veterinarian motions dorsal to ventral through the sacroiliac joint plane (45 degrees to the horizontal plane) to induce increased extension of the sacroiliac joint.

Restriction in Extension of the Pelvis Bilateral, Bilateral Dorsal Tuber Coxae Contacts

Upon motion palpation, the veterinarian finds restriction in extension of the pelvis bilaterally. The horse's position is standing. The veterinarian's position is standing on a stable elevated surface, next to the horse's pelvis on either side of restriction facing toward the horse and cranially with a slight fencer's stance. The veterinarian contacts the horse at the bilateral, dorsal aspect of the tuber coxae with both hands, with pisiform, thenar, or calcaneal contacts. The stabilization of the horse is inherent in the pelvis and sacroiliac joint ligaments. The veterinarian motions dorsal to ventral, through the lumbosacral joint plane, to induce increased extension of the lumbosacral and sacroiliac joints.

Restriction in Flexion of the Pelvis Unilaterally, Tuber Coxae Contact

Upon motion palpation, the veterinarian finds restriction in flexion of the pelvis unilaterally. The horse's position is standing square. The veterinarian's position is standing next to the horse's pelvis, on the ipsilateral side of restriction, facing toward the horse's pelvis in a fencer's stance facing caudally and medially. Note that the veterinarian needs to get down low in fencer's stance to get the correct line of correction. The veterinarian contacts the horse at the ventral aspect of the tuber coxa, ipsilateral to the affected tuber coxa with the caudal hand, with calcaneal or thenar contacts. The stabilization of the horse is inherent in the pelvis and sacroiliac joint ligaments. The veterinarian motions ventral to dorsal and cranial to caudal and lateral to medial, through the sacroiliac joint plane (45 degrees to the horizontal plane) to induce increased flexion of the sacroiliac joint.

Sacroiliac Joint or Lumbosacral Joint, Restriction in Extension of the Lumbosacral Joint or Dorsoventral Movement of the Sacral Base (S2 Spinous Process)

Upon motion palpation, the veterinarian finds restriction in extension of the lumbosacral joint or dorsoventral movement of the sacral base (S2 spinous process). The horse's position is standing square. The veterinarian's position is standing on a stable elevated surface, next to the horse's trunk, on either side of the restriction, facing toward the horse with a slight fencer's stance, facing cranially. The veterinarian contacts the horse at the dorsal aspect of the second sacral (S2) spinous process with his caudal hand, pisiform, calcaneal, or thenar contacts with fingers directed cranially. The stabilization of the horse is inherent in the pelvis and sacroiliac joint ligaments. The veterinarian motions dorsal to ventral and caudal to cranial, along the axis of the second sacral spinous process (caudal inclination) to induce increased flexion of the lumbosacral joint.

Restriction in Rotation Movement of the Sacrum

Upon motion palpation, the veterinarian finds restriction in rotation movement of the sacrum. The horse's position is standing square. The veterinarian's position is standing on a stable elevated surface, next to the horse's pelvis, on the ipsilateral side of the restriction, facing towards the horse, facing cranially and medially at 45 to 65 degrees. The veterinarian contacts the horse at the dorsally over the median sacral crest, lateral to the second sacral vertebra, ipsilateral to the affected articulation with his hand. The stabilization of the horse is inherent in the pelvis and sacroiliac joint ligaments. The veterinarian motions dorsal to ventral and medial to lateral through the sacroiliac joint plane (45 degrees to the horizontal plane) to induce increased sacral rotation motion of the sacrum.

Restriction in Lateral Bending Movement of the Sacrum

Upon motion palpation, the veterinarian finds restriction in lateral bending movement of the sacrum. There is unilateral pain to sacroiliac joint challenge. The horse's position is standing square. The veterinarian's position is standing next to the horse's pelvis, on the ipsilateral side of restriction, facing toward the horse's pelvis, in a fencer's stance. The veterinarian contacts the horse at the lateral aspect of the sacral apex, ipsilateral to the affected articulation with the caudal hand, with pisiform contact. The stabilization of the horse is obtained by holding the dorsal aspect of the opposite tuber sacrale with the cranial hand, with fingers over the top. The veterinarian motions lateral to medial, along the horizontal plane, to induce increased lateral bending motion of the sacral apex.

Gastrointestinal Medicine

Katharina L. Lohmann,

Noah D. Cohen

Gastrointestinal diseases are common among horses, including older horses. Colic was the most common cause of death among horses in the United States aged 5 to 20 years, and was second to old age as the leading cause of death among horses older than 20 years of age.[1] Of adult horses evaluated in the study, the overall colic incidence did not vary significantly among different age categories and the annual incidence for horses 20 years of age and older was 4.2 events per 100 horse years.[1]

The purpose of this chapter is to review medical gastrointestinal disorders of greatest relevance to older horses. A brief discussion of age-related alterations in gastrointestinal function and general considerations regarding diagnostic and therapeutic approach to geriatric patients presenting for colic or weight loss is provided at the beginning. The reader is also referred to the discussion of dental diseases, neoplasia, and surgical conditions in separate chapters.

Alterations in Gastrointestinal Function with Age

Structural and functional alterations of the equine gastrointestinal tract with age have not been evaluated extensively. While some age-dependent conditions such as wave-mouth formation and tooth loss are readily evident, other more subtle changes such as altered gastrointestinal motility or nutrient absorption are not sufficiently understood at this time and their potential effect on susceptibility to disease has not been thoroughly investigated. In the human medical literature, the overall opinion is that true age-associated alterations in gastrointestinal function are of little clinical significance and that most conditions initially attributed to older age are in fact the result of underlying disease processes.[2] The extent to which age-related changes in laboratory animals or human beings can be extrapolated to equine patients is unknown, and further equine-specific studies are necessary.

Dental abnormalities including tooth loss are a well-recognized and potentially severe problem in geriatric horses and are likely responsible for many cases of anorexia and weight loss, esophageal obstruction, and impaction colic. The role of age-related alterations in esophageal function is less well understood, as most cases of dysphagia in horses are attributable to obstruction or anatomic changes such as stricture. Dysphagia in geriatric human patients was originally attributed to changes in esophageal function such as altered contractility and sphincter relaxation; however, most of these changes are now thought to result from concurrent diseases, including diabetes mellitus or neurologic disorders.[2] Certain age-related anatomic changes such as decreased upper esophageal sphincter pressure resulting in delayed relaxation after swallowing are, however, recognized and may contribute to dysphagia in some cases.[2] The effect of alterations in glucose metabolism due to pituitary adenoma on esophageal function in horses has not been evaluated, but one may speculate about its potential impact in horses repeatedly suffering from esophageal obstruction in the absence of anatomic abnormalities. Age-dependent alterations in gastric mucosal integrity appear to be mostly related to decreased protective mechanisms rather than increased secretion of gastric acid or pepsin. Decreased bicarbonate secretion with age is a common feature in human beings and laboratory animals and may affect basal and/or stimulated secretion, thereby resulting in a lower gastric pH.[2] Gastric mucosal proliferation in response to injury also decreases with age, which may delay healing of ulcers and erosions.[2] The effect of aging on gastric blood flow appears controversial at this time, with atherosclerotic changes resulting in microcirculatory failure being the greatest concern in human patients. In horses, blood supply to the gastric mucosa should not be significantly affected by aging per se; however, the potential for side effects of frequent administration of nonsteroidal anti-inflammatory drugs (NSAIDs) in geriatric horses with health problems should be considered. Aging apparently does not affect gastric emptying in human patients.[2] Gastric emptying in horses has not been evaluated sufficiently to establish normal ranges of emptying parameters, and the effect of aging on emptying time in horses remains unknown.

Aside from dental abnormalities, decreased small intestinal absorptive function is often suspected when older horses show problems maintaining adequate weight. Possible reasons for decreased nutrient absorption in aged patients include altered intestinal motility, reduced intestinal enzymatic activity (maldigestion), and reduced absorptive capacity of mucosal enterocytes (malabsorption). Experimentally, delayed maturation and expression of brush border enzymes in senescent small intestinal villus epithelial cells during crypt-to-villus migration has been demonstrated.[2] Despite these observations, nutrient absorption is generally not impaired in geriatric human patients,[2] although changes in micronutrient absorption have been observed in some animal studies. Absorption of vitamin D, folic acid, vitamin B12, calcium, copper, zinc, fatty acids, and cholesterol has been found to be decreased in some studies, whereas absorption of vitamin A and glucose appeared increased.[2] In aged horses, reduced apparent digestion of crude protein and phosphorus in alfalfa pellets as well as lower digestion of fiber was observed.[3] These changes were similar to those observed in horses that have undergone large colon resection, which suggests that absorptive changes in older horses might be related to altered colonic function.[3]

Changes of small bowel motility in aged human patients appear to be minor and are not thought to be of clinical significance. Findings regarding large bowel motility are somewhat controversial; however, some studies show age-associated reduction in neuron number within the colonic myenteric plexus as well as decreased release of acetylcholine from these neurons.[2]

A cause-and-effect relationship of these finding with an increased occurrence of constipation in geriatric human patients is proposed. It is unknown to what extent similar changes occur in aged equine patients and how they may be related to an increased incidence of impaction colic in geriatric horses.

Evaluation and Treatment of Geriatric Patients Presenting for Colic

The diagnostic work-up of a geriatric horse presented for colic should be in most respects similar to that for any other adult horse, and, generally, the same differential diagnoses should be considered. Not many causes of colic have a proven age-specific distribution, and most often, the distinction between foals—including yearlings—and adult horses older than 1 year of age is more important than the distinction between different age groups of adult horses. Certain specific conditions, such as intestinal strangulation caused by pedunculated lipoma, however, are known to occur with significantly higher frequency in older horses and, as mentioned above, an increased occurrence of dental abnormalities may predispose geriatric horses to problems related to impaction colic.

When evaluating the aged horse with colic, it should be kept in mind that these horses might experience as well as exhibit pain to a lesser degree than younger horses. In people, decreased pain perception in geriatric patients is a well-established phenomenon. Possible explanations include increased production of endogenous opiates, decreased nerve conduction, and mental depression.[4] The extent to which these observations are applicable to horses is unknown; however, the stoic old horse is not an uncommon anecdotal observation. In these patients, evaluation of clinical signs of pain as an indicator of lesion severity obviously has to be ranked lower than other variables (such as heart rate or mucous membrane color) in the process of deciding whether surgical exploration is necessary. Clinicopathologic data appear to not differ considerably between aged and young horses and, therefore, normal ranges for laboratory values should be applicable to the evaluation of geriatric colic patients.

Some neoplasias such as gastric squamous cell carcinoma, which may result in colic signs, occur with higher frequency in aged horses. Although the overall occurrence of gastrointestinal neoplasia is low, this possibility should be considered in evaluating the geriatric colic patient. Rectal examination, abdominal ultrasonography, peritoneal fluid analysis, and evaluation of biopsy specimens are helpful in detecting abdominal neoplasia in horses; however, surgical exploration of the abdomen may be required in some cases to evaluate the entire intestinal tract and obtain representative biopsy specimens. Because gastric squamous cell carcinoma is one of the most common gastrointestinal neoplasias in horses, suspicious-appearing ulcerative lesions observed during esophagoscopy and gastroscopy should be sampled for microscopic analysis.

Healthy geriatric horses undergoing inhalant anesthesia are generally not thought to be at increased risk of anesthetic complications as compared to other adult horses. In geriatric horses with colic, however, especially those that are debilitated overall, the risk of prolonged general anesthesia may be considerable. Attempts should be made to stabilize the patient as much as possible prior to surgery. Dehydration and cardiovascular compromise should be addressed by administration of intravenous fluids. In severely hypovolemic patients, administration of hypertonic saline solution (4 mL/kg of a 7.5% solution) followed by volume expansion with crystalloid fluids is often helpful. Endotoxemic patients may benefit from administration of plasma or lipopolysaccharide-binding drugs such as polymyxin B (1000–6000 U/kg intravenously). Because of the potential for nephrotoxicity of polymyxin B, adequate fluid therapy must be ensured in azotemic patients, and the benefits of the drug need to be weighed against the risks in horses in which adequate renal function is questionable. Aside from the anesthetic risk itself, aged horses, especially those with chronic musculoskeletal problems or generally debilitated animals, may also have more difficulty standing after general anesthesia. A hoist or body sling can be very helpful to temporarily support these horses after surgery.

Geriatric horses, especially if in moderate to poor body condition at the onset of colic, may tend to lose weight more rapidly and have more difficulty recovering adequate body condition after a colic episode. Depending on the cause of colic, nutritional support should, therefore, be considered as part of the treatment protocol and, if indicated, should be instituted early on to prevent excessive weight loss from occurring. Parenteral nutritional support may be necessary in horses showing contraindications to enteral feeding such as gastric reflux and ileus. Enteral feeding on the other hand, aside from being easier and cheaper to implement, promotes intestinal motility and improves nutrient supply to enterocytes. Daily weighing of geriatric horses with colic, especially those having undergone surgery, is recommended to objectively monitor body weight.

Evaluation and Treatment of Geriatric Patients Presenting for Weight Loss

Weight loss is a common concern in geriatric patients and a number of possible causes need to be considered (Fig. 10-1). Weight loss can be caused by an absolute insufficiency of intake, digestion or absorption of nutrients; relative insufficiency of nutrient supply due to increased metabolic requirements and catabolic body states; nutrient loss. Often, categories will overlap; for example, a horse with intestinal neoplasia, which has increased nutrient requirements due to a catabolic body state, has an altered small intestinal absorptive capacity due to infiltrative disease and in addition is anorexic, resulting in an absolute lack of feed intake. Treatment of horses suffering from weight loss will, therefore, have to address various aspects of the problem.

Evaluation of diet and feeding regimen is an important part of the diagnostic investigation and will be discussed in more detail in a separate chapter. If feed intake overall is inadequate, it needs to be determined whether dysphagia or anorexia is present or whether the horse simply does not receive enough feed. As mentioned previously, early institution of nutritional support should be considered in anorexic geriatric horses to avoid excessive weight loss, even if duration of anorexia is expected to be limited. Appropriate treatment of the underlying condition is a prerequisite for recovery of appetite and lost body weight. Dysphagia can be caused by abnormalities of the oral cavity and teeth, laryngeal and pharyngeal dysfunction, esophageal disorders, or gastric disorders such as squamous cell carcinoma affecting the cardia. Thorough oral examination, endoscopy, radiography including contrast studies, ultrasonography, and surgical exploration may be necessary to identify the exact cause of dysphagia.

If dysphagia and anorexia secondary to disease unrelated to the gastrointestinal tract can be ruled out and the horse loses weight in the face of adequate feed intake, alterations in nutrient digestion and/or absorption or

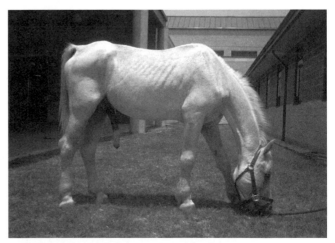

Figure 10-1 Geriatric horse with severe weight loss caused by protein-losing enteropathy. Notice the peripheral limb edema due to hypoproteinemia.

nutrient loss need to be considered. The diagnostic work-up for these patients is often extensive and may include clinical pathologic evaluation of blood and peritoneal fluid, fecal examination, rectal examination, gastroscopy, abdominal radiography and ultrasonography, absorption tests, and rectal biopsy. Exploratory abdominal surgery may be necessary to gain adequate access to all portions of the intestine and obtain representative biopsy samples. Any clinical signs in addition to weight loss need to be identified, as they may help to pinpoint the affected organ or organ system. Horses suffering from intestinal malabsorption due to inflammatory bowel disease including lymphosarcoma will often show anemia, leukogram changes consistent with acute or chronic inflammation, hyperfibrinogenemia, and hypoproteinemia and hypoalbuminemia. A decreased immunoglobulin M fraction has been associated with lymphosarcoma in some horses; however, this test appears to lack sensitivity and specificity, which limits its clinical value.

Chronic intestinal parasitism (Fig. 10-2) is thought to occur frequently in geriatric horses[5]; therefore, fecal examination should be performed and the deworming regimen should be evaluated. Horses with pituitary adenoma may suffer from chronic parasitism more frequently than healthy geriatric horses. Sedimentation of a fecal sample and radiography may be used to investigate sand accumulation within the intestine, which can result in chronic mucosal irritation and impaired digestion and absorption. Rectal examination may identify conditions such as chronic gastric, colonic, or cecal impaction, which result in weight loss in some horses. Rectal examination should further include evaluation of bowel wall thickness, serosal surfaces, and mesenteric lymph nodes to detect neoplastic or chronic inflammatory changes and of the cranial mesenteric artery to detect

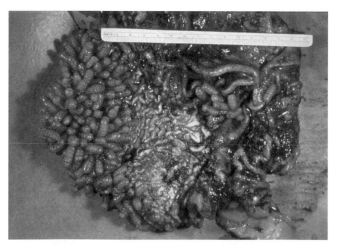

Figure 10-2 Severe infestation of the stomach with *Gastrophilus* larvae. Geriatric horses with pituitary dysfunction may be predisposed to chronic parasitism. (Courtesy of Dr. Michelle H. Barton, University of Georgia.)

lesions consistent with verminous arteritis. Abdominal ultrasonography is useful to assess bowel wall thickness, size and texture of abdominal organs, and the presence, amount, and echogenicity of peritoneal fluid. Peritoneal fluid analysis may help to identify abdominal neoplasia or chronic abdominal inflammation due to abscessation. However, only 44 percent of neoplasias and 20 percent of abdominal abscesses were diagnosed by peritoneal fluid analysis in one study, and repeated analysis may be necessary to obtain a positive finding.[6] Rectal biopsy is often recommended to identify infiltrative bowel diseases such as neutrophilic, basophilic, lymphocytic-plasmacytic, and eosinophilic enteritis as well as lymphosarcoma and is particularly indicated if abnormalities of bowel wall structure have been detected upon rectal or ultrasonographic examination. In 27 of 38 horses (71%) with significant intestinal lesions found at necropsy, pathologic changes were observed in rectal biopsy specimens.[7] Although changes observed in rectal biopsy specimens may not be diagnostic for a specific condition, abnormal findings such as simple proctitis may, therefore, prompt further investigation, repetition of rectal biopsy at a later time, or acquisition of further specimens by means of exploratory laparotomy. Absorption tests (glucose or xylose absorption) help to identify malabsorption due to small intestinal disease. Because geriatric horses may show alterations in glucose metabolism due to pituitary adenoma, the xylose absorption test, which is less influenced by metabolic and endocrine activity, may be preferable.[8] Hourly sampling and determination of plasma glucose or xylose concentration is recommended for 6 hours after carbohydrate administration.[9] For glucose absorption, a peak glucose concentration of at least 85 percent over the baseline concentration is expected at 120 minutes after administration (1 g/kg body weight as a 10-20% solution). Peak D-xylose concentrations are expected at 60 to 90 minutes after administration (0.5 g/kg body weight as a 10% solution); however, discriminative values for absolute peak concentrations have not been established.[9] Although abnormal results appear to fairly reliably indicate small intestinal malabsorption,[8] potential influencing factors such as the rate of gastric emptying, intestinal motility, intraluminal bacterial overgrowth, renal clearance, and dietary history should be considered. For example, prolonged anorexia can alter the gastric emptying rate, and flatter D-xylose absorption curves and a slower decrease in plasma D-xylose concentration were shown in horses after 72 to 96 hours of feed deprivation.[10] Although absorption test findings may be normal in early stages of disease and abnormalities may not be detected initially, transient malabsorption has also been described in horses.[11] In the absence of a definitive diagnosis, for example one achieved by intestinal biopsy, repetition of the absorption test after a period of treatment or dietary modification may therefore be useful. Repeatedly abnormal absorption test results are often associated with a poor prognosis.

Treatment of weight loss must address the primary cause, and prognosis for improvement or recovery will vary greatly depending on the underlying disorder. Often, such as in cases of chronic infiltrative bowel disease due to neoplasia, palliative treatment may be the only viable option and only temporary improvement is to be expected. Treatment of specific conditions particularly important to geriatric horses will be discussed in the following sections. In addition to medical or surgical treatment, dietary modification to increase nutrient intake and/or enhance palatability will almost always be indicated.

Esophageal Disorders

Esophageal disorders encountered in adult horses include esophagitis and esophageal ulceration, intra- or extraluminal esophageal obstruction, stricture, perforation, megaesophagus, and esophageal diverticula. In most retrospective studies, a wide range of ages is observed in affected horses and age is not always identified as a risk factor in the development of esophageal conditions.[12] Aged horses, however, may be predisposed to intraluminal obstruction by swallowing poorly chewed feed boluses due to poor dentition, dental disease, or dental loss and to neoplasia. Intraluminal esophageal obstruction most frequently occurs in the cervical esophagus, less frequently at the thoracic inlet, and rarely in the intrathoracic portion of the esophagus.[13] In addition to dental abnormalities, esophageal feed impaction has been associated with poor-quality feed, sudden feed changes, rapid ingestion (bolting feed), and dehydration. Aside from feed impaction, acute intraluminal esophageal obstruction can result from ingestion of bulky feed items such as carrots, apples or beets,[12,14] or foreign bodies. Circumferential stricture, diverticulum formation, or extraluminal compression of the esophagus by space-occupying lesions can further predispose the horse to recurrent intraluminal obstruction and dysphagia. The most common esophageal neoplasia in horses is squamous cell carcinoma, which should be considered in cases of recurrent obstruction as it more commonly affects older horses.[13] When evaluating horses with dysphagia, the true definition of the term as "difficulty in eating"[15] should be kept in mind, and abnormalities of prehension, pharyngeal transport, swallowing, and esophageal transport should be considered as differential diagnoses to esophageal obstruction. These include obstructive, infectious, inflammatory or traumatic lesions of the pharynx, larynx, or esophagus, megaesophagus, neurologic disorders such as forebrain disease (including rabies), or cranial nerve dysfunction (cranial nerve IX, X, or XII), guttural pouch disease, or stylohyoid osteopathy.[13]

Dysphagia in horses with esophageal obstruction typically manifests as frequent attempts to swallow, stretching of the neck and retching, coughing, salivation, nasal regurgitation of feed mixed with saliva (Fig. 10-3), and potential aspiration of food into the airways.[13-15] The time lag between swallowing and regurgitation may provide valuable information regarding the location of obstruction, with more distal obstructions showing a greater delay between swallowing and regurgitation. Obstruction of the cervical esophagus may result in a palpable enlargement[13] that appears to be especially common in cases of esophageal diverticula.[12] Additional clinical signs may include depression or restlessness, anorexia, tachycardia, and tachypnea, which are often attributable to discomfort and anxiousness. They may, however, also result from complications such as cellulitis secondary to esophageal perforation or aspiration pneumonia and should prompt thorough investigation of these potential sequelae. Esophageal rupture should be suspected in the event of observing subcutaneous swelling or emphysema, pain and heat upon palpation, or fistulous tracts. Saliva and feed may be seen to drain from these tracts after eating.[13] Clinical pathologic abnormalities are generally attributable to inflammation, anorexia, and salivary losses. Dehydration, metabolic alkalosis, hyponatremia, and hypochloremia may be recognized.[13] Hyperfibrinogenemia, neutrophilia with or without left shift, or neutropenia indicate acute (esophageal perforation, aspiration pneumonia) or chronic (abscessation, neoplasia) inflammatory processes.

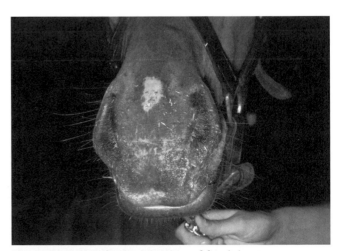

Figure 10-3 Nasal regurgitation of feed due to esophageal obstruction. (Courtesy of Dr. Michelle H. Barton, University of Georgia.)

In cases of recurrent obstruction, identification of the underlying cause can present a diagnostic challenge. Although there may be relief of the obstruction, careful endoscopic examination is required to assess the extent of esophageal damage, identify potential underlying problems, and detect potential complications early on. Plain and contrast-enhanced radiography, as well as ultrasonography may also used for evaluation. Because some morphologic lesions such as stricture may be detectable only by endoscopy or radiography, respectively, both procedures have been recommended for diagnostic evaluation of every horse with recurrent esophageal obstruction.[14] Passage of a nasogastric tube should be performed with great care to avoid new damage to the esophageal mucosa or worsening of existing damage. In some cases of feed or foreign body obstruction, but particularly in cases of incomplete obstruction due to a neoplasm, it might be possible to pass the tube past the obstruction and into the stomach.[13] Although resistance is often encountered in these cases, it might be mistaken for cardiac sphincter spasms. Endoscopy may identify type and extent of the obstruction and is invaluable in assessing mucosal damage such as ulceration or perforation. The degree of esophageal dilatation and the quality of motility further provide information about the chronicity of an obstruction.[16] Esophageal motility disorders are recognizable by extreme distention of the esophageal lumen before and after air insufflation, absence of normal peristaltic waves, and impaired clearance of swallowed materials.[16] If functional abnormalities are suspected, it is advisable to not sedate the horse before examination, as sedation will interfere with normal swallowing and esophageal motility. Prior to esophagoscopy, it might be useful to evaluate the trachea for evidence of feed contamination; however, evidence of tracheal contamination does not appear to correlate with development of aspiration pneumonia.[14] Extraluminal obstructions, perforations, and esophageal dilatation may be difficult to detect by endoscopy, and radiography with or without contrast enhancement is recommended in these cases.

Lateral survey radiographs of the head, neck, and thorax are useful for evaluation of pharyngeal swelling or masses, emphysema (extraluminal radiolucency) indicating esophageal rupture, persistent air accumulation within the esophagus, intraluminal feed impaction (dense granular pattern), foreign body obstruction, extraluminal masses causing obstruction, pneumomediastinum, or esophageal displacement.[12,13,16] Barium sulfate is the most commonly used contrast material for esophageal radiography. Its use should, however, be avoided if perforation of the esophagus has not been ruled out; a water-soluble iodinated, less irritating contrast medium can be used in these cases. To avoid aspiration, it is preferable to administer the contrast media via a nasogastric tube (ideally cuffed) that is passed just past the larynx as opposed to giving it orally. Disorders that may be recognized using single contrast studies include intraluminal obstruction, mural neoplasms, extensive esophageal compression, perforations, and some strictures.[13] Double contrast studies—that is, administration of a contrast medium to coat the esophageal mucosa, followed by air distention—may be helpful to demonstrate extraluminal obstructions and intramural masses causing compression of the esophageal lumen, strictures, esophageal rings, diverticula, and megaesophagus.[12,13] Strictures, diverticula, large ulcers, and extrinsic compression may further be documented by administration of a larger volume of contrast material (500 mL) under pressure.[16] A cuffed nasogastric tube should be used for this procedure. Ultrasonography may be helpful to assess cervical swellings and space-occupying lesions and to detect fluid and/or gas accumulations and foreign bodies.[13]

Because of the potential for serious sequelae, esophageal obstruction should initially be regarded as an emergency.[13] On the other hand, simple cases of intraluminal feed impaction, although often dramatic in their presentation, are rarely life-threatening, and some will resolve either without treatment[16] or with fluid therapy alone. Because harm can be done by a too aggressive attempt at relieving an obstruction, the benefit of any therapeutic intervention has to be carefully weighed against its potential risks. The goals of treatment are resolution of the obstruction, maintenance of homeostasis, and prevention of complications.[16] Supportive medical treatment should address dehydration, electrolyte imbalances, and acid-base disturbances, provide pain relief and anti-inflammatory therapy, and ensure adequate nutrient intake, particularly in chronic cases or those with severe damage to the esophagus, in which oral feed intake is anticipated to be restricted for a longer period of time. For esophageal obstruction caused by extraluminal compression, or for chronic recurrent cases of intraluminal obstruction due to anatomical or functional abnormalities, treatment approach depends on the underlying disorder. Prognosis for chronic recurrent cases is generally guarded to poor, while most cases of simple intraluminal obstruction can be successfully treated.

With very early cases of esophageal obstruction by feed impaction (especially pelleted feed), withholding of feed, sedation, and pain relief may in some cases lead to sufficient calming of the horse and muscle relaxation to allow the obstruction to resolve. Acepromazine (0.05 mg/kg) has been recommended for sedation,[13] but xylazine (0.25-0.5 mg/kg) or detomidine

(0.01-0.02 mg/kg) may also be used. The horse should be monitored closely and an adequate level of sedation needs to be maintained. If it appears that the obstruction has resolved, free passage of a nasogastric tube into the stomach should be ensured before the horse is introduced to any type of feed. If the obstruction does not resolve within 4 to 6 hours, the risk of drying of the impacted material, progressive proximal dilation, and loss of motor function exists[16] and a more aggressive treatment approach has to be taken. Careful lavage can be performed with the horse standing, but general anesthesia may be required in severe cases to allow more forceful lavage.[13] Documentation of any preexisting damage not only may change the therapeutic approach but may also be of legal relevance in certain cases. During lavage, care should be taken to keep the horse's head lowered and to protect the airway. Under general anesthesia, the trachea should be protected by a cuffed endotracheal tube. For standing procedures, a cuffed nasotracheal tube may be inserted prior to passing a tube (or tubes) into the esophagus. Alternatively, a small-diameter cuffed endotracheal tube can be passed into the esophagus and a smaller nasogastric tube can be inserted through its lumen for lavage. In the latter case, care needs to be taken to prevent damage to the esophageal mucosa caused by excessive cuff pressure. Warm water is generally recommended for lavage. Although lubricants such as carboxymethylcellulose can be helpful in relieving esophageal obstruction, they should only be used if prevention of aspiration can be ensured. Lubricants and softeners such as mineral oil or dioctyl sodium succinate carry the risk of severe chemical pneumonia if aspiration occurs and should be avoided.[13] The use of oxytocin (0.11-0.22 IU/kg IV) in uncomplicated cases of esophageal obstruction has been proposed.[17] Its effect is attributed to short-term reduction of striated muscle tone resulting in reduced intraluminal pressure.[17] Recent in vitro studies, however, indicate little effect on skeletal muscle and suggest centrally mediated mechanisms of action.[18] Potential side effects of oxytocin include abdominal discomfort and abortion, and use in pregnant mares is contraindicated. If medical therapy and lavage are unsuccessful at relieving an obstruction, a surgical approach via esophagotomy is indicated.

Because of the significant risk of aspiration pneumonia subsequent to esophageal obstruction, and the difficulty in predicting its occurrence in individual horses, some authors recommend antimicrobial therapy for every case of esophageal obstruction.[14] Broad-spectrum coverage, including for anaerobic infections, can be provided by combination therapy with, for example, penicillin, gentamicin, and metronidazole.[16] Aspiration pneumonia typically results from aspiration of feed material before the obstruction is relieved; however, aspiration can also occur after resolution of an obstruction if the horse is fed before inflammation and pain have subsided enough to allow unimpaired swallowing. Removal of all feed and bedding as long as obstruction is existent and careful refeeding after obstruction are, therefore, important. Treatment of aspiration pneumonia should follow general principles of antimicrobial and anti-inflammatory treatment and ideally should rely on culture and sensitivity testing of a tracheobronchial aspirate. Aspiration pneumonia apparently has a good prognosis with early treatment.[14]

Feeding of horses after esophageal obstruction has to be designed on an individual basis with consideration of the cause and severity of the obstruction, the extent of mucosal damage, the condition of the horse's teeth, the overall condition of the horse, and owner compliance. Horses should not be offered feed as long as signs of dysphagia persist.[13] If feeding appears safe, based on endoscopic evaluation, one should start by offering small amounts of a mash or pellet slurry, fresh grass, or soaked hay. If these are tolerated well, the horse can be slowly returned to normal feeding over the next several days. Offering of soft feed has been correlated with decreased occurrence of stricture after obstruction and should therefore be continued for a longer time (several weeks) in cases with more severe mucosal irritation.[19] In horses with poor dentition, or in those with esophageal diverticula, soft feed may further be required indefinitely to prevent recurrence of obstruction. Patients in whom severe mucosal damage has occurred may show prolonged esophageal dysfunction due to trauma and inflammation, and parenteral nutrition or feeding via an esophagostomy tube can be considered. Long-term esophageal intubation, however, has attendant sequelae, including pressure necrosis of the pharyngeal and esophageal mucosae. Enteral feeding via esophagostomy may further temporarily allow maintenance of patients with incurable problems such as neoplasia. Even after the introduction of feeding, however, electrolyte supplementation may be necessary to correct for salivary loss and to prevent abnormalities such as hyponatremia and hypochloridemia from recurring. Serious commitment on the part of the owner and diligent care of the esophagostomy site is a prerequisite for longer term maintenance of horses in this manner.

Recurrence of obstruction typically indicates functional or morphologic abnormalities and should prompt thorough investigation of possible causes. Esophageal stricture (Fig. 10-4) can develop after severe mucosal damage due to long-standing feed obstruction, or obstruction by a foreign body exerting extreme pressure on the mucosa. Medical treatment of strictures has been described,[19] but a surgical approach is warranted in

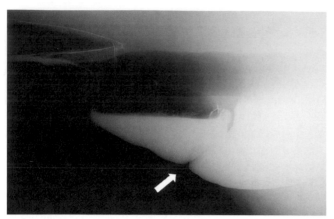

Figure 10-4 Contrast esophagogram of a horse with esophageal stricture, left lateral view. The stricture site is indicated by an arrow. Notice esophageal dilatation anterior (left) to the stricture site and pooling of contrast material. Esophageal dilatation posterior to the stricture site suggests a second stricture site more distally; however, this portion of the esophagus could not be visualized radiographically. The horse was managed by being placed on a gruel diet indefinitely. (Courtesy of Dr. Michelle H. Barton, University of Georgia.)

severe cases and those of longer duration (>60 days). A life-long gruel diet may be considered for cases for which surgical management is not considered an option. Esophageal perforation may occur due to severe mucosal trauma caused by external trauma and extension of infection from surrounding areas, intraluminal obstruction (chronic feed impaction or perforating foreign body), or iatrogenically by aggressive use of a nasogastric tube. The treatment approach varies depending on the individual case, with both surgical closure and open wound management being an option. The site of perforation may also be used to introduce an esophagostomy tube for feeding until adequate healing has occurred.[12] Treatment of esophageal diverticula depends on the severity of clinical signs and can include dietary modification (feeding of soft feed and pellet slurry) or surgical repair.

Gastroduodenal Ulceration

Gastric ulceration is highly prevalent among horses and can lead to overt clinical signs of colic as well as more insidious changes such as a loss of body condition and a decrease in performance. While the prevalence of gastric ulceration approaches 100 percent in Thoroughbred racehorses, the incidence specifically in geriatric horses has not been reported. In human patients, the prevalence of gastric ulcer disease increases with age.[4] Potential reasons for this observation in human beings are increasing injury to the gastric mucosa with age from sources such as more frequent use of NSAIDs, an increased prevalence

of *Helicobacter pylori* infection, and decreased defense mechanisms such as decreasing mucosal prostaglandin levels.[4] Although there is only scant evidence at this time that *H. pylori* infection occurs in horses (D. Scott, personal communication, ACVIM 2002), decreased protective mechanisms and potential drug-induced gastric injury should be considered when evaluating the geriatric equine patient for suspected gastric ulceration.

The occurrence of squamous ulceration does not correlate with that of glandular ulceration, which suggests that the two entities differ with regard to their pathophysiology.[20] Overall, however, the central pathophysiologic event is thought to be an imbalance between protective and aggressive factors that affects mucosal integrity.[21] Protectors of gastric mucosal integrity encompass a mucus-bicarbonate barrier overlying the glandular epithelium, mucosal blood flow, prostaglandin E_2, cell restitution and renewal, growth factors such as epidermal growth factor, bicarbonate secretion in saliva to buffer gastric acid, and normal gastric emptying.[21,22] Many of these protective mechanisms are absent in the squamous portion of the stomach, which makes it more sensitive to injury.[21] Protective mechanisms specific for the squamous mucosa include intercellular mucopolysaccharide glycoconjugates, intercellular tight junctions, intercellular buffering of acid by bicarbonate, and intracellular buffering mechanisms.[21] The main aggressors are hydrochloric acid secreted on the luminal side of parietal cells via an H^+/K^+-ATPase (or proton pump), and pepsinogen released from chief cells, which is subsequently activated to pepsin by the acidic intraluminal environment of the stomach. Stimuli for acid secretion are manifold,[22] including vagal input initiated by anticipation, feed prehension, chewing and swallowing, and gastric distension; gastrin released from G cells within the gastric glands; and histamine, which is released from enterochromaffin-like cells after their stimulation by gastrin and vagal afferents and stimulates the histamine type 2 (H_2) receptors on parietal cells. Acid secretion in horses is continuous and independent of feed intake. Mucosal and submucosal blood is important to provide nutrients, oxygen, and bicarbonate to epithelial cells and remove back-diffused gastric acid.[22] Compromised blood flow, resulting for example from suppression of prostaglandin E_2 production by NSAID treatment is, therefore, a potentially important factor in the development of gastric ulceration. NSAID use may be a factor of increased importance in geriatric horses that suffer from chronic disease such as arthritis or laminitis and require frequent administration of these analgesic and anti-inflammatory drugs. The extent to which absorption, distribution, and metabolism of NSAIDs are different among geriatric horses has not been determined, but it is possible that they might be predisposed to NSAID intoxication if such differences occur. Anorexia due to any disease process is a risk factor for the development of gastric ulcers because it results in increased acidity of stomach contents. Stress, physiologic as well as psychological, is a well-known risk factor for gastric ulceration in people. Although the influence of psychological stress is difficult to determine in horses, physiologic stress such as that due to chronic disease needs to be considered in geriatric horses. It is unclear whether horses with pituitary dysfunction (equine Cushing's disease), a condition more common among older horses, are predisposed to gastric ulceration.

Clinical signs commonly seen in horses with gastric ulceration include acute or recurrent colic, which can vary considerably in its severity; loss of body condition; reduced appetite; decrease in performance; and attitude changes such as increased nervousness or reluctance to be handled.[21] Because all of these clinical signs can also be caused by a number of other disease processes (many of which may result secondarily in gastric ulceration), it may at times be difficult to determine whether gastric ulceration is the primary cause of disease or whether ulceration occurred secondarily. In some cases, it may be necessary to treat gastric ulcers to determine their clinical significance relative to the observed clinical signs. The owner should be advised that further diagnostic testing might become necessary if clinical signs persist after successful treatment of gastric ulcers.

Diagnosis of gastroduodenal ulceration is made by endoscopy. An effort should be made to evaluate the entire gastric mucosa, including that of the cardia, antrum, and pylorus, as well as the proximal duodenum. Most gastric ulcers of the squamous mucosa occur adjacent to the margo plicatus (Fig. 10-5). Isolated ulceration of the glandular mucosa of the body of the stomach is rarely observed in adult horses, but 58 percent of horses in a recent study were found to have erosions or ulcers in the antrum or pylorus.[20] Fecal occult blood analysis and contrast radiography are considered unreliable for diagnosis of gastroduodenal ulceration.[21] Recent evidence indicates that sucrose permeability testing may be useful for identifying gastric ulceration.[23]

To allow adequate visualization of the entire gastric mucosa, including the pylorus, most horses need to be fasted for 16 to 20 hours before endoscopy, and an endoscope of 2.5 to 3 m in length should be used. The stomach should be sufficiently inflated with air to allow smoothening of mucosal folds. The introduced air should be suctioned as completely as possible before withdrawal of the endoscope to avoid discomfort associated with gastric distention. With some practice, one can manage to "loop" the endoscope around the inside of the stomach to view the pyloric sphincter in most horses. A fluid level

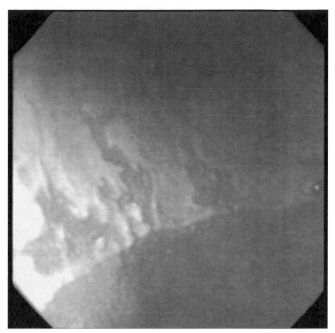

Figure 10-5 Endoscopic view of the margo plicatus in a horse with gastric ulceration. The lighter (ulcerated) portion represents squamous gastric epithelium, the darker portion glandular epithelium.

may be present in the ventral stomach and pyloric region despite fasting and may interfere with visualization of the pyloric sphincter. During the endoscopic examination, ulcer location and severity should be recorded for reference at follow-up examination, but the ability to accurately diagnose ulcer severity has recently been challenged. In a study comparing endoscopic ulcer scores of yearling horses with subsequent necropsy findings and histopathologic diagnosis, the presence of glandular ulcers was significantly underestimated, whereas observation of squamous lesions was accurate. Furthermore, severity, especially depth, of nonglandular lesions was underestimated.[24] These findings may offer one explanation for the fact that endoscopically observed ulcer severity does not appear to correlate with the severity of clinical signs in many cases. In horses with severe ulceration and/or atypical appearance of ulcers, and if ulcers fail to respond to treatment, biopsy to rule out neoplastic changes (most commonly squamous cell carcinoma) is recommended. If a biopsy instrument is not available, smears of brushings of the lesion can be useful, if there is sufficient exfoliation of neoplastic cells. The duodenum and the major duodenal papilla of the pancreatic duct can be viewed in smaller horses by experienced examiners. The esophageal mucosa is best viewed upon retraction of the endoscope from the stomach and under careful inflation with air.

Successful management needs to treat existing ulcers and address any underlying cause or predisposing factors for gastric ulceration. The primary objective in treating gastric ulceration is to raise gastric pH. This can be achieved by neutralization of stomach acid, blockade of H_2 receptors, or blockade of the proton pump. Antacids are rarely used in adult horses because they must be administered frequently (every 2-3 hours) and in large volumes. In some cases, however, antacids may be helpful as an adjunct treatment, such as to reduce inappetence.[21] Administration of an adequate volume of antacids may also give some indication of the clinical significance in horses showing signs of colic. H_2 antagonists used in horses include cimetidine, ranitidine, and famotidine, all of which have been shown to successfully resolve gastric ulceration and associated clinical signs.[21] Suggested oral dosages are 6.6 mg/kg every 8 hours for ranitidine, 20 to 30 mg/kg every 8 hours for cimetidine, and 3.3 to 5 mg/kg every 8 hours for famotidine. Individual variation in bioavailability and treatment response has been noted, and adjustment to an effective dose may be necessary in certain cases.[21] Duration of treatment with H_2 antagonists depends on the rate of ulcer healing; at least 14 to 21 days of treatment are required in most cases. Omeprazole (GastroGuard, Merial) is a proton pump blocker approved by the Food and Drug Administration and available in paste form for once-daily administration to horses. At a dose of 4 mg/kg, omeprazole has been shown to increase gastric pH to above 4 for at least 12 hours after administration.[25] Dosage recommendations are 4 mg/kg once daily for 4 weeks followed by 2 mg/kg once daily for prevention of recurrence. Several compounded generic omeprazole preparations are available, apart from the Food and Drug Administration approved paste. These preparations differ in their characteristics such as vehicle pH and not all can be expected to perform satisfactorily.[25] Sucralfate is thought to adhere to ulcerated glandular mucosa and may be beneficial in the treatment of glandular ulceration, especially if combined with antacid therapy such as H_2 antagonists.[21] Additional effects of sucralfate include stimulation of mucus secretion, enhanced prostaglandin E synthesis, and concentration of growth factor at the site of ulceration.[21] The recommended dose of sucralfate is 20 to 40 mg/kg every 6 to 8 hours, and the drug can be administered concurrently with the H_2 antagonists.[21] Misoprostol is a synthetic prostaglandin E analogue whose effects include inhibition of acid secretion and mucosal cytoprotection. Although some practitioners eschew this drug because of concerns for gastrointestinal side effects, in the authors' experience, oral administration at a dose of 2 to 5 μg/kg every 6 to 12 hours has not been associated with colic or other intestinal side effects. The drug is contraindicated in pregnant mares because of its potential to induce uterine contractions and abortion. Gastrointestinal prokinetic drugs may be useful in horses with suspected gastric emptying delay

or esophageal ulceration indicating reflux of stomach acid into the lower esophagus that is not associated with a physical obstruction to gastric emptying. Recommended agents and dosages include metoclopramide, a dopamine antagonist, at 0.1 to 0.25 mg/kg IV, PO, or SC every 6 to 8 hours, and bethanechol, a cholinergic agonist, at 0.025 to 0.03 mg/kg SC every 3 to 4 hours, followed by an oral maintenance dose of 0.35 to 0.45 mg/kg every 6 to 8 hours.[21] Because metoclopramide may result in serious side effects such as sudden neurologic excitation, administration of a test dose (e.g., 0.1 mg/kg) over 60 minutes as a continuous drip has been recommended.[21] Bethanechol appears to be associated with fewer side effects, which may include diarrhea, salivation, inappetence, and colic.[21]

Feeding, with regard to both the type of feed and the feeding schedule, is an important contributor to gastric mucosal health. Experimentally, a feeding-fasting interval program will induce gastric ulceration, which underscores the importance of constant and regular feed intake. Roughage intake in particular is associated with increased chewing time, increased saliva production, and improved buffering of stomach contents. In any horse, therefore, but particularly in those with gastric ulceration, free-choice access to roughage should be provided to decrease the length of time during which the horse's stomach is empty and intragastric pH is low. With specific regard to geriatric horses, regular dental care is important to maintain a horse's ability to consume an adequate amount of roughage. Aside from the benefits of roughage intake for gastric health, the intake of small amounts of feed during large parts of the day more closely resembles natural equine behavior than ingestion of two large meals with a high proportion of concentrate.

Disorders of the Small Intestine

Strangulating Lipoma

Intestinal strangulation by a pedunculated lipoma has consistently been associated with older age. Different reports have stated median or average ages observed in horses with pedunculated lipoma as 14 years (median age),[26] 16.6 years (average age),[27] and 17.6 years (average age).[28] Obstruction by pedunculated lipoma mostly involves the small intestine, most often results in strangulation, and typically carries a guarded prognosis.[28] Cases of obstruction by pedunculated lipoma of the small colon and rectum have also been described. An increased incidence of strangulation by lipoma in geldings as compared to mares and stallions has been reported.[27,28] Certain breed dispositions may also exist, with one investigation of 75 cases stating a significantly increased risk for ponies and a decreased risk for Thoroughbreds.[28] A genetic predisposition due to differences in fat metabolism and management factors, including overfeeding, were proposed as possibly contributing to the increased risk in ponies.[28] In another study, an increased risk of strangulation by pedunculated lipoma was found for ponies, Quarter horses, Arabians, and male horses.[29]

It is reasonable to assume that strangulation becomes more likely with increased length of the pedicle and increased weight of the attached lipoma. The exact mechanism of strangulation development is, however, unknown and has to be regarded as accidental.[28] Intra-abdominal lipomas are occasionally an incidental finding during abdominal surgery or necropsy. Based on investigation of the distributions of the sizes of asymptomatic lipomas and those causing intestinal obstruction, it has been recommended to remove all but the smallest lipomas surgically when they are encountered as an incidental finding.[28]

Clinical signs of small intestinal strangulation by lipoma are those of small intestinal obstruction in general and include persistent abdominal pain, gastric reflux (the amount of which depends on the location and duration of blockade), absence of borborygmi, and cardiovascular compromise manifested by tachycardia, altered mucous membrane color, signs of dehydration (e.g., dry mucous membranes, skin tenting) and weakened pulse quality. Gastric rupture may occur as a result of retrograde accumulation of intestinal contents and ongoing intestinal secretion, in which case abdominal pain typically subsides and the horse rapidly develops signs of severe endotoxic shock. Rectal examination reveals small intestinal distention, which can also be detected by transcutaneous ultrasonographic examination of the flank regions and ventral abdomen. Small intestinal loops typically appear edematous and amotile if a mechanical obstruction is present.[30] Ultrasonographic examination may also be helpful in cases of suspected gastric rupture to assess the amount of free peritoneal fluid. Peritoneal fluid analysis reflects the degree of intestinal compromise; bacterial organisms and/or feed material in the peritoneal fluid are consistent with gastric rupture.

Treatment necessitates exploratory laparotomy, removal of the lipoma, and in most cases resection and anastomosis of the affected portion of intestine. Prognosis depends on the amount of intestine involved in the strangulation, its degree of compromise, the promptness with which surgical intervention occurs, and the degree of cardiovascular compromise. In a retrospective study of 75 horses undergoing surgery for small intestinal strangulation by pedunculated lipoma, 36 horses survived short-term (7 days postoperatively), and of 19 horses for which long-term information was available, 15 survived to at least 1 year postoperatively, although colic episodes recurred in 2 horses.[28]

Epiploic Foramen Entrapment

Aside from strangulation by a pedunculated lipoma, entrapment of small intestine in the epiploic foramen is often suggested to be associated with advanced age in horses. Atrophy of the right liver lobe is given as a reason for the purportedly increased incidence of this problem in aged horses.[31] Recent evidence, however, refutes an increased occurrence of epiploic foramen entrapment with age.[32] With regard to liver atrophy, it appears to be an incidental finding in aged as well as younger horses and its occurrence does not appear to be associated with increased size of the epiploic foramen or entrapment.[33,34]

Disorders of the Large Intestine

Large Colon Impaction

The higher risk of impaction colic in aged horses has been primarily attributed to poor dentition resulting in inadequate chewing of feed. Large colon impaction may further be caused by dehydration, intake of coarse feed, sudden feeding changes, management changes such as moving a horse from pasture to stall confinement, changes in exercise routine, concurrent disease such as lameness resulting in prolonged stall confinement, and migrating parasite larvae causing mucosal damage and altering motility.

Clinical signs are variable and can range from inappetence, reduced fecal output, and mild discomfort to more severe abdominal pain, abdominal distention, absence of borborygmi, gastric reflux, and varying degrees of cardiovascular compromise. Clinical signs often develop over several days and horses may continue to eat between episodes of discomfort. If feces are passed, they are often dry and covered with mucus.[35] Clinicopathologic data are generally normal or only slightly altered and nonspecific. Increased packed cell volume and total protein concentration indicating hemoconcentration are the most common abnormalities.[35] Diagnosis is generally achieved by rectal examination and detection of a variably compressible mass within the ascending colon, frequently the pelvic flexure, and colonic gas distention. Gastric reflux in the absence of small intestinal distention may be caused by pressure on the stomach exerted by the distended colon as well as generalized intestinal stasis. Differential diagnoses primarily include causes of secondary feed impaction such as colonic displacement, enterolithiasis, and foreign body obstruction. Concurrent sand impaction may be detected by abdominal radiography, sedimentation of sand from a fecal sample, and auscultation of the characteristic "waves on the beach" sound of intestinal borborygmi when the stethoscope is placed on the ventral abdomen.

Treatment of large colon impaction generally involves feed restriction, pain management, administration of oral fluids and mineral oil (2-4 L via nasogastric intubation) and, if necessary, overhydration by intravenous fluids. Laxatives such as docusate sodium (dioctyl sodium succinate, 6-12 g/500 kg) and magnesium sulfate (0.1 mg/kg given in 2-4 L of water) are also frequently employed[35]; however, care should be taken with repeated administration of such laxatives because of the potential for side effects such as dehydration, mucosal irritation, and hypermagnesemia. The rate of intravenous fluid administration depends on the degree of dehydration and the severity of impaction; rates of two to five times the maintenance rate, or 4 to 10 mL/kg/hr have been recommended. Evidence exists that intragastric administration of fluids can be as or more effective than intravenous fluid administration for increasing fluid in intestinal luminal contents.[36] Feed should be withheld initially; however, handwalking and grazing of small amounts of fresh grass may be beneficial to stimulate intestinal motility and to allow some exercise. Feeding small amounts also may help to maintain normal intestinal flora, because diarrhea may occur after resolution of long-standing impactions, particularly those treated with repeated administration of oral laxatives. Feed impaction of the large colon only rarely has to be resolved using a surgical approach; however, surgery should be considered in cases refractory to medical treatment for more than 48 to 72 hours, or in those suspected to represent impactions secondary to a condition meriting celiotomy for diagnosis or treatment.

Large Colon Volvulus

Colonic volvulus or torsion purportedly occurs with increased frequency in older broodmares just before or after foaling,[37] although horses of all ages and both sexes can be affected. The exact cause of colonic torsion is unknown, but decreased intestinal motility and excess intestinal gas accumulation has been implicated in the initiation of torsion.[37] Clinical signs in cases of colonic torsion involving the cecum do not differ from those observed with torsion of the colon alone.[37]

Clinical signs are typically dramatic and occur suddenly. Severe abdominal pain, which often is nonresponsive to administration of sedatives or pain medication, and abdominal distention predominate. Horses may show signs of cardiovascular compromise and endotoxemia such as dehydration, elevated heart rate, and pale or congested mucous membranes. The degree of compromise correlates with the duration of torsion. Gastric reflux may be present and is likely attributable to pressure on the pylorus or proximal duodenum exerted by the distended colon. Extreme colonic distention can further result in respiratory compromise, and respiratory acidosis may be detected by blood gas examination.[37] Rectal examination, if possible, reveals a tightly distended large colon, which is frequently oriented horizontally across the pelvic inlet due to distention and elongation of the colon or rotation on the mesenteric axis.[37] In many cases, rectal examination is difficult and dangerous to both the horse and examiner because of the unrelenting pain of the horse. Results of a complete blood cell count and serum biochemistry panel are typically nonspecific but may reveal hemoconcentration and electrolyte abnormalities. Peritoneal fluid analysis reflects the degree of intestinal compromise; however, the degree of abdominal pain is usually sufficient to indicate the need for exploratory laparotomy. With severe abdominal gas distention, some clinicians choose to trocarize the cecum or large colon prior to surgery. Treatment is almost exclusively surgical and includes evacuation of the colon, resolution of the torsion, and, if necessary, colonic resection. Successful outcome mostly depends on the promptness of surgical intervention and the degree of intestinal wall compromise, but the prognosis is, in general, guarded to poor. Because of the risk of recurrence, colopexy or partial colonic resection is sometimes performed in affected horses.[37]

Cecal Impaction

Of the cecal diseases, primary cecal impaction has been reported to occur with increased frequency in older horses.[38,39] Possible factors predisposing older horses to impaction of the cecum include, alone or in combination, poor dentition or dental disease leading to insufficient chewing of roughage, general debilitation, intestinal motility disorders, intestinal parasite infestation, concurrent disease, and NSAID use.[39,40] Cecal impaction is also recognized as a postanesthetic complication in horses of all ages. Clinical signs of cecal impaction frequently include reduced fecal output, anorexia, and mild, recurrent abdominal pain associated with slow deterioration of vital parameters and clinicopathologic values.[39] Passage of small amounts of feces, gas, and administered mineral oil may persist and can occasionally protract the decision for more aggressive treatment. Vital parameters, clinicopathologic data, and results of peritoneal fluid analysis are often initially normal. Changes in peritoneal fluid appearance and analysis parameters indicate compromised bowel wall integrity and progression of the disease to a point where the prognosis, even with surgical exploration, has to be guarded. Although success rates as high as 90 percent have been reported for medical therapy,[39] surgical exploration should be strongly considered in horses in which medical therapy has not resolved a cecal impaction within 24 to 48 hours.

Diagnosis of cecal impaction relies on history, physical examination including clinicopathologic analysis, rectal examination, and response to therapy. Rectal examination is reportedly helpful in diagnosing cases of cecal impaction, although typical findings of a taut ventral band and firm ingesta within the organ may not be present in all cases. Cecal impaction due to disruption of normal motility and/or outflow has been described as presenting a large, ingesta-filled cecum of fluid consistency upon rectal palpation.[41] Options for medical therapy include overhydration with oral and/or intravenous fluids; intragastric administration of fecal softeners and laxatives such as mineral oil, magnesium sulfate, and docusate sodium; and pain control. Feed should be withheld initially but it may be advisable to offer small amounts of easily digestible feeds such as grass or pellets once improvement is noted and passage of feces has resumed. In horses that are repeatedly given laxatives and fecal softeners, diarrhea may ensue, and feeding of small amounts may help to maintain normal intestinal flora. Consequently, administration of probiotics can be considered, although sufficient scientific evidence for their effectiveness is lacking and a recent investigation found most available veterinary products to be inaccurately labeled, to not contain the indicated amount of viable organisms, or to even contain organisms not considered to be probiotics.[42]

Prognosis for cecal impaction is good to guarded, depending on the severity, duration, and therapeutic approach. Primary impactions that are treated early and respond within 24 hours generally carry a good prognosis, whereas more protracted disease or impactions occurring postoperatively have a more guarded prognosis.[43] The most common complications of cecal impaction are failure to resolve, recurrence, and cecal rupture. Failure to resolve with medical therapy alone within 24 to 48 hours should prompt surgical exploration to assess cecal wall integrity and associated problems and to resolve the impaction via typhlotomy. Recurrence of impaction is likely associated with primary motility disorders, and such cases may require surgical bypass of the cecum. Some authors suggest a bypass procedure in any case of protracted cecal impaction because of the risk of an associated outflow disorder and inability to differentiate simple impaction from cecal dysmotility.[40,41] Cecal rupture after impaction is a serious concern and was reported in 12 of 21 horses in one study.[38] Cecal rupture is associated with a grave prognosis. Some authors suggest immediate surgical management for cases of cecal impaction to decrease the risk of cecal rupture.[38]

Descending (Small) Colon Disorders

Aged horses appear to be predisposed to diseases of the small colon.[44] An increased occurrence of small colon dis-orders has been proposed for Arabians, miniature horses and ponies, and mares.[45] Conditions affecting the small colon in adult horses include intraluminal obstruction by feed impactions, enteroliths, fecaliths, phytobezoars, trichobezoars, or foreign bodies; strangulation caused by lipomas or entrapment through mesenteric rents; volvulus; herniation; rectal and vaginal tears; intramural hematomas; submucosal edema; and intussusception.[44] The origin of intramural hematoma formation in the small colon is insufficiently understood. Some hematomas communicate with the bowel lumen whereas others do not.[46] Hematomas have been found in association with chronic mucosal ulceration and likely develop due to submucosal infection and extension of cellulitis resulting in vascular damage and localized hemorrhage; some cases may result from trauma subsequent to rectal palpation.[46]

Horses with obstructive lesions of the small colon frequently show mild, chronic signs of colic, unless distention of the intestine proximal to the obstruction results in more acute signs.[44] It is not uncommon for horses with small colon obstruction to pass small amounts of loose feces or diarrhea as well as gas, which prevents proximal distention from occurring. In these cases, colitis must be ruled out. Small colon disorders requiring surgical intervention often show a protracted course of disease and may not be associated with physical and hematologic abnormalities.[44] Repeated analysis of peritoneal fluid appears to be especially helpful in assessing the horse's need for surgical exploration.[44,45] Intramural hematomas of the small colon appear to cause severe pain, which has been attributed to distention of the hematoma, intestinal ischemia, and intestinal distention proximal to the obstruction.[46] Additional clinical signs observed in horses with intramural hematomas are abdominal distention and intestinal tympany, lack of auscultatable borborygmi, tachycardia, gastric reflux, and signs consistent with endotoxemia.

Despite the location of the small colon in the caudal abdomen, specific diagnosis of small colon disorders by rectal examination is often difficult due to the organ's mobility. Of the obstructive lesions, simple impactions are the easiest to identify, whereas enteroliths are often missed.[44,45] In one reported case of intramural hematoma, a hard mass was palpable in the ventral abdomen but could not definitively be associated with the small colon.[46] Peritoneal fluid analysis may provide evidence of hemorrhage in some cases of intramural hematoma, and increased total protein concentration and nucleated cell count represent evidence of intestinal wall compromise. Results of complete blood cell count and serum biochemistry are unlikely to provide specific information about the cause of colic but should nevertheless be performed to assess the horse's hydration, serum electrolyte, and acid-base status.

Simple feed impaction of the small colon is treated in accordance with general principles of treatment of impaction colic. Administration of enemas may be useful for distal impactions; however, great care should be taken to avoid damaging the mucosa of the rectum and small colon. Enemas should not contain potential mucosal irritants such as dioctyl sodium succinate. Feed impaction that is nonresponsive to medical therapy, foreign body obstruction, and strangulating obstruction requires surgical intervention. Owing to the severity of pain associated with most cases of small colon hematoma, exploratory surgery will most likely be performed for this condition as well. Access to the small colon via flank laparotomy may be suitable in certain cases as an alternative to ventral midline celiotomy. Prognosis depends on the degree of intestinal compromise and lesion location but is generally fair to good for simple intraluminal obstruction.[45] Prognosis in cases requiring resection and anastomosis depends on the accessibility and extent of the lesion and the promptness with which surgical correction is achieved.

Intestinal Neoplasia

In people, the prevalence of neoplasia as a cause of intestinal tract disease increases dramatically with age. In human patients presenting with acute abdominal crisis, cancer as a causative factor occurs in approximately 25 percent of patients older than 70 years, while it recognized as a cause in only 1 percent in those younger than 50 years.[4] Reports of intestinal tract neoplasia in horses are rare, with lipoma, lymphosarcoma, and squamous cell carcinoma (Figs. 10-6 and 10-7) being the most common reported conditions. Although lipoma and squamous cell carcinoma occur more frequently in older horses, the alimentary form of lymphosarcoma is more commonly found in younger horses.[47] Other reported tumors of the abdominal cavity include leiomyoma and leiomyosarcoma, adenocarcinoma, and fibroma and fibrosarcoma. Cecal neoplasia is rare and appears to be associated with older age and chronic weight loss; clinical signs of abdominal pain are often absent. Cecal neoplasias include leiomyoma, hemangiosarcoma, and papillary adenoma.[39]

In older horses with complaints of chronic colic, particularly if associated with weight loss and debilitation, intestinal tract neoplasia should be considered as a differential diagnosis.[48] Weight loss in patients with neoplasia is often attributed to cancer cachexia, which may result from inadequate caloric intake, impaired digestion and absorption, nutrient loss, tumor-host competition for nutrients, and increased energy requirements of the host.[48] Successful treatment of neoplasia is a prerequisite for reversing cancer cachexia.[48]

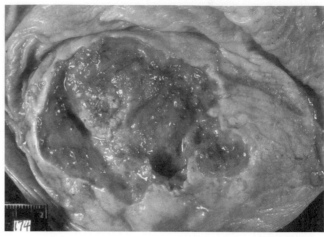

Figure 10-6 Gastric squamous cell carcinoma in a geriatric horse. The tumor perforated the gastric wall. (Courtesy of Dr. Michelle H. Barton, University of Georgia.)

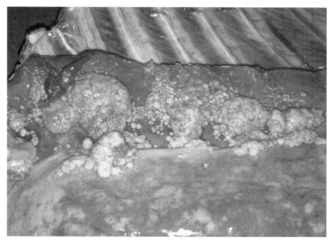

Figure 10-7 Metastasis of a gastric squamous cell carcinoma (same horse as in Figure 10-6) to the thorax in a geriatric horse. Note the extensive neoplastic spread to the serosal surfaces. The horse also had serosal metastases within the abdominal cavity. Metastasis was most likely due to direct extension of the primary tumor, which perforated the gastric wall, and lymphatic spread. (Courtesy of Dr. Michelle H. Barton, University of Georgia.)

The diagnostic approach to intestinal neoplasia should include a detailed history, thorough physical examination, evaluation of clinicopathologic data including analysis of peritoneal fluid, rectal examination, abdominal ultrasonography, and, if indicated, gastroscopic examination. Surgical exploration of the abdominal cavity via flank laparotomy or midline celiotomy will be necessary in many cases to obtain a definitive diagnosis. Neoplasia of abdominal organs other than the intestine, such as the kidneys, urinary bladder, liver, spleen, or ovaries, can manifest with signs similar to those of intestinal neoplasia and should be considered. In metastasizing neoplasias, intestinal and extraintestinal organs may be affected.[48] In some cases, metastatic changes such as involvement of mediastinal lymph nodes may be more readily detected than the primary tumor.

Summary

Geriatric horses are at increased risk for certain conditions (e.g., strangulating lipoma and dental disease) affecting the alimentary tract and are affected by many alimentary tract disorders that occur in horses of all ages. This chapter has provided a review of those alimentary tract disorders for which older horses are at increased risk or for which there may be special considerations for geriatric horses.

REFERENCES

1. National Animal Health Monitoring System (NAHMS): Equine '98 Part I: Baseline reference of 1998 equine health and management, N280.898. United States Department of Agriculture (online). Available at http://www.aphis.usda.gov/vs/ceah/cahm. Posting date 1998.
2. Hall KE, Wiley JW: Age-associated changes in gastrointestinal function. In Hazzard WR, Blass JP, Ettinger WH, et al, eds: Principles of Geriatric Medicine and Gerontology, 4th ed. New York, McGraw-Hill, 1999.
3. Ralston SL, Squires EL, Nockels CF: Digestion in the aged horse. J EqVet Sci 9:203, 1989.
4. Tepper RE, Katz S: Overview: Geriatric gastroenterology. In Tallis RC, Fillit HM, Brocklehurst JC, eds: Brocklehurst's Textbook of Geriatric Medicine and Gerontology, 5th ed. New York, Churchill Livingstone, 1998.
5. Ralston SL: How I treat chronic weight loss in geriatric horses. Comp Cont Ed PractVet 21:655, 1999.
6. Zicker SC, Wilson WD, Medearis I. Differentiation between intra-abdominal neoplasms and abscesses in horses, using clinical and laboratory data: 40 cases (1973–1988). JAVMA 196:1130, 1990.
7. Lindberg R, Nygren A, Persson SG: Rectal biopsy diagnosis in horses with clinical signs of intestinal disorders: a retrospective study of 116 cases. EVJ 28:275, 1996.
8. Brown CM: The diagnostic value of the D-xylose absorption test in horses with unexplained chronic weight loss. Br Vet J 148:41, 1992.
9. Roberts MC: Small intestinal malabsorption in horses. EVE 12:214, 2000.
10. Freeman DE, Ferrante PL, Kronfeld DS, et al: Effect of food deprivation on D-xylose absorption test results in mares. AJVR 50:1609, 1989.
11. Church S, Middleton DJ: Transient glucose malabsorption in two horses: fact or artefact? AustVet J 75:716, 1997.
12. Craig DR, Shivy DR, Pankowski RL, et al: Esophageal disorders in 61 horses: results of non-surgical and surgical management.Vet Surg 18:432, 1989.
13. Murray MJ: The esophagus. In Reed SM, Bayly WM, eds: Equine Internal Medicine. Philadelphia,WB Saunders, 1998.
14. Feige K, Schwarzwald C, Fuerst A, et al: Esophageal obstruction in horses: a retrospective study of 34 cases. CanVet J 41:207, 2000.
15. MacKay RJ: On the true definition of dysphagia. Comp Cont Ed Pract Vet 11:1024, 2001.
16. Green EM: Esophageal obstruction. In Robinson NE, editor: Current Therapy in Equine Medicine, 3rd ed. Philadelphia,WB Saunders, 1992.
17. Meyer GA, Rashmir-Raven A, Hlems RJ, et al: The effect of oxytocin on contractility of the equine oesophagus: a potential treatment for oesophageal obstruction. Equine Vet J 32:151, 2000.
18. Woolridge AA, Eades SC, Moore RM, et al: In vitro effects of oxytocin, acepromazine, detomidine, xylazine, butorphanol, terbutaline, isopro-

19. Todhunter RJ, Stick JA, Trotter GW, et al: Medical management of esophageal stricture in seven horses. JAVMA 185:784, 1984.
20. Murray MJ, Nout YS, Ward DL: Endoscopic findings of the gastric antrum and pylorus in horses: 162 cases (1996–2000). JVIM 15:401, 2001.
21. Murray MJ, Gastroduodenal ulceration. In Reed SM, Bayly WM, eds: Equine Internal Medicine. Philadelphia,WB Saunders, 1998.
22. Crawford JM: The gastrointestinal tract. In Cotran RS, Kumas V, Collins T, editors: Pathologic Basis of Disease, 6th ed. Philadelphia,WB Saunders, 1996.
23. O'Conor M, Roussel AJ, Steiner J, et al: Sucrose permeability as a marker for equine gastric ulceration [abstract]. In Proceedings of the 7th International Colic Research Symposium, Manchester, UK, July 14–16, 2002.
24. Andrews FA: Inability of endoscopic examination to predict gastric ulcer severity in horses [abstract]. In Proceedings of the 7th International Colic Research Symposium, Manchester, UK, July 14–16, 2002.
25. Merritt AM, Sanchez LC, Burrow JA, et al: Bioavailability of "Gastrogard" vs. three generic compounded omeprazole preparations in mature horses [abstract]. In Proceedings of the 7th International Colic Research Symposium, Manchester, UK, July 14–16, 2002.
26. Tennant B, Keirn DR, White KK, et al: Six cases of squamous cell carcinoma of the stomach of the horse. EVJ 14:238, 1982.
27. Blikslager AT, Bowman KF, Haven ML: Pedunculated lipomas as a cause of intestinal obstruction in horses: 17 cases (1983–1990). JAVMA 201:1249, 1992.
28. Edwards GB, Proudman CJ: An analysis of 75 cases of intestinal obstruction caused by pedunculated lipomas. EVJ 26:18, 1994.
29. Schmid A, Freeman DE, Schaeffer DJ: Risk by age, breed and gender for common forms of small intestinal strangulation obstruction in horses [abstract]. In Proceedings of the 7th International Colic Research Symposium, Manchester, UK, July 14–16, 2002.
30. Klohnen A, Vachon AM, Fischer AT: Use of diagnostic ultrasonography in horses with signs of acute abdominal pain. JAVMA 209:1597, 1996.
31. Rooney JR: Equine Pathology. Ames, Iowa State University Press, 1996.
32. Freeman DE, Schaeffer DJ: Age distributions of horses with strangulation of the small intestine by a lipoma or in the epiploic foramen: 46 cases (1994–2000). JAVMA 219:87, 2001.
33. Jakowski RM: Right hepatic lobe atrophy in horses: 17 cases (1983–1993). JAVMA 204:1057, 1994.
34. Schmid A, Freeman DE, Baker GJ: Anatomy of the epiploic foramen and the effect of age and body weight on size [abstract]. In Proceedings of the 6th Equine Colic Research Symposium, Athens, 1998.
35. Jones SL, Snyder JR, Spier SJ: Obstructive conditions of the large intestine. In Reed SM, Bayly WM, eds: Equine Internal Medicine. Philadelphia,WB Saunders, 1998.
36. Lopes MAF, White NA II, Donaldson L, et al: Treatments to promote colonic hydration: enteral fluids, I.V. fluids, magnesium sulphate and sodium sulphate [abstract]. In Proceedings of the 7th International Colic Research Symposium, Manchester, UK, July 14–16, 2002.
37. Sullins KE: Diseases of the large colon. In White NA, editor: The Equine Acute Abdomen. Philadelphia, Lea & Febiger, 1990.
38. Campbell ML, Colahan PC, Brown MP, et al: Cecal impaction in the horse. JAVMA 185:950, 1984.
39. Dart AJ, Hodgson DR, Snyder JR: Caecal disease in equids. Aust Vet J 75:552, 1997.
40. Collatos C, Romano S: Cecal impaction in horses: causes, diagnosis and medical treatment. Comp Cont Ed PractVet 15:976, 1993.
41. White NA: Epidemiology and etiology of colic. In White NA, editor: The Equine Acute Abdomen. Philadelphia, Lea & Febiger, 1990.
42. Weese JS: Microbiologic evaluation of commercial probiotics. JAVMA 220:794, 2002.
43. Snyder JR, Spier SJ: Disorders of the large intestine associated with acute abdominal pain. In Smith BP, editor: Large Animal Internal Medicine. Philadelphia,WB Saunders, 1996.

44. Dart AJ, Snyder JR, Pascoe JR, et al: Abnormal conditions of the equine descending (small) colon: 102 cases (1979–1989). JAVMA 200:971, 1992.
45. Snyder JR, Spier SJ: Abnormal conditions of the descending (small) colon. In Smith BP, editor: Large Animal Internal Medicine. Philadelphia, WB Saunders, 1996.
46. Speirs VC, van Veenendaal JC, Christie BA, et al: Obstruction of the small colon by intramural hematoma in three horses. Aust Vet J 57:88, 1981.
47. Carlson GP: Lymphosarcoma in horses. In Smith BP, editor: Large Animal Internal Medicine. St. Louis, Mosby, 1996.
48. Traub JL, Bayly WM, Reed SM, et al: Intraabdominal neoplasia as a cause of chronic weight loss in the horse. Comp Cont Ed Pract Vet 5:S526, 1983.

CHAPTER 11

Abdominal Surgery in the Geriatric Equine

A. T. Fischer Jr.

A bdominal surgery in the equine geriatric patient has seemingly become more common in the last decade. Many owners tend to treat their older horses as pets or even members of the family and are more willing to pursue diagnostics and therapeutics on older horses.[1] Today's increased attention to the human-animal bond as compared with previous generations may be in part responsible for this. Horses are no longer looked at as only useful while being able to be used but are considered pets or family members and provided with health care for as long as necessary and reasonable. Some owners will question the advisability of operating on older horses but I feel that this is a personal question for them to consider after they have the facts about the prognosis for their individual horse. The age of the horse at admission for colic surgery has not been shown to have a consistent link with mortality.[2]

Preoperative Assessment

Older horses presenting with colic may have other concurrent medical conditions that need attention or that will dictate differing strategies for anesthesia, surgery, and postoperative management. Subclinical liver or renal disease may be present. Equine Cushing's disease with its associated problems is more frequent in the older horse. Owners are frequently surprised at how thin a horse with a long hair coat is when it is clipped for an ultrasonographic examination. Osteoporosis may be present along with equine Cushing's disease or by itself. Degenerative joint disease and its associated lameness or reduced range of joint motion in one or more joints is frequently present.

Abnormalities of dentition leading to poor nutritional status, impactions, or even sinusitis may be present. Physical examination findings, interview of the owner for evaluation of previous or current medical problems, and a complete diagnostic evaluation for the presenting problem of colic are necessary.

Laboratory Evaluation of the Older Horse with Colic

In our clinic, all horses presenting with colic undergo the same basic laboratory diagnostic testing. A complete blood cell count with fibrinogen and serum biochemistry panel are obtained and abdominocentesis is performed and is analyzed for cytologic findings, total protein, and cell counts. Older horses present more frequently with anemia and this must be factored in when looking at their packed cell volume (PCV). A PCV of 40 percent in an older horse may indicate significant dehydration if that horse's normal PCV is in the low 20s range normally. Assessment of total protein will hopefully lend some clues to this, as the total protein will be elevated higher than one expects with a PCV of 40 (i.e., >8). Assessment of previous laboratory work (if available) when the horse was healthy may offer some clue that this is occurring. Clinical examination with assessment of skin turgor can help confirm or refute this. Hypernatremia and hyperchloremia are also indicators of dehydration and free water loss. Dehydration and electrolyte abnormalities should be corrected prior to surgery if possible. Examination of serum biochemical panel may indicate current subclinical renal or hepatic disease.

Physical Examination and Other Diagnostic Testing for Older Horses with Colic

Most horses presenting with colic undergo a very similar work-up in our hospital. A physical examination is performed, with particular attention paid to the gastrointestinal tract including evaluation of teeth, cursory evaluation of the sinuses, abdominal palpation per rectum, and abdominal auscultation. The evaluation of the horse for the presence of external tumors (squamous cell carcinoma or other malignancies) should also take place. A brief examination of the musculoskeletal system should be performed to ascertain whether there is any previous evidence of laminitis or other significant degenerative processes that may adversely affect the recovery from anesthesia or discourage the owner from pursuing exploratory surgery.

Abdominal radiography is performed in all horses presenting for colic looking for the presence of enteroliths or sand. In some horses, sand will be present with enteroliths, making the definitive diagnosis difficult. Sand accumulations tend to follow the shape of the bowel and have a straight dorsal line, whereas enteroliths are frequently round or triangular in profile. Abdominal ultrasonography is also performed and the entire abdominal cavity is imaged. The stomach is evaluated for the presence of fluid or masses. The small intestine is evaluated for mural thickness (normal <3 mm) and the presence of motility. Horses with small intestinal strangulation obstructions tend to have dilated loops of small intestine with increased wall thickness and minimal evidence of motility. The large intestine is evaluated similarly. Attention should be paid to the peritoneal surface and other internal organs looking for the presence of intra-abdominal neoplasia or metastatic lesions. The liver and kidneys should be assessed for normal architecture and the absence of calculi. Marked peritoneal effusion should make one suspicious of peritonitis or malignancies. Peritonitis is usually described by increased wall thickness of the small intestine with normal to decreased motility patterns. Horses with peritoneal effusion should also have their thorax examined ultrasonographically for the presence of masses or effusion.

Decision for Surgical Exploration

After appropriate evaluation of the horse with colic, a decision is usually made to continue treating the horse medically, to euthanize the horse, or to pursue exploratory surgery. The owners should be advised of the risks and advantages of each procedure and informed consent should be obtained. Intractable pain remains one of the most accurate indicators for the need for exploratory surgery. Older horses subjectively seem more stoic than younger horses and sometimes make the decision-making process harder. When a horse has been administered xylazine for analgesia and becomes painful again within the next 60 to 90 minutes, surgical exploration is typically recommended. Longer-lasting analgesics (detomidine or butorphanol) require adjusting the time frame for re-evaluating pain, and their use is avoided in preoperative colics in our clinic. Increasing heart rate and clinical signs of endotoxemia are another indication for surgical exploration if nonsurgical causes for these signs have been ruled out (e.g., colitis). The presence of edematous small intestine without motility is another indication for surgical exploration. Peritoneal effusion or evidence of peritonitis is an indication for surgical exploration of the abdomen. Controversy over the necessity for exploratory surgery for peritonitis remains, however. The presence of an enterolith on abdominal radiographs is another absolute indication for exploratory surgery.

Anesthesia

After appropriate stabilization and preparation, the horse is anesthetized. Older horses tend to require lower doses of anesthetic for induction. Lower doses of intravenous induction agents (e.g., 0.4 mg/kg of xylazine versus 1.0 mg/kg) should be attempted.[3] If more sedation is needed, additional xylazine may be administered. Induction is typically with ketamine (2.2-3.0 mg/kg) and Valium (0.05 mg/kg) or guaifenesin 5 percent solution until the horse becomes unstable, and then a bolus of ketamine (1.5 mg/kg) is administered. Supportive therapy during anesthesia is similar to that in younger horses but more vigilance is necessary because older horses subjectively seem to exhibit hypotension more frequently. After surgery is complete, the horse is placed in recovery with a nasopharyngeal or orotracheal tube until standing. Supervision of recovery or assistance should be provided. Subjectively, older horses seem to be more at risk for catastrophic fractures in recovery, and this may be due to osteopenia from old age or equine Cushing's disease; however, I am unaware of any specific equine literature supporting this observation.

Surgery

Abdominal exploratory surgery in the geriatric horse is identical to exploratory surgery in the younger horse. Older horses may have a thicker ventral midline due to chronic dermatitis, making the approach more difficult. Excessive accumulations of fat are also often present. Once entry to the abdomen is obtained, a thorough exploratory surgery is indicated, as concurrent lesions seem more frequent in older horses. Horses undergoing surgery for simple lesions such as enteroliths may have pediculated lipomas in their small intestinal or small colon mesentery that have the potential to create a strangulation obstruction in the future, and these should be addressed. Conversely, horses presenting with a pedunculated lipoma may have enterolithiasis concurrently. Congenital anomalies such as mesodiverticular bands may be present without having any effect for the horse's entire life but are removed as a matter of course during an exploratory celiotomy.

Specific Conditions Encountered in Older Horses Undergoing Exploratory Celiotomy

Neoplasia

Gastric squamous cell carcinoma may be recognized during an exploratory celiotomy. Most of these horses tend to present as weight loss cases and are diagnosed prior to a laparotomy by endoscopy or ultrasonography or laparoscopy. Other neoplasias such as lymphoma, melanomas, adenocarcinomas, and fibromas have all been encountered during exploratory celiotomy. If the mass is individual and resectable, it is removed. If there are multiple or nonresectable masses, they should be biopsied if possible. Use of intra-abdominal ultrasonography facilitates biopsy by demonstrating the nature of the mass and the presence of vascular structures that should be avoided during the biopsy procedure. Intra-abdominal neoplasia (excluding lipomas) in horses undergoing exploratory celiotomy for colic in our practice has been relatively rare (<2%) (AT Fischer, unpublished data, 2003, Chino, CA). Part of the low frequency of intra-abdominal neoplasia may be due to the fact that most horses with intra-abdominal neoplasia are diagnosed with a combination of laparoscopy and abdominal ultrasonography, precluding the need for an exploratory celiotomy.

Stomach

Lesions of the stomach are uncommon and include neoplasia or impactions. Gastric impactions may be either primary or secondary to a distal lesion. Gastric impactions are typically managed by frequent administration of oral fluids by nasogastric intubation after surgery until clearance of the impaction is confirmed by endoscopy. Surgical evacuation of the stomach appears to be impractical at this point owing to the massive contamination of the abdominal cavity that occurs.

Small Intestinal Lesions

Pedunculated lipomas causing a strangulation obstruction appear to be the most common cause of strangulation obstruction of the small intestine in the geriatric equine undergoing colic surgery. In some horses, reduction of the incarceration may be difficult due to the tightness of the incarceration and the relative shortness of the stalk of the lipoma. I have found it useful to sever the stalk of the lipoma within the abdomen to allow reduction of the incarceration. Mesenteric blood vessels may be in proximity to the stalk and may be injured doing this. The mesentery where the lipoma originated as well as the rest of the involved mesentery must be assessed for damage after this. Once the strangulation obstruction is reduced, the affected bowel is removed and the appropriate anastomosis created. It is important to examine the rest of the mesentery to make sure that there are no other lipomas present. If other lipomas are present, they should be removed at this time, if possible.

Other forms of small intestinal strangulation such as epiploic foramen entrapments, gastrosplenic entrapments and volvulus do occur but less frequently in the geriatric horse than pedunculated lipomas (AT Fischer, unpublished data, 2003, Chino, CA). Intussusceptions also occur and may be due to an intramural tumor such as a leiomyoma or other causes of mural damage and decreased motility. The treatment of these lesions is the same as in the younger horse.

Cecum

Primary lesions involving the cecum are not that common in the older horse. Carcinomas involving small parts of the cecum have been diagnosed as incidental findings and resected. Despite their aggressive histologic grade, spread has not been recognized. Typhlitis may occur, as may cecal impactions. Cecal impactions are initially managed by typhlotomy and evacuation. If they recur, cecal bypass techniques are employed.

Large Colon

Obstructing enteroliths are one of the more common reasons to pursue an exploratory celiotomy in geriatric horses in our practice. Most horses with enterolithiasis are identified by radiography and then exploratory surgery is planned after appropriate preoperative stabilization of the horse. The large colon is usually evacuated by introduction of a hose through a pelvic flexure enterotomy to remove the bulk of the digesta oral to the enterolith and allow mobilization of transverse or right dorsal colon enteroliths. The enteroliths are then removed through the pelvic flexure enterotomy if small enough or more commonly through a right dorsal colon enterotomy.

Sand obstructions are commonly seen in older horses in our practice. Medical management is usually first tried for sand obstructions if the horse is not too uncomfortable and there are not signs of clinical deterioration indicating compromise to the bowel wall. Intravenous rehydration combined with oral fluids and the administration of psyllium and mineral oil via nasogastric tube are usually selected as medical therapy. In horses that cannot be treated medically, an exploratory celiotomy is performed and the pelvic flexure is carefully exteriorized. The sand-impacted large colon is very heavy and prone to rupture if not manipulated carefully. Water is carefully introduced and then siphoned off to allow removal of the sand and ingesta admixture. This procedure can be very time consuming and is usually terminated once fluid is felt to be flowing through the transverse colon. It is not necessary to remove all sand from the colon but merely to reinstate the flow of ingesta so the colon can be cleansed by medical methods.

Obstructions by fecaliths are managed similar to enteroliths. The large colon is evacuated by a pelvic flexure enterotomy and the obstructing fecalith is mobilized if possible and removed. Some fecaliths will have to be broken up in situ and then removed if too large. Colonic displacements and torsions also occur, but less frequently in the older population. The management of these lesions is similar to that of young horses.

Small Colon

Fecaliths and enteroliths are the two most common obstructions of the small colon in the older horse. Fecaliths may occasionally be broken down without an enterotomy, but more frequently, an enterotomy is performed directly over the obstructing fecalith to allow its removal. Enteroliths are removed by an enterotomy directly over the site of obstruction. In some horses, the enterolith has damaged the bowel necessitating resection and anastomosis. Pedunculated lipomas may cause strangulating obstructions of the small colon. The lipoma's stalk is transected, allowing reduction of the strangulation obstruction and a segmental resection and anastomosis is created. The blood supply to the small colon is difficult to visualize due to the fat within the mesocolon, making this procedure more difficult than small intestinal resection. Transillumination of the fat with a fiberoptic light source or the use of intraoperative ultrasonography may be used to help locate the vessels.

Postoperative Supportive Therapy

The older horse seems to have less reserve than the younger horse and requires vigilant postoperative monitoring and support. Complications should be treated early and aggressively. Normal postoperative support consisting of broad-spectrum antibiotics are continued for 48 hours after surgery, and nonsteroidal anti-inflammatory drugs are administered throughout hospitalization. Intravenous fluids are administered as necessary based on serial monitoring of PCV, total protein, electrolyte balance, and acid-base status. Plasma from hyperimmunized horses is used to combat endotoxemia and replace protein loss if needed. Return to food is allowed as soon as possible based on the individual horse. Grazing is started as soon as the horse shows an interest in food. Return to full diet then takes place over the next several days. Anorexia appears to be more common in older horses and should be treated early before the horse becomes more catabolic. If there is no problem with motility, force-feeding of a slurried complete feed by nasogastric tube is tried in gradually increasing volumes. For horses that have reflux or motility problems, partial parenteral nutrition can be used.[4] Horses that are able and willing to eat may be supplemented with high-fat supplements to provide increased caloric content to their diet.

Colic surgery in the geriatric equine can be very rewarding for the horse and client, but it is not without complications. The owners should be adequately informed of the procedures necessary and of the appropriate prognosis and financial considerations and should make the appropriate decision for themselves and their horse.

REFERENCES

1. Paradis MR: Demographics of health and disease in the geriatric horse. Vet Clin North Am Equine Pract 18:391, 2002.
2. Proudman CJ, Smith JE, Edwards GB, French NP: Long-term survival of equine surgical colic cases. Part 2: Modelling postoperative survival. Equine Vet J 34:438, 2002.
3. Matthews NS: Anesthetic considerations of the older equine. Vet Clin North Am Equine Pract 18:403, 2002.
4. Zimmel DN: Postoperative parenteral nutritional support for colics. Proc Am Coll Vet Surg 12th Annual:65, 2002.

CHAPTER 12

Geriatric Musculoskeletal Disorders of the Horse

Julie Cary,

Tracy Turner

The aging process confounds healing and exacerbates musculoskeletal disorders in the older horse. Geriatric patients tend to be slower to heal, have less elasticity in soft tissues, and have a diminished capacity for tissue regeneration.[1] Most conditions encountered in the older horse are a culmination of years of athletic activity and are confounded by the horse's individual conformational faults. As such, they are managed and not cured. This chapter discusses the effects of aging on the musculoskeletal system and options for management of the geriatric athletic. As there is limited literature on equine geriatric musculoskeletal disorders, information has been extrapolated from clinical experience and research in other geriatric species.

Diagnosis of problems and determination of effective treatment and management can be challenging in geriatric horses. There is significant interconnectedness in the musculoskeletal system. Damage or degeneration in one area alters the biomechanical forces on the skeletal and soft tissue structures. As an illustration, geriatric horses may show alterations in their gait or balance, which may originate from a variety of locations and causes. The underlying pathology could be muscle weakness due to atrophy, or from neurologic impairment secondary to impingement of spinal nerves from arthritic changes in the axial skeleton. A geriatric horse may also show an altered gait from arthritic conditions in the appendicular skeleton or from altered elasticity and strength in tendons and ligaments. A vicious cycle of overstressing and exacerbating degenerative changes can be initiated. Maintaining a geriatric horse's physical condition, strength, and flexibility is crucial to help promote a functional and comfortable athlete or companion.

Effects of Aging on the Musculoskeletal System

Muscle

A commonly recognized change in older horses is a decrease in muscle mass. Maintaining healthy geriatric horses requires understanding of changes that occur related to musculature with aging. The most obvious cause of a decline in muscle condition is lack of activity. However, research in humans has shown that the age-related decrease in muscle mass with aging is complicated by factors in addition to a decline in physical activity.[2,3]

The change in body composition of geriatric patients relates to their function. The average loss of lean body mass in geriatric humans has been calculated to be 0.24 kg/yr,[3] which could be similar to that of older horses. Body fat progressively increases in older humans,[3,4] although the likelihood of this trend in horses is unknown. It has been noted that males had a greater decline in lean body mass than did females,[3] which is likely related to the effects of testosterone on muscle mass. It would be interesting to note whether a trend between stallions, geldings, and mares could be identified. Exercise dampens but does not halt this decline. Several studies of aged humans indicate that dynamic (running, swimming, cycling) and resistance training can prevent or reduce some of the age-induced decrease in muscle function.[5]

Muscle volume, muscle strength, and aerobic capacity decline with age in a parallel fashion[2] and are reduced by an estimated 20 percent in humans by the age of 65 years.[1] The decline in muscle mass seems closely related to the reduction in the number of muscle fibers. Over an average human lifespan, the loss of muscles fibers is estimated to be one third of the original numbe.[2] This loss appears to be a gradual change in muscle composition until a point (mid-70s) where more dramatic changes are seen. Fast twitch fibers (type II) are reduced in cross-sectional area more than slow twitch fibers. Because fast twitch muscle is about two times the diameter of slow twitch, the decline in muscle volume can be attributable to the loss of fast twitch fiber diameter. Histopathology demonstrated a change in the muscle fiber related to an increase in the denervation and reinnervation process.[2] An active life-style has been recognized to slow the effects of aging on musculature, but exercise does not entirely prevent this age-associated loss of muscle tissue.

In addition to a loss of muscle mass and decreased fiber size, aging in humans is associated with a decrease in capillary numbers and shifts in muscle fiber performance as well as a decline in the enzymes and substrates associated with aerobic exercise.[6] A small but functionally significant reduction in muscle respiratory capacity may be an inevitable consequence of aging.[7] Blood flow to working muscle is a major determinant of working ability. A decrease in the number of capillaries supplying a muscle will contribute to a decline in athletic performance. The degree of capillarity of muscle can be maintained to muscle by vigorous physical activity, which has been shown in studies of elite human masters athletes.[4] However, decreased vascular compliance resulting from changes in vessels with age may limit exercise capacity by limiting blood flow to working muscles.[6] Lehnhard and colleagues found similar changes in the horse related to decreased muscle mass and a shift in muscle fiber profile with a change in the myosin heavy chain resulting in less aerobic capacity.[8]

Endurance capacity declines in a variety of geriatric mammals, although the exact cause is speculative and likely multifactorial, including loss of muscle mass. Attenuated endurance capacity of old age is accompanied by more rapid glycogen depletion during exercise. Endurance training can ameliorate this. The fatigability of elderly muscle is dependent on the recovery period and the efficacy of blood flow. In one study, old rats depleted hepatic and muscle glycogen more slowly during exercise after an endurance training program than before training and had improved endurance.[9]

Along with availability of energy substrate, utilization of adenosine triphosphate may affect exercise capabili-

ties. Research into the amount of mitochondria in muscle of older versus younger patients has been controversial,[2] although a decline in mitochondrial concentration in muscle mass would provide an explanation of decreased endurance capacity. Little is known about the effects of age on the metabolic response of skeletal muscle to exercise in humans and even less is understood in horses. Analysis of working geriatric rat muscle demonstrated a greater depletion of adenosine triphosphate and phosphocreatine and glycogen as well as a greater accumulation of lactate during electrical stimulation of associated nerve fibers stimulating work activity over their younger counterparts.[7] This finding would indicate that energy substrates in muscle were consumed more rapidly in older animals, resulting in a decline in exercise capacity.

Muscle weakness coupled with impaired gait and balance is a problem in humans but has not been documented to occur in older horses, although individual clinical cases may be affected by mild ataxia. Elderly muscle is weaker, more slowly contracting, and more fatigable than young muscle.[10] The loss of contraction force with age is in part due to a decline of functioning motor units and a decrease in type II fiber area.[10] Exercise can effectively postpone functionally important thresholds for loss of function for 10 to 20 years in humans.

Joints

Arthritis is the most common source of musculoskeletal pain,[11] especially in elderly horses. The increasing lifespan of horses increases the chance of injury during its life. Unfortunately, the progression of osteoarthritis in geriatric horses has not been as well defined as in younger horses and in elderly humans. The degeneration of joints from years of use may be exacerbated by conformational faults, previous trauma, joint sepsis, or repetitive microtrauma. Furthermore, shoeing problems, training protocols, and environmental conditions (e.g., poor footing) can speed progression of osteoarthritis. Unattended osteochondral fragments within the joint, precipitated either by trauma (chip fracture) or developmental orthopedic disease (osteochondritis dissecans), result in physical damage to the cartilage, diminishing the resilience of the joint. Failure to address problems early in the progression can lead to osteoarthritis.

The hallmark pathologic feature of osteoarthritis is progressive deterioration of articular cartilage. Signs range from superficial fibrillation of the cartilage to complete erosion. Synovitis and a decrease in joint fluid quality is almost always present in horses with osteoarthritis.[12] Other features include osteophyte formation and subchondral bone sclerosis. Furthermore, osteoarthritis is progressive due to a complex cascade of biochemical and biomechanical alterations. In addition, repetitive microtrauma with inadequate recovery or an abnormal load on the joint can cause inflammation cascading to osteoarthritis.

This progressive deterioration of articular cartilage and the resultant cascade of events further exacerbates problems for geriatric horses. Loss of joint congruity and stability leads to fibrosis of the joint capsule and pain. This results in limited range of motion, which is particularly common in geriatric horses (Figs. 12-1 and 12-2). Sclerosis of subchondral bone results in a signifi-

cant loss of shock absorption, leading to increased trauma to other areas of the limb. Chronic inflammation can diminish the quality of synovial fluid, further decreasing the shock-absorptive capacity in a geriatric joint. Loss of shock-absorptive capacities of the joint fluid may also contribute to the progression of arthritis. It has been shown in humans that the synovial fluid viscosity decreases with age.[1]

Full-thickness cartilage defects repair themselves with fibrocartilage. Fibrocartilage is inferior in its ability to withstand the trauma to weight-bearing areas; however, in many areas of partial or non-weight-bearing,

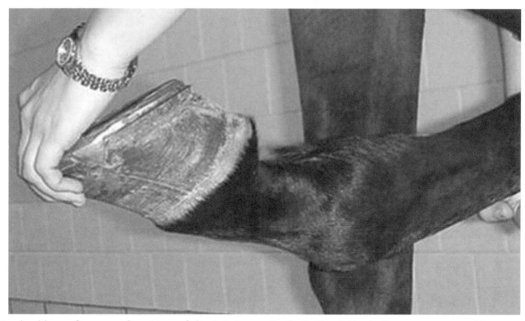

Figure 12-1 Gradual loss of range of motion of the joints, particularly the fetlocks is a common problem seen with aging horses. This is an early case.

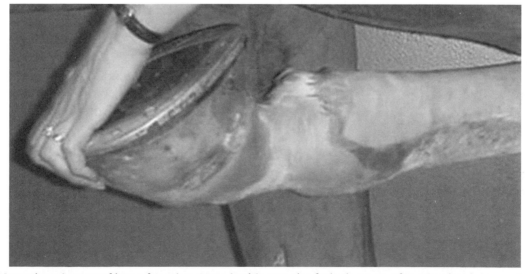

Figure 12-2 More chronic case of loss of motion. Note in this case the fetlock range of motion has been reduced to 10 degrees.

it functions adequately. In humans, advancing age may further affect the cartilage response to damage because the ability to synthesize and assemble matrix micromolecules declines with age.[12]

Osteophytes are considered a hallmark feature of osteoarthritis. The proposed causes of osteophyte formation include wear and tear, mechanical instability, proliferation secondary to synovitis, and response to stretching to synovial membrane at its insertion.[12] Osteophytes can be seen in horses with chemically induced synovitis and in those without evidence of articular cartilage damage. Their removal is generally not justified unless it is interfering with the movement of the joint or has fractured from the parent bone. Additionally, removal of osteophytes may contribute to joint instability.[11]

Understanding of the effects of chronic pain in geriatric patients is at an early stage. Chronic arthritis is known to be a painful condition that can significantly affect the quality of life for human geriatric patients (Fig. 12-3). The pain from osteoarthritis joints originates from multiple areas within the joint and surrounding tissues. Potential sources of pain include the articular cartilage, synovial membrane, joint capsule, and articular ligaments as well as the periosteum, subchondral bone, and changes in intramedullary pressure.[13] Understanding the various sources of pain associated with osteoarthritis allows better understanding of the underlying pathologic condition as well as the best analgesia management options.

The control of pain and inflammation resulting from osteoarthritis, and a subsequent return to soundness, is important to help decrease stress and strain on other parts of the geriatric athlete's musculoskeletal system. Chronic

pain can create significant physiologic and mental stress on a horse. Managing the arthritic conditions in geriatric horses is vital in providing components necessary for an adequate quality of life. Although the most common locations of arthritis include the lower joints of the hock, the pastern, fetlock, carpus, and stifle, it is also possible to see this condition affecting other joints, including the coffin joint, elbow, shoulder, and hip. Few campaigners avoid being plagued by this condition, which dictates that the veterinarian have an appropriate arsenal of treatment and management options.

It must be cautioned that there can be nonprogressive degenerative changes that are incidental findings. It is vital that the clinician be able to determine lesions that are of clinical significance over those that are merely the jewelry of a decorated athlete. For further information, the authors recommend several well-written articles and texts on the pathophysiology of joint disease.[12, 13]

Tendons and Ligaments

The effects of aging on the structure and integrity of tendons and ligaments in geriatric patients are currently being elucidated. There is a recognized trend for reduced connective tissue elasticity[1] and subsequent alterations in tendon strength and ability to store energy.[14] Progressive deterioration of the matrix structure also occurs, increasing the risk of damage to the tendon or ligament. Additionally, the repair of tendons or ligaments resulting in dystrophic calcification rather than collagenous tissue will further decrease the tissue's resilience, elasticity, and strength.

In the horse, the superficial digital flexor tendon and suspensory ligament are the most commonly studied ligamentous structures (Fig. 12-4). The superficial digital flexor tendon matures early in life, and with advancing age seems to have a limited ability to adapt to stress and undergoes progressive deterioration.[14-16] This is probably most confined to the central portion of the tendon, where focal hypocellularity, collagen fibril degeneration, and alteration in the noncollagenous matrix are noted.[15] The tendon increases in stiffness with age, which is thought to be related to the progressive elimination of the crimp within the fascicles of the tendon[15] as well as the presence of more rigid crosslinks and decreasing fascicle size.[15] As horses age, there are increasing areas in the tendon which become avascular,[17] which may further exacerbate other degenerative changes seen within the tendon.

Progressive degeneration of the suspensory ligament in the hind limbs has been noted in geriatric horses, particularly older broodmares (Figs. 12-5 and 12-6).[18] It has been associated with straight hock conformation with or without hyperextension of the fetlocks. Affected horses appear to have an aberrant healing response within the

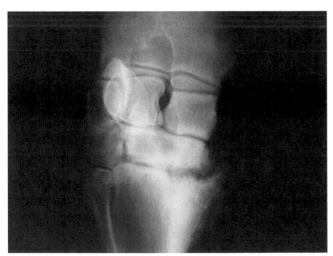

Figure 12-3 Carpometacarpal disease in an aged Arabian mare. The disease can affect any breed but is seen more commonly in Arabians. Onset usually begins in the middle to late teens and gradually becomes worse. The cause is not known but it always starts between the C2/MC2 articulation.

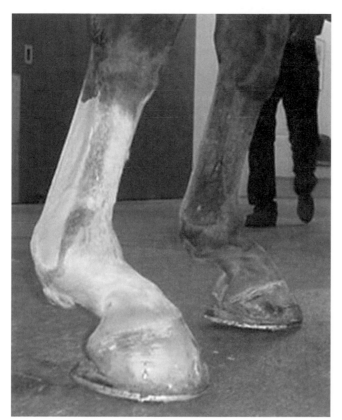

Figure 12-4 Degenerative suspensories in the front limbs of an older horse. The condition is almost always bilateral, affecting front limb and rear limbs with the same frequency.

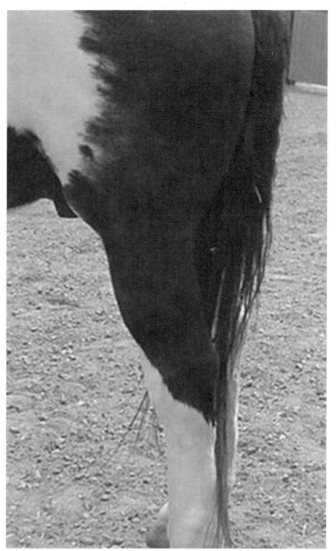

Figure 12-5 In many older horses, the rearlimb conformation gradually becomes straighter through the hock and stifle. This precedes the suspensory degeneration seen in Figure 12-6.

suspensory ligament.[16] During the degenerative process, individual bundles of collagen fuse. The fibroblasts in the center of the resultant large bundles have a diminished blood supply, which results in death or transformation into chondrocytes, resulting in cartilage-like tissue filling the defect.[16] Eventually, the ligament becomes inelastic and has less ability to provide support, leading to progressive sinking of the fetlock,[16] leading in turn to abnormal stresses and diminished support of the joint.

The ability of the tendon to adapt to musculoskeletal stresses declines dramatically after maturity.[15] Tendon matrix appears to undergo age-related degeneration. This is seen as patchy acellularity within the tendon matrix fibrillation, chondroid metaplasia, chondrome formation, neovascularization, and fibroplasia.[15] Cartilage oligomeric matrix protein is thought to play a role in the structure of tendons and has been shown to undergo an age-related decrease in concentration.[15,17] The ability to heal and the quality of repair of tendon injuries may be related to the levels of cartilage oligomeric matrix protein.

Further strain on the tendon can be caused by fatigue, lack of fitness, or loss of muscle tone in the older horse. Continued, regular exercise can modify some of the deleterious effects of aging on tendons and ligaments in geriatric mammals.[19]

Axial Skeleton

Pathologic changes to the axial skeleton in older equine patients are not uncommon. Spondyloarthropathy in Equidae was one of the most common forms of arthritis recognized in fossils from 40 million years ago.[20] Erosive spondyloarthropathy has been determined to be increasing in frequency by three to six times since antiquity, which leads to some speculation that its persistence may provide evidence that spondyloarthropathy may actually provide some type of evolutionary benefit.[20] Osteoarthritis progressing to ankylosis of the spinal column is noted in many geriatric patients, although the clinical significance of this condition is not completely understood.

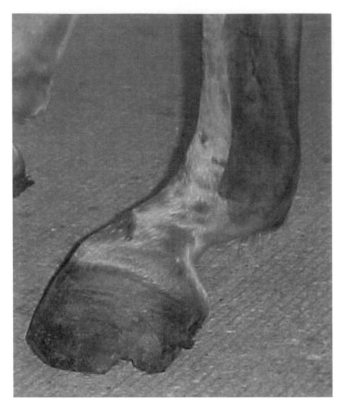

Figure 12-6 Rear lower limb conformation of an older horse suffering from degenerative suspensory desmitis. Note the severe "dropping," hyperextension of the fetlock.

The occurrence of spondylosis deformans seems to be relatively frequent in the older equine population. Ankylosis or degenerative disease of vertebral joints results in large osteophytes, which span the intervertebral disk between vertebral bodies. The equine thoracolumbar spine is predisposed to chronic proliferation at the ventrolateral vertebral body margins.[21,22] This is likely a result tearing of the outer annular fibers and degeneration of the annulus fibrosis and periarticular tissues from microtrauma. Spondylosis deformans at this site can result in compression of nerve roots or impingement on the spinal cord. The change in structure also results in altered transfer of normal forces through the vertebral column. Spondylosis is initially insidious and subclinical unless the bone callus fractures, causing pain, or an episode of inflammation resulting in spinal cord or nerve impingement occurs. The occurrence of spondylosis deformans has been thought to exist in mares more frequently than geldings or stallions, although this is of questionable occurrence.

Articular process osteoarthritis can also be seen in the geriatric horse most commonly in the lumbar region. Osteoarthritis in this area may significantly alter the biomechanics of the vertebral column. However, there is debate on the significance of this condition in the horse. Articular process osteoarthritis is recognized as a significant course of pain in humans.[21] Degeneration of the articular facets and articular processes in the cervical region of older horses has been recognized as a significant source of pain and, depending on the degree of proliferation, may even contribute to impingement on the spinal cord, resulting in neurologic deficits.[21]

The sacroiliac region can undergo changes related to advancing age in the horse. Degenerative changes of the sacroiliac ligament are common and can cause pain and alter the biomechanics of the way the horse moves. Fusion of the sacrum to the first caudal vertebrae can also occur in older horses with regular frequency, although the clinical significance of this is unknown.

Other changes that have been seen in geriatric horses include intervertebral disk degeneration. Owing to the structure of the intervertebral disks, herniation of disk material is believed to be relatively rare. Changes in musculature and soft tissue attachments, as well as a predisposition to the problem in relation to the skeletal shape or a career as a brood mare can contribute to the development of lordosis. The classic "sway-back" horse does not show clinical signs related to the abnormal shape of the back. The significant alteration of biomechanics caused by lordosis is likely underestimated and epaxial musculature strengthening exercises should be regularly utilized to slow the progression. Lordosis may increase the strain on the sacroiliac joint.

Overall, the morbidity of axial skeleton degenerative changes in the geriatric horse is unknown. These types of changes are known to be a source of significant pain in humans and can contribute to perceived quality of life significantly. Close scrutiny of our geriatric patients may reveal a higher incidence of clinically significant back and neck problems.

Exercise Programs as Therapy for Old-Age Related Changes

It is vital to maintain overall fitness in older horses. Creating a balance between endurance, strength, and flexibility can help maintain geriatric patient's quality of life and functional ability beyond that of their less active counterparts. The interconnectedness of the muscles, ligaments and tendons, bones, and joints cannot be overstated. A weakness in one part of the musculoskeletal system may predispose a horse to injury in another part. As an example, an imbalance in muscle strength can ultimately cascade to pain. Muscle or ligamentous strain across a joint has been reported as a major cause of osteoarthritis. Pain in a peripheral joint acts centrally to alter the horse's way of going, which can cascade into further imbalance and pain. As research has convincingly shown in humans, regular exercise can increase the average lifespan of individuals, as well as the quality of life, while postponing critical functional thresholds.[2]

Inactivity can be the most traumatic event in a geriatric lifespan. The functional changes that take place with inactivity can be more detrimental than those that coincide with the aging process. Functional changes associated with inactivity include reduced aerobic fitness, loss of postural reflexes, altered lipid metabolism, negative energy balance, loss of muscle mass, and osteopenia in humans.[1] Complete stall rest should be avoided, and when unavoidable, a return to exercise should take place as soon as possible.

In one human study, by the age of 80 years, 1 to 2 years of additional life had been attributed to exercise.[1] The idea of lengthening the lifespan of horses through exercise is interesting. Although horses do not tend to make the poor life-style choices that their human counterparts do, remaining active late into life will help improve muscle tone and flexibility. Physical adaptations that are made with exercise include increased bone density, improved flexibility and range of motion, increased muscle tone and strength, and improved coordination.

Training can improve not only muscle strength but also the quality of muscle function, although some degree of age-related degeneration is inevitable. Endurance exercise helps promote capillary migration into muscle tissue, which can provide better blood supply for more optimal function of the muscle tissue. Maintenance of good muscle tone and strength will help absorb forces that would be absorbed by joints, tendons, and ligaments and by the axial skeleton. Muscle mass, muscle respiratory capacity, metabolic responses, and exercise performance is different between young and older trained men, suggesting that endurance training cannot completely prevent changes in these variables.[7]

The inclusion of an exercise prescription or training program in the veterinarian's care of geriatric equine patients should be considered. It is important to tailor this program to each individual horse with consideration of other conditions occurring in the horse such as chronic obstructive pulmonary disease, cardiac problems, or musculoskeletal conditions. The exercise program should be tailored to each patient and to the owner's expectations and abilities.

An exercise prescription should begin with a pre-exercise assessment, which includes identifying the goals of the exercise program, performance expectations, and a medical history including pertinent information on any lameness concerns. Critical information for the exercise prescription is obtained thorough a physical and lameness examination and an assessment of the fitness level. Annual re-evaluation should be employed to optimize the effect of the prescription without creating undue stresses on other parts of the musculoskeletal system. Any lameness or physical problem noted should be addressed as quickly as possible to avoid creation of further areas of pain or stiffness as compensation for the primary site.

The exercise prescription should include recommendations on the intensity, duration, frequency, mode, and progression of exercise.[1] Intensity generally will be a subjective measurement of perceived exertion on the part of the rider or trainer. The use of heart rate monitors can improve the accuracy of determining intensity, as can measuring heart rate immediately after exercise to help minimize overexertion. In general, the duration of a given activity that is being performed should be inversely related to the intensity of activity. It has been recognized that in elderly human athletes, there may be a greater benefit of shorter bouts of exercise (5-10 minutes) at a lower intensity performed on a more frequent basis.[1] This is probably a good rule of thumb for the older equine athlete. Free exercise with a herd of similar horses may allow this type of exercise to occur naturally. Frequency of exercise is variable in the geriatric population and is dependent on many management and intrinsic factors. The final component of exercise prescription is progression. The dynamic process of the exercise plan includes three stages: initial conditioning, improvement, and maintenance.

Older horses have a diminished capacity to recover from exercise and their need for adequate warm-up, cool down, and stretching routines cannot be overemphasized. Stretching to improve flexibility is important in any exercise prescription, and the exercises should be performed at least three times weekly. Good warm-up in geriatric horses is vital, as it enhances blood flow to the muscles providing increased levels of oxygen and energy substrate,[23] which is especially critical in muscle that is undergoing aging-related changes.

When designing programs, it is important to remember that exercise programs that are appropriate for younger animals may not be appropriate for older equine athletes. Currently, there are almost no data regarding the adjustments in training programs that might be warranted in aged horses. Good communication between the veterinarian, owner, and trainer is important to optimize the exercise program for geriatric horses.

Nutrition

Optimal nutrition is important to help maintain geriatric equine athletes. Unfortunately, relatively little attention has been paid to optimal diets of geriatric athletes. Each horse is an individual. Some horses simply require a high-quality hay diet to maintain body condition, whereas others need special considerations. A complete blood cell count and full biochemical panel should be performed on geriatric horses on a regular basis to rule out renal or hepatic dysfunction before making feeding recommendations.[24] Horse with evidence of pituitary dysfunction (Cushing's disease) should also be identified and fed a lower level of carbohydrates and sweet feed in an attempt to avoid complications such as laminitis. Geriatric horse may require age-specific formulated feedstuffs that are designed for easy digestibility if there are dentition or digestion concerns.

The National Research Council nutritional recommendations are general guidelines for the average horse and may not accurately reflect the needs of geriatric athletes.[25] Individual variation occurs as well as changes in each individual secondary to extrinsic and intrinsic factors. Supplementation of geriatric athletes with a high-quality vitamin and mineral supplement formulated to complement their feeding regimen is recommended. Specific nutritional therapies may include increased supplementation of vitamin E if there is muscle pathology or glucosamine and vitamin C for osteoarthritic changes.[25]

Levels of vitamin C (plasma ascorbic acid) are low in geriatric horses.[26] Vitamin C plays a role in collagen synthesis and in protecting against the free-radical damage to joints.[25] As a potentially important component in the development of osteoarthritis, there is evidence that vitamin C should be supplemented in the geriatric horse's diet. Two recommendations for supplementation were found that included 10 grams twice daily[24] or 30 to 40 mg/kg daily.[27] Antioxidants may have a protective role in the control of arthritis, as free radicals may play a part in the development of arthritis. If the horse is fed fresh grass or good-quality fresh hay, there should be ample antioxidants in the diet to provide protection from free radicals. Examples of antioxidants that may be needed include Mn, Cu, Se, Zn, vitamin C, vitamin A, vitamin E, and beta carotene.[25] Additional recommendations for the addition of supplemental vitamin E have been made for protection of muscle tissue.

Alternative energy sources such as fat provide a good energy source for the geriatric athlete without carrying the risk of laminitis or exacerbation of endocrine-associated problems. Palatability is an important consideration in geriatric diets, especially if there is a decreased appetite as a result of chronic pain. Chronic pain can change the metabolic demand of a horse as well as exacerbate problems with the diet,[24] and the practitioner should pay special attention to relieve suffering.[28]

Pain Management and Other Treatment Options

Pain is a major hallmark feature of osteoarthritis, as well as some of the other changes associated with aging. Because most aging changes are currently thought to be irreversible, the majority of treatment options are focused on palliation of pain and on slowing the progression of the disease condition. Control of pain reduces the detrimental physiologic effects of pain, prevents changes in behavior such as depression, and therefore reduces the morbidity associated with painful degenerative conditions such as osteoarthritis. In addition to controlling the pain, other treatment goals including optimizing function of the athlete as well as attempting to ameliorate the degenerative process, and as technology advances, aiding in the repair process or reversing the degeneration.

A staple of management of pain-inducing musculoskeletal disorders in the horse includes the use of nonsteroidal anti-inflammatory drugs (NSAIDs). In addition to phenylbutazone, aspirin, ibuprofen, flunixin meglumine, ketoprofen, carprofen, etodolac, and meloxicam are options for treatment of geriatric arthritic conditions.[11,29] While NSAIDs can be used judiciously without serious side effects for years, it must not be forgotten that there are potential detrimental consequences with their use, including oral, gastric, and duodenal ulceration; colitis; and renal papillary necrosis as well as altered clotting times.[29] These complications may be amplified in the geriatric horse. Certainly, it may be indicated to use gastrointestinal protective agents in an attempt to avoid the complications of NSAID administration. Most importantly, an attempt should be made to use the lowest effective dose of an NSAID necessary to control pain in geriatric horses, as their metabolism for the drug can be altered, and individual patient variation must be accounted for. As more specific cyclooxygenase inhibitors become available, the treatment of musculoskeletal pain in geriatric horses will become safer. Unfortunately, cyclo-oxygenase (COX)-2 selective compounds still inhibit the physiologically important COX-1 at various levels and may still result in adverse side effects.[29]

In most situations, NSAIDs are effective at controlling pain. However, adjunctive therapies are available to optimize the athletic function of a geriatric horse. Intra-articular therapy is a viable method of treating pain caused by progressive osteoarthritis. Along with providing palliation from pain, it is also possible to improve the joint environment with intra-articular medication. Options for intra-articular medications include steroids and chondroprotective agents. Additionally, other nutraceuticals and herbs are available for treatment of musculoskeletal disorders in geriatric horses.

Steroids can exert a protective effect in diminishing the amount of inflammation present in a joint, thereby decreasing the inflammatory mediators, which contribute to cartilage breakdown. The use of methylprednisolone acetate is supported by clinical findings. Unfortunately, in a high motion osteochondral fragment model trial, the use of methylprednisolone acetate intra-articularly failed to demonstrate a significant clinical improvement and resulted in deleterious effects on the cartilage in the joint.[11] In a similar clinical trial, triamcinolone was found to have a favorable effect on the lameness score while proving to be chondroprotective.[11] The authors feel that methylprednisolone acetate is a good option for low motion joints where the goal is not preservation of the articular cartilage. Triamcinolone is considered a superior steroid option for high motion joints when used judiciously and often in combination with hyaluronic acid. The possibility of steroid-induced arthropathy, laminitis, or exacerbation of other medical conditions in the geriatric patient must be considered and weighed against the benefits of the intra-articular administration of steroids. The recommended dose of methylprednisolone acetate is 40 to 80 mg/site and triamcinolone 3 to 12 mg/site with a maximum of 16 mg for the entire horse.

The use of chondroprotective agents, such as hyaluronic acid and polysulfated glucosaminoglycan, in geriatric horses is somewhat controversial. The substances are commonly used as "insurance" for the cartilage and joint environment. Although there are no known side effects, it is not always possible to determine whether the agents are providing a protective or reparative role in the joints. These substances are able to decrease inflammation, although less effectively than steroids or NSAIDs, while providing the necessary constituents for the matrix of the components of the joint, synovial fluid, and tendons and ligaments.[25] Hyaluronan has analgesic properties with an unknown mechanism of action,[12] and polysulfated glucosaminoglycan may have a similar effect in ameliorating pain. Intra-articular hyaluronan has been found to be chondroprotective and provides viscosupplementation.[11] Intravenous hyaluronan has been found to decrease the severity of clinical lameness both in experimental models and in clinical cases without any adverse side effects.[11] Polysulfated glucosaminoglycans have historically been used to provide the components of matrix for cartilage repair. The potential for joint flares and the potentiation of subclinical infections when used intra-articularly has convinced many practitioners to restrict its use to intramuscular administration.

Oral supplementation with good-quality glucosamine and chondroitin provides the building blocks required for the synthesis of GAGs. Human trials have demonstrated a decrease in pain and improved range of motion of joints with the use of oral joint supplements over placebo.[11] Geriatric horses likely benefit from the administration of these substances as the production of glucosaminoglycans likely declines with age, which may be one reason that older joints are more prone to arthritis. Ligaments and tendons may also benefit from the basic matrix components supplied in the joint protectants. Additionally, as was mentioned previously, there is evidence that joint lubrication declines with age. The administration of substances containing GAGs is thought to improve the quality of joint fluid, which is of benefit to geriatric equine athletes.

Other ingredients that may be beneficial in joint supplements include manganese, copper, vitamin C, yucca, perna mussel, and MSM (methyl sulphonyl methane), which is a derivative of dimethyl sulfoxide (DMSO). The gold standard in veterinary medicine among the oral supplements is Cosequin, which is a combination of glucosamine hydrochloride, chondroitin sulfate, manganese, and vitamin C. There are a huge number of products available to treat joint conditions in horses. The authors recommend that owners treat horses with oral supplements for a minimum of 3 months to determine whether a noticeable change occurs. Unfortunately, it may be difficult to detect whether the administration of joint supplements is beneficial to the articular environment and potentially increasing the longevity of the joints.

As an adjunctive analgesic therapy, Devil's Claw (*Harpogophytum procumbens*) is an herb included in several different formulations intended to provide pain relief to horses. The herb is used as both an anti-inflammatory and an analgesic. The herb has been noted to have dramatic effects on many horses in the authors' practice, who were unable to tolerate chronic administration of NSAIDs. Of the principal constituents of the Devil's Claw, the iridoid glycosides have been investigated, focusing in particular on the anti-inflammatory effects. Little documented research is available on the use of this herb in the management of geriatric musculoskeletal issues, although anecdotally there is support for its use.

Capsaicin, a substance found in hot peppers, has been used to manage musculoskeletal pain. The substance excites C fibers leading to the release and subsequent depletion of substance P from afferent nerves. Prolonged exposure leads to analgesia due to lack of neurotransmitter. Topical application can help focal sources of pain in geriatric horses.[30]

Acupuncture, massage, and chiropractics can potentially be of benefit to geriatric equine athletes. Acupuncture is effective in providing pain relief by normalizing pain hypersensitivity, balancing energy flow, and providing endogenous opioid release.[30] Chiropractics is focused on the interaction between neurologic mechanisms and the biomechanics of the spine.[31] Massage addresses the musculoskeletal system by increasing circulation, releasing scar tissue, balancing muscle function, and providing relaxation.[32] Each of these modalities addresses the entire horse and may provide significant benefit in terms of function and comfort of the athlete. The authors recommend that individuals become trained in acupuncture, massage, or chiropractics, or to refer cases to trained individuals for treatment.

Recent attention has been focused on the analgesic and reparative benefits of extracorporeal shock wave therapy. While there is significant anecdotal evidence of its effects on musculoskeletal concerns such as distal hock joint arthritis and proximal suspensory injuries, at the time of this writing no definitive research efforts have been made to determine the mechanism and effectiveness of analgesia.

Good-quality shoeing with attention to support and ease of breakover will benefit many horses with arthritis or other orthopedic conditions. Often, close attention to regular trimming and hoof care will be all that is required to provide optimal farrier care to geriatric equine athletes. An extended heel shoe may be required to support the limb of a horse with suspensory degeneration. By the time full support from a patten shoe is required, the horse's athletic career has ended.

Surgical intervention in geriatric horses is rarely indicated. Arthrodesis of low motion joints, such as the proximal interphalangeal and distal tarsal joints may improve the functional life of a horse with significant arthritic changes in these areas. It should be cautioned that geriatric horses may be slower to heal, increasing the length of time to return to work. Twelve to 18 months of convalescent time may prove to be detrimental to the older athlete due to the significant inactivity that occurs during this time. Arthroscopy may be indicated in cases in which an acute change in the joint is causing significant problems. Uncommonly, osteophytes may fracture off the parent bone and become osseous fragments within the joint, leading to a worsening of arthritic changes. In such a situation, retrieval of the fragment via arthroscopy may be in the horse's best interest. If there is significant inflammation within a joint or tendon sheath, significant clinical improvement may be seen simply with a thorough lavage to the joint removing detrimental inflammatory mediators.

The creation of a balanced pain management program for geriatric equine athletes should include a veterinarian's evaluation. The synergistic effects of NSAIDs, chondroprotective anti-inflammatory agents, and regular exercise and stretching as well as massage, acupuncture, and chiropractics in addition to veterinary administered adjunctive therapies will help ensure optimal longevity in athletic activity and quality of life. With our current understanding of the adverse effects of chronic pain and the analgesic agents available, no geriatric horse should be without a veterinary-based pain management plan.

REFERENCES

1. Barry HC, Eathorne SW: Exercise and aging: Issues for the practitioner. Med Clin North Am 78:357, 1994.
2. Grimby G: Physical activity and muscle training in the elderly. Act Med Scand Suppl 711:233, 1986.
3. Forbes GB, Reina JC: Adult lean body mass declines with age: Some longitudinal observations. Metabolism 19:653, 1970.
4. Pollock ML, Foster C, Knapp D, et al: Effect of age and training on aerobic capacity and body composition of master athletes. J Appl Physiol 62:725, 1987.
5. McKeever KH, Malinowski K: Exercise capacity in young and old mares. AJVR 58:1468, 1997.
6. White T: Skeletal muscle structure and function in older mammals. In Lamb DR, Gisolfi CV, Nadel E, editors: Perspectives in Exercise and Sports Medicine. Vol 8, Exercise in Older Adults. Carmel, IN, Cooper Publishing, 1995.
7. Coggan AR, Abduljalil AM, Swanson SC, et al: Muscle metabolism during exercise in young and older untrained and endurance-trained men. J Appl Physiol 75:2125, 1993.
8. Lehnhard RA, McKeever KH, Kearns CF, et al: Myosin heavy chain is different in old versus young Standardbred mares. Med Sci Sports Exer 32:S13, 2001.
9. Cartee GD, Farrar RP: Exercise training induced glycogen sparing during exercise by old rats. J Appl Physiol 64:259, 1988.
10. Davies CTM, Thomas DO, White MJ: Mechanical properties of young and elderly human muscle. Acta Med Scand Suppl 711:219, 1986.
11. McIlwraith CW: Diseases of joints, tendons, ligaments, and related structures. In Stashak TS, editor: Adam's Lameness in Horses, 5th ed. Philadelphia, Lippincott Williams & Wilkins, 2002.
12. McIlwraith CW: General pathobiology of the joint and response to injury. In McIlwraith CW, Trotter GW, editors: Joint Disease in the Horse. Philadelphia, W.B. Saunders, 1996.
13. Palmer JL, Bertone AL: Joint biomechanics in the pathogenesis of traumatic arthritis. In McIlwraith CW, Trotter GW, editors: Joint Disease in the Horse. Philadelphia, W.B. Saunders, 1996.
14. Gillis C, Sharkey N, Stover SM, et al: Effect of maturation and aging on material and ultrasonographic properties of equine superficial digital flexor tendon. Am J Vet Res 56:1345, 1995.
15. Dowling BA, Dart AJ, Hodgson DR, et al.: Superficial digital flexor tendonitis in the horse. Equine Vet J 32:369, 2000.
16. Pool RR: Pathologic changes in tendinitis of athletic horses. In Rantanen NW, Hauser ML, editors: Proceedings of the 1st Dubai International Equine Symposium, Dubai Equine International Symposium, United Arab Emirates, 1996.
17. Smith RKW, Gerard M, Dowling B, et al: Correlation of cartilage oligomeric matrix protein (COMP) levels in equine tendon with mechanical properties: A proposed role for COMP in determining function-specific mechanical characteristics of locomotor tendons. Equine Vet J Suppl 34:241, 2002.
18. Dyson SJ, Arthur RM, Palmer SE, et al: Suspensory Ligament Desmitis. Vet Clin North Am 11:177, 1995.
19. Nielsen HM, Skalicky M, Viidik A: Influence of physical exercise on aging rats. III. Life-long exercise modified the aging changes of the mechanical properties of limb muscle tendons. Mech Ageing Dev 100:243, 1998.
20. Rothschild BM, Prothero DR, Rothschild C: Origins of spondyloarthropathy in Perissodactyla. Clin Exp Rheumatol 19:628, 2001.

21. Haussler KH: Osseous spinal pathology. Vet Clin North Am 15:103, 1999.
22. Jeffcott LB: Disorders of the thoracolumbar spine of the horse—a survey of 443 cases. Equine Vet J 12:197, 1980.
23. Rokuroda S, Lawrence L, Pratt S, et al: Metabolic effects of warm-up on exercising horses. In Pagan JD, Geor RJ, editors: Advances in Equine Nutrition II. Nottingham, UK, Nottingham University Press, 2001.
24. Ralston SL: Management of geriatric horse. In Pagan JD, Geor RJ, editors: Advances in Equine Nutrition II. Nottingham, UK, Nottingham University Press, 2001.
25. Kendall RV: Basic and preventative nutrition for the cat, dog, and horse. In Shoen AM, Wynn SG, editors: Complementary and Alternative Veterinary Medicine. St Louis, Mosby, 1998.
26. Ralston SL, Nockels CF, Squires EL: Differences in diagnostic test results and hematologic data between aged and young horses. Am J Vet Res 49:1387, 1988.
27. Saastamoinen MT: Vitamin requirements and supplementation in athletic horse. In Pagan JD, Geor RJ, editors: Advances in Equine Nutrition II. Nottingham, UK, Nottingham University Press, 2001.
28. Pugh DG: Feeding the geriatric horse. AAEP Proc 48:21, 2002.
29. Moses VS, Bertone AL: Nonsteroidal anti-inflammatory drugs. Vet Clin Equine 18:21, 2002.
30. Fleming P: Equine acupuncture. In Shoen AM, Wynn SG, editors: Complementary and Alternative Veterinary Medicine. St Louis, Mosby, 1998.
31. Willoughby S: Chiropractic care. In Shoen AM, Wynn SG, editors: Complementary and Alternative Veterinary Medicine. St Louis, Mosby, 1998.
32. Porter M, Bromley M: Massage therapy. In Shoen AM, Wynn SG, editors: Complementary and Alternative Veterinary Medicine. St Louis, Mosby, 1998.

CHAPTER 13

Neoplasia

Beth A. Valentine

The reported incidence of neoplasia in the horse varies depending on the type of study. Cotchin[1] reported an incidence of approximately 1 percent to 3 percent in horses undergoing surgery and 11 percent in horses examined at slaughter. Kerr and Alden[2] reported an incidence of 26 percent in biopsy material and 4.4 percent in necropsy studies, with a combined incidence of 12.6 percent. The four most common equine neoplasms reported by Kerr and Alden[2] were sarcoid (39.9%), squamous cell carcinoma (12%), melanoma (5.7%), and lipoma (5.7%). All of these tumors except sarcoid occurred most often in horses older than 9 years of age.

In all species, increasing age is clearly a factor that increases susceptibility to neoplasia. In part, this is due to the multistep pathogenesis that underlies most neoplastic processes. With increasing age, there is greater exposure to potential carcinogens, greater likelihood of a genetic alteration within a dividing cell that could lead to neoplasia, and diminished cellular DNA repair capacity. It is difficult, however, to determine what defines "geriatric" as it applies to equine neoplasia. If this discussion were confined only to those tumors occurring almost exclusively in horses older than 15 years of age, this would be a short section indeed. Pituitary and thyroid adenomas and intra-abdominal lipomas are among the few tumors that occur only in aged horses. For many neoplastic processes in the horse, "tumor age" is achieved by 6 to 8 years of age. Rather than trying to define "geriatric" as it applies to equine neoplasia, this section focuses on tumors that occur in middle-aged to aged horses. In some cases, reference is made to identical or related tumors in young horses.

Descriptions are given with an emphasis on clinical and clinicopathologic findings. Although the gross appearance of a tumor may be strongly suggestive of a particular diagnosis, it is vitally important to submit excised masses for pathologic evaluation. When it comes to tumors, looks can be deceiving.

Tumors and Tumor-Like Lesions of the Skin, Subcutis, and Skeletal Muscle

Tumors involving the skin, subcutis, and skeletal muscle are clearly the most common form of equine neoplasia. They are also the most obvious tumors, causing visibly and palpably apparent lesions. Those involving skin and subcutis are generally accessible to diagnostic testing, including cytologic and histopathologic evaluation. Those involving deeper skeletal muscle present more of a diagnostic and surgical challenge.

Melanocytic Tumors

Aged gray horses are prone to development of a unique form of melanoma. The dermal melanoma of aging gray horses can occur as one to several discrete masses, or as multiple confluent nodular masses, a condition known as *melanomatosis* (Fig. 13-1).[3] These tumors typically occur in gray horses older than 6 years of age and are most common in breeds such as Arabian, Thoroughbred, Andalusian, Lipizzaner, Percheron, Irish Draught, Shire, and Welsh pony in which gray hair color is common. Most studies find no sex predisposition.

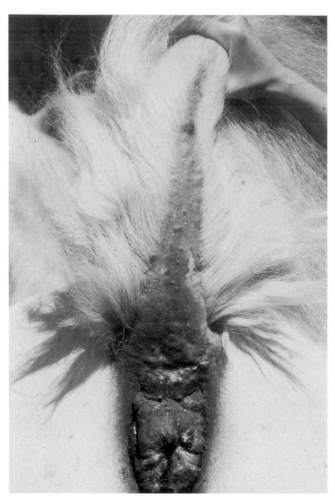

Figure 13-1 Multiple cutaneous melanomas characteristic of melanomatosis on the underside of the tail and perineal region of an aged gray horse. (Courtesy of Dr. Betsy Graham.)

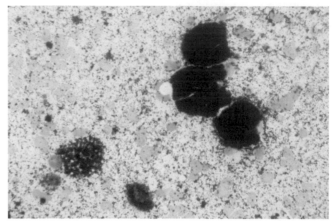

Figure 13-2 Cytologic findings of melanin-pigmented cells and background melanin granules are characteristic of melanoma of aging gray horses.

Gray horse melanomas typically occur in one or more specific areas, including the perineum, underside of the base of the tail, prepuce, commissure of the lips, and in the parotid gland region. Tumors are covered by pigmented alopecic skin, and are often not freely moveable due to invasion into deeper tissues. Dark brown to black melanin pigment is readily appreciated on section and on cytologic (Fig. 13-2) and histopathologic preparations. Melanin can also stain green in cytologic preparations stained with Wright stain.

Although slowly growing, these tumors are locally invasive and, if given enough time, will often metastasize to muscle fascia and internal organs. Metastasis, however, may or may not be associated with clinical signs of organ dysfunction. Many aged gray horses with metastatic melanoma die of causes unrelated to their tumors. Depression, weight loss, colic, and peripheral edema are the most common clinical signs in horses with metastatic melanoma.[4] Rectal palpation and ultrasonography are useful for detection of internal tumors. The finding of melanin pigmented cells, which may be either neoplastic

melanocytes or associated melanophages, in biopsy or cytology samples of internal masses, or in cytologic preparations of thoracic or abdominal fluid, confirms the diagnosis of metastatic melanoma.

Surgical excision, when possible, is the treatment of choice. Excision of discrete tumors can be curative.[3] Only debulking may be possible when very large tumors are present, and complete surgical excision is not possible in cases of melanomatosis. Cryonecrosis can result in reduction in the size of large melanomas. Oral cimetidine (2.5 mg/kg tid),[5] or preparation of a melanoma vaccine prepared from an excised tumor (Dr. K. Ann Jeglum, West Chester, PA), have been advocated as potentially useful treatments of gray horse melanomas that are not amenable to surgical excision. But the cost of these treatments is fairly high, and the efficacy is questionable. Such treatments may be best reserved as a "last ditch effort" for owners who are willing to pay the cost and who also realize that a positive response is by no means guaranteed. Continued research into therapy for gray horse melanoma is clearly needed.

An aggressive variant of equine melanoma occurs most commonly in aged non–gray horses, although aged grays may also be affected. These tumors often occur in sites considered atypical of gray horse dermal melanoma, are rapidly growing and invasive, and frequently metastasize early and widely. When present in skin, ulceration is common. Cytologic and histopathologic evaluation will reveal a pleomorphic population of often poorly pigmented melanocytes with frequent mitoses. Epithelial invasion is typical. To date, neither surgical excision nor medical therapy appears to be effective, and the prognosis for such horses is poor.

Squamous Papilloma

Papillary proliferations of epidermis in geriatric horses occur almost exclusively on the genitalia, including the penis, vulva, vestibule, and clitoral fossa. As opposed to papillomas of young horses, tumors in older horses are less likely to express papillomavirus antigens with immunohistochemical testing,[6] and they do not undergo spontaneous regression. In one study of 21 genital papillomas, tumors were most common in males, occurring at a mean age of 11.6 years (range, 7-16 years). Genital papillomas in mares occurred at a slightly younger age, with a mean of 8.7 years (range, 7-10 years).[6]

Tumors are raised, plaque-like or warty, single or multiple unpigmented masses that can be secondarily infected. The characteristic histologic feature of squamous papilloma is proliferative epithelium forming papillary projections with only moderate dysplasia and with no evidence of invasion. Although histologically benign, they are considered to be capable of malignant transformation, and wide surgical excision is the treatment of choice.

Squamous Cell Carcinoma

Squamous cell carcinoma is most common on the genitalia and in the ocular region, oral cavity, and nasal sinuses (see Tumors and Tumor-Like Lesions of the Head) of middle-aged to older horses. Genital squamous cell carcinoma is more common in males than in females, with a mean age at diagnosis of 10.6 years (range, 5-25 years) for males and 12.8 years (range, 8-23 years) for females.[6] In rare cases, squamous cell carcinoma arises in chronic nonhealing skin wounds.

Squamous cell carcinoma appears as a raised or flattened fleshy mass that is often ulcerated and secondarily infected. Cytologic preparations can be difficult to interpret if there is marked inflammation. Many squamous cell carcinomas are very well differentiated, and the distinction between reactive squamous epithelium in the face of inflammation, and neoplastic squamous epithelium with secondary inflammation, can be difficult or impossible to make. Clusters of markedly atypical epithelial cells with variable nuclear to cytoplasmic ratios and presence of atypical keratinocytes are characteristic cytologic features (Fig. 13-3). Histologic features are a formation of cords and nests of invasive and atypical squamous epithelium. Cases with marked cytologic atypia within plaques of thickened epithelium, in the absence of invasion, may be diagnosed as a preneoplastic lesion or as carcinoma in situ.

Cutaneous and genital squamous cell carcinomas are markedly locally invasive and destructive but slow to metastasize. In one study, only approximately 10% of equine cutaneous squamous cell carcinoma exhibited distant metastasis.[2] Wide surgical excision is often curative. Partial penile amputation may be employed for horses with invasive or with multiple penile tumors. Topical treatment with cisplatin and injection of

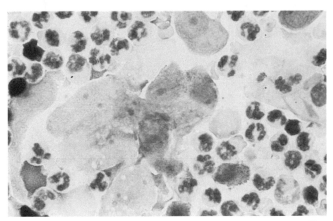

Figure 13-3 Clusters of atypical squamous epithelial cells admixed with neutrophils are characteristic cytologic features of squamous cell carcinoma with secondary inflammation. (Photograph by Dr. Sue Tornquist.)

cisplatin in an oily emulsion into small tumors or after tumor excision have proven to be useful for treatment of equine cutaneous squamous cell carcinoma.[7]

Sarcoid

Equine sarcoid is a fibroblastic tumor associated with bovine papillomavirus. Although most common in horses up to 6 years of age, these tumors can occur at any age. In areas of high sarcoid prevalence, the occurrence of this tumor in an aged horse is not uncommon. The appearance of sarcoids varies from raised and wart-like masses to flattened plaques within the dermis. Histologic patterns vary considerably, and equine sarcoid may be misdiagnosed as fibroma, fibrosarcoma, neurofibroma, schwannoma, or even hemangiopericytoma. Although there are descriptions of the differentiating features of fibroma and sarcoid in equine skin, it is this pathologist's experience that a true, nonviral fibroblastic tumor (fibroma or fibrosarcoma) is very rare in the horse. It is often difficult for the pathologist to distinguish an extensively ulcerated and secondarily inflamed sarcoid from exuberant granulation tissue.

Sarcoid is often insidiously locally invasive and frequently recurs after excision. Sarcoid can also be multicentric. Wide surgical excision, when possible, is the treatment of choice. Cryotherapy of the area has proven useful in some cases. Various local therapies have been employed for treatment of primary or recurrent sarcoid, including injection of immunostimulants and application of various topical formulations. Injection of cisplatin has also proven to be useful in the treatment of equine sarcoid.[7]

Cutaneous Lymphoma (Lymphosarcoma)

Equine lymphoma can manifest with primarily or exclusively cutaneous and subcutaneous involvement.

The vast majority of horses with cutaneous lymphoma are older than 6 years of age, although younger horses can be affected. Subcutaneous involvement is most common, although rare cases are confined within the epidermis and dermis, a form known as *epitheliotropic lymphoma* ("mycosis fungoides"). Superficial lymph nodes may or may not be involved in horses with cutaneous lymphoma. Tumors occur as multifocal raised plaques and nodules of varying size. Most tumors are not alopecic or ulcerated, although epitheliotropic lymphoma can result in ulceration. Rare cases have had extensive periarticular involvement.[8]

Progressive weight loss is common. Fever of unknown origin, hypercalcemia, anemia, and pruritus are possible paraneoplastic disorders associated with equine cutaneous lymphoma.[9] Peripheral white blood cell counts and differentials are typically normal.[10] Selective IgM deficiency can be seen, but this is not a consistent or specific finding in horses with lymphoma.

Cytologic diagnosis of equine cutaneous lymphoma can be extremely difficult, as these tumors often contain an admixture of small lymphocytes and histiocytes (so-called lymphohistiocytic lymphoma), mimicking reactive lymphoid tissue or inflammation. Similarly, histopathologic evaluation of small samples may not be conclusive, because only by recognizing the pattern of tissue infiltration can a pathologist be certain of the diagnosis of equine cutaneous lymphoma. Immunocytochemistry to evaluate for lymphocyte markers can be useful for differentiating neoplasia from a reactive process and for determining the neoplastic cell type. Most equine cutaneous lymphomas prove to be T-cell–rich B-cell lymphomas, with the exception of epitheliotropic lymphoma, which is a T-cell neoplasm.

Cutaneous lymphoma in many horses can have a protracted and indolent course, with waxing and waning of tumor masses over a course of several years. Occasional cases of spontaneous remission have occurred. One interesting report documents regression of cutaneous lymphoma following excision of an ovarian tumor in a mare.[11] Chemotherapy with a combination of cytosine arabinoside, cyclophosphamide, and prednisolone has been shown to have promise in therapy of equine lymphoma.

Mast Cell Tumor

Cutaneous mast cell tumors are relatively uncommon in horses. They occur in horses of all ages but are most common in horses older than 6 years of age. The trunk and head are the most common sites,[12] although the limbs can be involved.[13] Mast cell tumors occur as nonulcerated, firm, raised, dermal to subcutaneous masses that either remain static after initial growth or only very slowly enlarge. Multicentric equine cutaneous mast cell tumor is

rare. Mineralization visible on radiographic[13] or ultrasonographic examination is common. On section, pale zones of granular, caseous-appearing material resembling equine eosinophilic granuloma (see Tumor-Like Lesions, later in this chapter) can be seen (Fig. 13-4). Cytologic preparations contain numerous relatively homogeneous and well-differentiated mast cells admixed with eosinophils. Necrotic cells and debris are common. Characteristic histologic features are nests or sheets of finely granulated, well-differentiated mast cells admixed with eosinophils, often with multifocal zones of tumor necrosis that may be partially mineralized. Wide surgical excision is the treatment of choice, as it is generally curative.[12] Occasional cases have spontaneously regressed.

Hemangiosarcoma

Vascular neoplasia in young horses is typically benign (hemangioma), but vascular neoplasia in older horses is almost always malignant (hemangiosarcoma). Hemangiosarcoma is relatively uncommon and can occur within the skin, subcutis, or skeletal muscle. Tumors manifest as localized soft swellings that may wax and wane. Superficial tumors often bleed. On section, these tumors are typically markedly hemorrhagic. Tumors deep within the muscle resemble hematoma and may be associated with lameness, limb edema, or peripheral nerve damage. Anemia, neutrophilia, and thrombocytopenia are common. Red blood cell abnormalities such as schistocytes, common in dogs with hemangiosarcoma, are not common in horses.[14] Paraneoplastic bullous stomatitis has been reported in association with intramuscular hemangiosarcoma in a horse.[15] Cytologic preparations often contain only blood, and multiple biopsy samples may be necessary to detect characteristic atypical endothelial cells lining irregular vascular channels. Surgical excision of superficial tumors can be attempted, but these tumors are often markedly invasive and frequently metastasize to lungs, liver, and other internal organs.

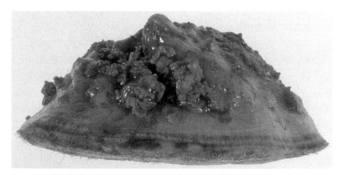

Figure 13-4 Equine cutaneous mast cell tumor with characteristic granular material visible on section. Equine eosinophilic granuloma has a similar appearance. (Photograph by Dr. Stan Snyder.)

Schwannoma

Tumors within the dermis composed of Schwann cells occur in horses but are relatively uncommon. Schwannomas most often occur in horses older than 10 years of age and present as discrete, raised, nodular, nonulcerated dermal masses that are firm and pale tan on section. Histologic evaluation reveals characteristic ovoid to spindle cells forming a vague neural pattern, often with prominent perivascular sclerosis. Confirmation of Schwann cell origin requires immunohistochemistry. These tumors may be mistaken for fibroma, fibrosarcoma, or equine sarcoid by pathologists unfamiliar with their characteristic nature. Wide surgical excision is curative.

Basal Cell Tumor

Basal cell tumors have been reported in horses from 4 to 26 years of age. Most have occurred in horses 6 years of age or older. Reported mean age at diagnosis varies from 10.6 years[16] to 16.8 years.[17] Tumors present as freely moveable, discrete dermal nodules that may be ulcerated. Basal cell tumors can occur on the eyelids, limbs, neck, trunk, vulva, or tail. Cytologic preparations contain small nests of relatively bland epithelial cells consistent with basal cells. Tumors are typically discrete, firm, and pale tan on section. Histologic appearance is variable and includes solid, adenoid, and medusoid patterns. Wide surgical excision is curative.[16,17]

Giant Cell Tumor of Soft Parts

A characteristic subcutaneous tumor occurs in adult horses, with a reported mean age of 6.8 years.[18] These tumors are raised, solitary masses firmly attached to subcutaneous tissues. Tumors occur on the neck, trunk, or legs. Cytologic preparations may contain large multinucleate cells admixed with smaller mononuclear cells and evidence of hemorrhage. Tumors are firm and mottled white and red on section. Histologic features are characteristic, with admixed multinucleate giant cells, mononuclear polygonal cells, fibroblasts, collagen, and multiple foci of hemorrhage. Mitoses are uncommon. Giant cell tumors of the subcutis in the horse are locally invasive and recur after incomplete excision, but wide excision is curative.

Rhabdomyosarcoma

Primary tumors of striated muscle are rare in horses. Rhabdomyosarcoma has been diagnosed in horses from 2 to 19 years of age[19] and has occurred within skeletal muscle of the limb and of the tongue, as well as within the mediastinum, urinary bladder, and uterus. Tumors are composed of pleomorphic ovoid to elongate cells that generally require immunohistochemistry for confirmation of skeletal muscle differentiation. Rhabdomyosarcoma is a locally invasive tumor that is also capable of metastasis.

Lipoma

Infiltrative lipoma occurs in the subcutaneous tissue of horses younger than 2 years of age. In older horses, multiple subcutaneous masses composed of mature adipose tissue can occur. Despite a rather bizarre physical appearance, these horses are otherwise clinically normal. Whether these represent true adipose neoplasia or atypical fat deposits is not known.

Tumor-Like Lesions

A variety of non-neoplastic disorders cause focal or multifocal superficial lesions in horses that can be mistaken for neoplasia. Equine eosinophilic granuloma (collagenolytic granuloma) is a common cutaneous nodular lesion in adult horses that is thought to represent hypersensitivity. Identification of eosinophils on cytologic preparations aids in making this diagnosis, but histopathologic confirmation is necessary to differentiate eosinophilic granuloma from mast cell tumor and from other eosinophil-rich inflammatory lesions. Cutaneous amyloidosis occurs in adult horses and results in multiple raised nonulcerated and nonpainful nodular growths within the skin. Biopsy reveals characteristic amyloid deposits with an associated granulomatous response. Persistent insect bite reactions in horses of any age cause nodular skin growths with dense lymphocytic infiltrates mimicking lymphoma. Careful evaluation of the pattern and type of cells present is often necessary to distinguish this pseudolymphomatous lesion from true lymphoma. Focal cutaneous fungal granulomas occur with some frequency in horses of all ages, especially in horses in the Pacific Northwest. Lesions are typically smooth, raised nodules not associated with pruritus or pain. Diagnosis is by histologic evaluation of excised nodules, which contain fragments of pigmented or nonpigmented fungal hyphae with associated dense granulomatous inflammation. Intramuscular desmoid tumors (musculoaponeurotic fibromatosis) occur occasionally in adult horses and are characterized by progressive infiltration of skeletal muscle by fibrosis. The cause is not known but may involve an atypical response to local trauma. When localized, surgical excision of desmoid tumors can be curative, but advanced lesions will exhibit marked invasion, making surgical excision impossible.

Tumors and Tumor-Like Lesions of Bone and Joint

Primary bone tumors are exceedingly rare in the horse, and primary tumors of synovium have not been reported. The pedal bone appears to be the most common site of primary bone neoplasia within the limbs of equids. Metastatic tumors to bone or joint occur in the horse but are uncommon. Clinical signs are of persistent or progressive lameness, and tumors involving bone can result in pathologic fracture. Depending on the site, there may be visible swelling of the area, or the bone lesion may only be visible on radiographs. Cytologic and histopathologic evaluation are necessary for diagnosis.

Primary Tumors of Bone

Osteochondroma is a benign tumor of bone arising from the bone surface. Multiple osteochondromas (cartilaginous exostoses) occur in young horses as an inherited disorder. Similar solitary tumors have been reported involving the radius of three horses from 4 to 8 years of age presenting with lameness and a characteristic sessile exostosis arising from the surface of the bone.[20] Surgical excision can be curative.

Chondrosarcoma in the radius was reported in a 20-year-old horse. Clinical signs were of progressive lameness, carpal and distal radial enlargement, and weight loss. Radiographs revealed an expansile, destructive bony lesion within the distal radius, with marked periosteal reaction. Histopathologic features were the presence of neoplastic cartilage without evidence of osteoid or osseous differentiation. Metastasis did not occur.[21]

Pedal osteosarcoma was reported in an 18.5-year-old donkey. Clinical signs were progressive lameness and an enlarging mass on the dorsal aspect of P3 causing distortion of the hoof wall. The mass was invasive and composed of pleomorphic mesenchymal cells forming islands of osteoid. Metastasis was not found.[22]

Secondary Tumors of Bone

A mast cell tumor occurred within P3 of a 6-year-old Quarter horse and was associated with lameness. Radiographs revealed a fracture of P3 associated with a large area of radiolucency.[23] Lymphoma involving bone occurs as part of a more generalized neoplastic process and can result in pathologic fracture. Radiographic features include osteopenia and bone lysis. Similar findings were reported in an 8-year-old horse with intraosseous involvement by fibrosarcoma involving multiple tissues.[24] Multiple myeloma (see Tumors of Bone Marrow) frequently involves bone and can result in lytic bone lesions that may or may not be associated with clinical signs of pain.

Tumors and Tumor-Like Lesions of Synovium

Synovial tumors are rare in horses. Biliary carcinoma causing joint effusion and lameness due to metastasis to synovium was reported in an 11-year-old horse.[25] Cartilaginous metaplasia of synovium mimicking neoplasia occurs occasionally.

Tumors of the Hoof and Coronary Band

Tumors involving the hoof wall and coronary band are more common than are tumors involving bone and joint. Tumors in these areas will cause persistent or progressive lameness. Depending on the site, a visible swelling or distortion of the hoof wall may be present. In some cases, lesions are only visible on radiography. Cytologic and histopathologic evaluation are necessary for definitive diagnosis.

Keratoma

The most common tumor of the hoof is keratoma. Keratoma is a benign tumor that can arise within the horn-producing cells of the coronary band, within the keratin-producing cells of the inner hoof wall, or within the solar corium. Keratoma has been reported in horses from 2 to 20 years of age.[26] When located at the coronary band, the mass is visible as a raised lesion on the dorsal or lateral hoof wall. The most common radiographic appearance is of a circular or semicircular radiolucent defect with sharp margins within P3. The mass may have an onionskin appearance on radiographs and on section (Fig. 13-5). At surgery, these tumors are discrete and encapsulated. Histologically, keratoma is composed of a wall of well-differentiated stratified squamous keratinizing epithelium with a core of keratin. Although described as tumors, it is likely that these are non-neoplastic lesions related to follicular and epidermal cysts of the skin. Hoof wall resection and surgical excision of keratoma is curative.[26]

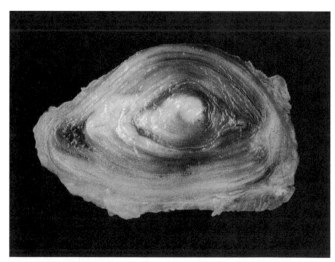

Figure 13-5 Keratoma of the hoof wall after surgical removal. The mass is an encapsulated nodular lesion with a central zone of lamellated keratin that is partially mineralized.

Squamous Cell Carcinoma

Squamous cell carcinoma is the second most common tumor of the equine hoof and occurs within the hoof wall of aged horses. The radiographic appearance is often similar to that of keratoma, but surgical exploration reveals an invasive fleshy tumor associated with lysis of P3. Eventual pathologic fracture of P3 is possible. Histopathologic diagnosis is based on characteristic cords and nests of atypical and invasive squamous epithelium. Complete surgical excision is generally not possible because of tumor invasion.

Malignant Melanoma

Less commonly, anaplastic malignant melanoma affects the hoof of aged horses, most often those older than 20 years of age. These tumors are not related to coat color and so often occur in non-gray horses. Anaplastic malignant melanoma can occur within the coronary band or within the hoof wall. Lameness, swelling, and osteolysis of P3 are typical, and hoof wall melanoma can result in draining tracts within the hoof wall or sole. The tumor tissue is often pigmented on gross examination. Characteristic pleomorphic and often poorly pigmented cells are identified on histologic sections. Marked invasion is typical, making complete excision difficult or impossible, and metastasis is also possible.

Tumors and Tumor-Like Lesions of the Head

There are multiple tissues within the head of the horse in which neoplasia can arise. These include ocular and periocular tissue, oral cavity, nasal, sinus, and guttural pouch mucosa, parotid region, larynx, and bones of the skull. Tumors are readily visible if on or near the surface, can cause bone distortion or nasal discharge if within nasal or sinus cavities, nasal discharge if within the guttural pouch, and difficulty breathing or abnormal respiratory sounds if tumors occlude airways. Tumors within the oral cavity can cause difficulty eating and may be associated with a foul odor if there is mucosal ulceration.

Ocular and Periocular Tissue

Squamous cell carcinoma is by far the most common tumor in this area. Although squamous cell carcinoma can occur in young horses, typically it is a disorder of older horses. One study of 44 horses with ocular squamous cell carcinoma reported tumors in horses from 4 to 22 years of age, with a mean age of about 11 years.[6] Tumors can arise in the nictitans, eyelid, limbus, conjunctiva, cornea, orbit, or a combination of these sites, and bilateral involvement either at the time of diagnosis or with time is common. Horses with ocular squamous

cell carcinoma can also have similar tumors at other sites, especially external genitalia.[27] Tumors are most common in horses with sun exposure of unpigmented skin in the ocular region, although Belgians are highly susceptible to ocular squamous cell carcinoma, particularly of the conjunctiva and nictitans. Early squamous cell carcinoma may be misdiagnosed as a wound or infection. Metastatic squamous cell carcinoma involving the sympathetic nerves causing bilateral Horner's syndrome has been reported.[28] Tumors within the eyelid are more likely to be invasive than those on the limbus or nictitans.[27] Biopsy of suspicious lesions early on is vital, as wide surgical excision is the treatment of choice. Histopathologic diagnosis is based on typical invasive cords and nests of atypical squamous epithelium. Early lesions may form a plaque-like lesion without evidence of invasion and are often designated as carcinoma in situ. Treatment is often successful, especially early on, as these tumors are more likely to be locally invasive than to metastasize. Successful treatment modalities include complete surgical excision, such as by removal of an affected nictitans, cryosurgery, and irradiation.[27] Intratumoral injection of cisplatin has also proven useful in therapy of periocular squamous cell carcinoma.[7]

Lymphoma often involves the eyes and periocular tissues and may be the first indication of generalized lymphoma. The age of affected horses has been reported to be 4 months to 21 years, with a median age of 11 years.[29] Lymphoma most commonly causes thickening of the eyelids and palpebral conjunctiva and is often associated with hyperemia and edema of affected tissue. Lymphoma can involve one or both eyes. Early lesions can easily be misdiagnosed as edema secondary to trauma. Occasionally, lymphoma involving only the nictitans occurs. Persistent uveitis or exophthalmos are less common manifestations. Diagnosis relies on cytologic or histopathologic evaluation. In the small number of cases in which lymphoma is confined to one or both nictitans, excision of the nictitans can apparently be curative. Most horses with lymphoma of the nictitans, however, also have generalized lymphoma.[29]

Conjunctival hemangiosarcoma occurs in aging horses. A study of four cases reported an age range of 9 to 17 years.[30] Tumors occur as poorly demarcated zones of firm, thickened tissue that is not always obviously vascular. Biopsy is required for diagnosis. Local invasion is typical, and recurrence and metastasis are common.

Intraocular and nonlymphomatous retrobulbar tumors are not common in the horse. Neuroendocrine tumors occur in aged horses, with a reported range of 13 to 29 years.[31] Rarely, older horses develop tumors within the optic nerve.[32] All such tumors manifest with exophthalmos as the primary presenting sign. Surgical removal of the affected eye and periocular tissue, and submission of samples for histopathologic evaluation, are necessary for diagnosis. Although long-term survival of a horse with an orbital neuroendocrine tumor after orbital exenteration has been reported,[31] the local invasion of most orbital and retrobulbar tumors, and the advanced stage when detected, warrant a guarded to poor prognosis after surgery.

Proliferative corneal or conjunctival lesions due to eosinophilic inflammation can resemble squamous cell carcinoma. Such lesions are considered a form of hypersensitivity reaction and are responsive to corticosteroid therapy. Similar lesions can also be caused by larval parasites. Diagnosis is based on characteristic cytologic and histopathologic findings.

Skull

Most tumors arising within bones of the skull are either localized or locally invasive but have a low metastatic potential. Wide surgical excision, when possible, can be curative.

Odontogenic (dental) tumors are the most common tumors involving the skull and arise in either the maxilla or the mandible. These tumors can occur in horses of any age, although they are most common in young horses. Histopathologic classification is based on the differentiation of the tissues involved in the tumor. Ameloblastoma (previously known as adamantinoma) is the least differentiated odontogenic tumor and is also the most commonly reported odontogenic tumor in older horses. Odontogenic tumors result in obviously expanded and distorted areas of bone, often with displacement or other abnormalities of tooth growth in the area. Ameloblastoma in the horse has been associated with hypercalcemia.[33] Radiographic evaluation will confirm the intraosseous nature of the tumor. The radiographic appearance of odontogenic tumors is variable, but most are found to be expansile tumors with variable associated mineralization within intact, although often thinned, cortical bone. Computed tomographic studies can also be useful. Diagnosis is based on characteristic histopathologic findings, although differentiation of ameloblastoma from carcinoma can be difficult. Wide surgical excision of odontogenic tumors is the treatment of choice, as it will be curative. These tumors will recur if incompletely excised.

Mesenchymal tumors involving bones of the skull include fibrosarcoma, osteosarcoma, osteoma, chondrosarcoma, and chondroma. These tumors are uncommon in the horse and can occur in young horses as well as in aged horses. In most cases, these are slowly growing tumors that only rarely metastasize. Radiographic or computed tomographic studies will aid in determining the nature and extent of the tumor, and histopathologic evaluation is necessary to determine the nature of the tumor cells. Wide excision, when possible, is the treatment of choice, as it can be curative. The local invasion of sarcomas, however, results in frequent recurrence.

Intraosseous epidermoid cyst causing a progressive expansile swelling has been reported in the mandible of a 21-year-old horse. This is a rare non-neoplastic lesion that can be cured by surgical excision.[34]

A peculiar bony proliferative lesion involving suture lines, known as suture line osteitis, occurs in the skull of adult horses. This condition has been referred to as the "unicorn syndrome," although the development of a single elongate mass is rare. The more recently adapted description of development of Klingon-like features in affected horses is much more accurate. These lesions are typically nonpainful and, after initial growth, remain static. Treatment is neither necessary nor recommended.

Oral Cavity

Tumors of the oral cavity can cause difficulty in eating, swelling of external tissue, and a foul mouth odor. Tumors in this location may be visible on oral examination of an awake horse. But, if they are located caudally, examination during general anesthesia may be necessary. Radiographic studies can help to determine the extent of tumors that involve underlying bone. Oral tumors are often ulcerated and secondarily infected, and histopathologic evaluation is often preferred to cytologic studies. Wide surgical excision of oral tumors in early stages can be curative. Unfortunately, it is often the case that by the time an oral tumor is recognized, the extent of tumor growth is such that surgical excision is not an option.

Squamous cell carcinoma is the most common tumor to involve the oral cavity of horses. Although oral and pharyngeal squamous cell carcinoma can occur in the head of young to young adult horses, most affected horses are older than 8 years of age. The average age of reported cases is approximately 15 years.[35] The behavior of oral squamous cell carcinoma varies depending on species. In the dog, this tumor is locally invasive but slow to metastasize, whereas in the cat, oral squamous cell carcinoma is highly metastatic. In the horse, local invasion and destruction are typical and metastasis to internal lymph nodes and lung is common. It is not known whether the high incidence of metastasis of squamous cell carcinoma in the oral mucosa of horses is due to inherent metastatic capability of the tumor, or whether it simply reflects the advanced stage most such tumors have reached by the time they are diagnosed. Cases of early metastasis of squamous cell carcinoma of the lip in horses suggest an inherent aggressive nature.

Myxomatous lesions, either myxoma or myxosarcoma, occur within the gingiva of older horses. Tumors form fleshy masses that may or may not be ulcerated.

Characteristic histopathologic features are of stellate cells in a myxoid matrix. These tumors are typically slowly growing but are often invasive. Surgical debulking may relieve signs of discomfort and difficulty in eating, but owners should be warned that recurrence is likely.

Benign proliferative lesions within the oral cavity of horses are uncommon and include squamous papilloma and gingival hyperplasia. Histopathology is necessary for diagnosis, and surgical excision is curative.

Nasal and Paranasal Sinuses, Pharynx, and Larynx

Tumors of the nasal and paranasal sinuses, pharynx, or larynx will result in clinical signs of a purulent unilateral or bilateral nasal discharge, often with hemorrhage and a foul odor. Tumors can cause distortion or destruction of bone associated with a soft tissue or bony mass that is evident on physical examination, endoscopic evaluation, or on radiographic or computed tomographic studies. Cytologic and histopathologic studies are necessary for definitive diagnosis.

Squamous cell carcinoma is the most common tumor to involve these areas in the horse. The average age of affected horses is 15 years. Dyspnea and inspiratory stridor are common in horses with laryngeal and pharyngeal involvement.[36] Squamous cell carcinoma of the paranasal sinus can also expand along the path of least resistance and present as a periocular mass.

Lymphoma involving the nasal sinus or pharyngeal region occurs in mature horses, with a reported range of 5 to 15 years.[37] Lymphoma in these areas can result in a nodular fleshy growth, or can cause diffuse thickening of affected tissue with associated ulceration. Similar to cutaneous lymphoma in horses, the typical mixture of neoplastic small lymphocytes with histiocytes makes interpretation of cytologic and histopathologic samples difficult. These tumors are often misinterpreted as chronic granulomatous inflammation.[37] In many cases, it is only at necropsy examination that the extent and true nature of the tumor are determined. Underlying lymphoma should be considered in any case of persistent ulcerative pharyngitis in an older horse. Surgical excision is not an option in these cases, although systemic chemotherapy may have some benefit. In one case of intranasal lymphoma, radiation therapy was apparently effective.[38]

Less common tumors involving the nasal and paranasal sinuses and the pharyngeal region of aged adult horses include mast cell tumor, melanoma, carcinoid tumors, and ethmoid adenocarcinoma. Cytologic and histopathologic samples help to differentiate these tumor types.

Of the tumor-like lesions that occur in the head of horses, progressive ethmoid hematoma is by far the most common. These vascular lesions result in recurrent or persistent epistaxis, and large lesions cause expansion and distortion of the overlying bone. That a simple hemorrhage could be progressive and cause bony changes boggles the mind, and it is this pathologist's opinion that ethmoid hematoma should be considered a low-grade vascular neoplasm. These lesions occasionally occur in young to young adult horses but are most common in older horses, with a reported mean age of 8 years[39] to 10 years.[40] Histopathologic features include evidence of chronic and active hemorrhage, frequent calcification of intralesional blood vessels, and formation of multinucleate giant cells apparently of macrophage origin. Recurrence after surgical excision is common, but successful resolution of ethmoidal hematoma has been achieved after single or multiple intralesional injection of 4 percent formaldehyde.[40] Less common lesions mimicking neoplasia are nasal amyloidosis and inflammatory nasal polyps. Histopathologic evaluation is needed for accurate diagnosis.

Parotid Region and Guttural Pouch

Melanoma of aging gray horses is the most common tumor to involve the parotid region and guttural pouch in horses. Involvement of the guttural pouch is most often by extension from the parotid gland. It is not clear whether melanoma of the parotid salivary gland represents primary parotid gland neoplasia or metastasis to the gland or associated lymph nodes. Cases in which only parotid region melanomas have been detected suggest that melanoma can be primary at this site.[41] Tumors in the parotid region present as progressive nonpainful swellings. Large tumors can cause compression of the airways and resultant dyspnea, respiratory stridor, and exercise intolerance. In cases of guttural pouch involvement, endoscopy will reveal melanotic lesions within the wall. The gross appearance of these brown to black pigmented tumors is characteristic, although histopathologic confirmation is still useful, especially in cases of poorly pigmented tumors.

Squamous cell carcinoma involving the guttural pouch is uncommon. Cases can be unilateral or bilateral and most often manifest with associated nasal discharge. Ulceration and secondary inflammation are common, making cytologic interpretation difficult. Histopathologic confirmation of squamous cell carcinoma is often necessary.

Tumors of Endocrine Glands

Nodular growths, either hyperplastic or neoplastic, within endocrine glands are common, occur almost exclusively in aged horses,[1] and can affect multiple glands. Equine endocrine tumors occur most often in the thyroid, adrenal, and pituitary glands. Tumors of other endocrine organs, such as aortic or carotid body tumors and parathyroid tumors, are extremely rare in the horse. With the exception of pituitary tumors, clinical signs associated with endocrine tumors in horses are uncommon. The vast majority of endocrine tumors in aged horses are benign. The diagnosis of malignant endocrine neoplasia most often relies on histopathologic features of capsular and local invasion by the tumor, rather than on cytologic features. A diagnosis of endocrine malignancy based on aspirated or needle biopsy samples should be confirmed with histopathologic examination of excised samples.

Thyroid

Nodular lesions within the thyroid glands of aged horses are the most common tumor reported in horses examined at slaughter.[1] Nodular lesions can be multifocal and can involve one or both lobes of the thyroid. Enlargement of the affected lobe can result in a visible or palpable mass. These tumors are not apparently associated with hypothyroidism and only rarely cause hyperthyroidism. In cases of functional thyroid adenoma or localized carcinoma, surgical excision of the affected lobe is curative. Metastasis of thyroid carcinoma can occur but is uncommon.

Adrenal

Adrenal tumors can arise either within the cortex or the medulla. Nodular growths within the adrenal cortex are described as either adenomas or foci of nodular hyperplasia. Given the common finding of multiple such lesions as an apparently incidental finding in older horses, it is this author's opinion that true adrenocortical neoplasia is rare in the horse. Pheochromocytoma arising within the adrenal medulla is an uncommon tumor occurring most commonly in horses older than 12 years of age.[42] Pheochromocytoma occurs as a soft, red, often hemorrhagic mass replacing part or all of the adrenal medulla. Tumors typically bulge from the surface on section, and characteristic nests of finely granulated basophilic endocrine cells are seen on histopathologic sections. Nonfunctional tumors can be found as an incidental finding at necropsy. Functional tumors produce catecholamines that can result in clinical signs of muscle tremors, colic, tachycardia, mydriasis, hypertension, and excessive sweating. Increase in the level of norepinephrine in EDTA blood samples aids in the diagnosis of functional pheochromocytoma, although the level of norepinephrine can also be increased in a normal horse due to excitement or stress.[42]

Pituitary

Pathologists often encounter benign nodular growths within the pars intermedia of the pituitary gland of aged horses. Nodular hyperplasia and adenomas are most common, and these lesions may or may not be associated with a history consistent with equine Cushing's disease. Laminitis, hirsutism, muscle atrophy, excessive sweating, polyuria, and polydipsia are the most common clinical signs associated with equine Cushing's disease. Hypertrophic osteopathy has also been reported in a pony with a pituitary adenoma.[43] Diagnosis of equine Cushing's disease can be difficult and is discussed at length in Chapter 7, as are treatment options. Invasive tumors characteristic of pituitary carcinoma are rare.

Tumors and Tumor-Like Lesions of the Thorax

In a 20-year review of 5629 horses examined at necropsy, Sweeney and Gillette[44] found an incidence of 0.62% for tumors involving the thoracic cavity. Clinical signs of intrathoracic tumors are quite variable. Weight loss and anorexia are common, and fever of unknown origin is possible.[45] Pleural effusion is a common finding in horses with intrathoracic neoplasia. Limb enlargement due to hypertrophic osteopathy can occur secondary to space-occupying masses of various types within the lung. Neoplasia involving the heart, most often metastatic disease, can cause arrhythmia or cardiac failure. Diagnosis of intrathoracic neoplasia can often be made using radiography, ultrasonography, endoscopy, and cytologic evaluation of tracheal wash fluid, bronchoscopy samples, or pleural fluid. Although it may be possible to identify neoplastic cells in thoracic fluid, it is not always possible to determine the exact cell type (Fig. 13-6). In most cases, the definitive diagnosis of thoracic mass lesions requires histopathology.

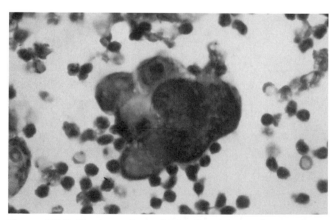

Figure 13-6 Clusters of atypical cells with varying nuclear to cytoplasmic ratio indicative of neoplasia within pleural fluid from a horse. The differential diagnoses for the findings in this case are carcinoma and mesothelioma. (Photograph by Dr. Sue Tornquist.)

Lymphoma

Lymphoma involving mediastinal lymph nodes, mediastinum, cranial thorax, or lung is the most common intrathoracic neoplasm in the horse. The mean age of reported cases ranges from 10 years[45] to 12 years.[44] Involvement of cardiac muscle can result in signs of cardiac dysfunction. Ventral edema is a common clinical sign, occurring in 80 percent of horses in one study.[44] Pleural effusion is variable but is often abundant, and in most cases neoplastic lymphocytes can be identified in cytologic preparations of pleural fluid (Fig. 13-7). Tumors occur as infiltrating soft to slightly firm pale tissue that may be multilobular or multinodular. Histopathologic evaluation of biopsy samples of affected tissue reveals characteristic sheets of neoplastic lymphocytes obliterating normal architecture. As with other forms of equine lymphoma, the prognosis for such horses has always been grave, although recent development of chemotherapeutic regimens offers some hope.

Mesothelioma

Neoplasia of thoracic mesothelium is rare and occurs in mature to aged horses. Marked pleural effusion results in severe respiratory distress. Ventral edema and fever also occur. Cytologic diagnosis of mesothelioma based on evaluation of pleural fluid is possible. But, given the wide range of reactive mesothelial cell morphology, this can be a difficult diagnosis to make even on histopathologic samples. Postmortem findings of disseminated visceral and parietal pleural thickening, with multifocal small firm nodules or villous projections, are characteristic of mesothelioma.

Lung

Pulmonary tumors can be primary or metastatic. Tumors involving airways and lung may or may not

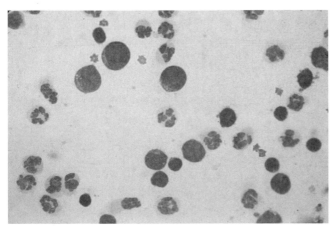

Figure 13-7 Large, atypical lymphocytes indicative of lymphoma admixed with neutrophils in pleural fluid from a horse. (Photograph by Dr. Sue Tornquist.)

result in signs of respiratory disease such as coughing, dyspnea, or nasal discharge. If pulmonary tumors are metastatic, clinical signs are often referable to the primary tumor site. Many types of pulmonary neoplasia are not associated with clinical signs referable to the respiratory system, and some are often found as incidental findings at necropsy.

Granular Cell Tumor: Pulmonary granular cell tumor occurs most often in horses older than 10 years of age.[46] Although no granular cell tumors were reported in two veterinary college studies of thoracic neoplasia involving a total of 73 horses,[44,45] this is the most frequently described pulmonary tumor of horses. The number of reports on what is actually a relatively uncommon tumor, with a reported incidence from 0.0015 percent to 0.01 percent of horses examined at slaughter,[47] stems in part from the mystery surrounding the cell of origin of granular cell tumor. Although it was originally described as granular cell myoblastoma, immunohistochemical studies point to origin from Schwann cells rather than from skeletal muscle precursor cells.[48] Granular cell tumors in horses can be associated with chronic coughing,[46,47,49] but these tumors are also encountered as incidental findings at necropsy or slaughter. Tumors can be single or multiple and are typically discrete nodular expansile masses. Tumors typically involve bronchi. Cytologic or histopathologic evaluation reveals relatively homogeneous round cells with abundant cytoplasmic granules that often stain positively with periodic acid-Schiff and Luxol fast blue stains. These are benign tumors that do not invade or metastasize, and recent reports of successful treatment by either complete lung resection[49] or transendoscopic electrosurgery[46] indicate that surgical treatment is possible.

Carcinoma and Adenocarcinoma: Pulmonary carcinoma or adenocarcinoma is quite rare and occurs in mature to aged horses. Clinical signs of dyspnea, anorexia, ventral edema, fever, and lethargy are common.[45] Pleural effusion frequently occurs, and evaluation of pleural fluid often reveals neoplastic cells. Necropsy reveals firm nodular masses that can involve pleura, heart, mediastinum, and lung. In some cases, origin from pulmonary parenchyma is obvious, whereas in others the exact site of origin is not clear.

A syndrome of multifocal fibrosing interstitial pneumonia causing chronic respiratory disease occurs in mature to aged horses and mules. Multiple irregular and often large zones of firm tissue occur throughout the lung lobes, without evidence of lymph node, pleural, or other tissue involvement. Lesions are typically evident on radiographic and ultrasonographic studies. Pleural effusion is not common. This syndrome can be mistaken for primary pulmonary carcinoma or adenocarcinoma due to the gross appearance and to the florid proliferation of type II pneumocytes, mimicking neoplasia, seen on histopathologic evaluation.

Metastatic Tumors: The majority of malignant epithelial neoplasms occurring within the lungs of horses represent metastatic disease. Hemangiosarcoma often metastasizes to the lungs of horses and can result in epistaxis and hemothorax.[44] Disseminated malignant melanoma can involve the lungs as well as other internal organs.

Thymus and Mediastinum

Nonlymphomatous thymic and mediastinal tumors, including thymoma and primary or metastatic carcinoma, are rare in the horse. Affected horses are mature to aged and most often present with ventral edema and signs referable to the respiratory system. Spread of tumor cells can result in palpable masses at the thoracic inlet. Radiology or ultrasonography reveals a soft tissue mass at the base of the heart. Definitive diagnosis requires histopathology.

Tumors and Tumor-Like Lesions of the Abdomen

Neoplasia involving abdominal organs in the horse is common, particularly in mature to geriatric horses. Intra-abdominal neoplasia is often a diagnostic challenge due to the fact that clinical signs are often nonspecific and to the fact that palpation and imaging of abdominal organs can be difficult in the horse. Two of the most common clinical signs of abdominal neoplasia, weight loss and colic,[42] are associated with a long list of differential diagnoses. Common abnormal findings on complete blood counts, such as anemia, hyperfibrinogenemia, and leukocytosis, are also nonspecific. Serum biochemistry can be useful if there are abnormalities indicative of specific organ dysfunction. Rectal palpation, ultrasonography, endoscopy, radiology, percutaneous organ biopsy and aspiration, and cytologic evaluation of abdominal fluid are often useful. Laparoscopic examination can aid in detection of equine abdominal neoplasia. In some cases, however, exploratory surgery is the best antemortem approach to diagnosis.

This section will focus on neoplasia involving the gastrointestinal tract, liver, spleen, and abdominal cavity as a whole. Tumors of the adrenal gland and of the urogenital system are described in other sections.

Lipoma

By far the most common intra-abdominal tumor of geriatric horses is lipoma arising in the mesentery or in the intestinal serosa. Reported mean age is about 17 to 19 years.[50-52] Geldings are at higher risk compared with stallions and mares,[50,52] and ponies are at higher risk than horses.[51] It is not at all clear whether increased body condition is associated with a higher risk of intra-abdominal lipoma. These tumors are most often multiple and are thought to arise as broad-based tumors that can eventually become pedunculated. Large tumors on thin stalks can undergo necrosis and even mineralization, and occasionally such a mass is found floating free in the horse's abdomen. The propensity to develop a stalk is what makes these otherwise benign tumors dangerous, as pedunculated lipomas are likely to wrap around portions of intestine, causing intestinal obstruction or strangulation (Fig. 13-8). More broad-based lipomas that periodically restrict movement of ingesta without intestinal compromise can also occur. Horses with intestinal obstruction due to lipoma can present with severe sudden-onset colic, or can present with a history of intermittent colic. Nasogastric reflux may or may not be present.[50] Given the physical nature of the tumors and of the intestines, the small intestine is the most common site of obstruction, followed by the small colon. Rectal palpation may reveal only markedly dilated loops of small intestine or of small colon. Surgery to remove the tumor, the affected intestine, and as many other large lipomas as possible is the only treatment. Long-term survival after surgery varies from 38 percent[51] to 50 percent.[50]

Lipomatosis is an unusual variant of lipoma in which a locally extensive expansile and invasive fatty tumor occurs within the abdomen.[42]

Lymphoma

Intra-abdominal lymphoma is not uncommon in the horse and occurs in young horses as well as aged horses.

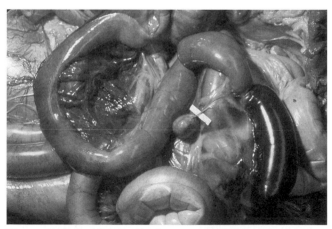

Figure 13-8 Small intestinal strangulation by a pedunculated lipoma. The affected intestine is markedly dilated with a large dark zone of ischemic necrosis. (Photograph by Dr. John King.)

Lymphoma is the most common tumor to involve the intestinal tract of horses.[42] Lymphoma can be restricted to the intestine as a localized or diffuse process, or it can be widespread, involving multiple abdominal organs. In cases of diffuse small intestinal mucosal involvement, chronic weight loss and hypoproteinemia due to protein-losing enteropathy are typical, and hypergammaglobulinemia is common. Diarrhea is uncommon unless there is extensive large intestinal involvement. Carbohydrate absorption tests are useful to confirm malabsorption but do not differentiate inflammatory from neoplastic intestinal disease. Neoplastic lymphocytes are not found in abdominal fluid of lymphoma confined to the intestinal wall but may be present in cases with more widespread involvement. Affected areas of intestine are thickened and the mucosa often has a corrugated appearance. Associated lymph nodes may or may not be enlarged. Lymphoma involving other organs typically results in either diffuse enlargement or nodular masses composed of soft to slightly firm, pale white to tan tissue. Histopathologic or cytologic evaluation of samples of affected organs is diagnostic. Rectal mucosal biopsies are useful when intestinal lymphoma extends to this area, but negative findings do not rule out lymphoma affecting other portions of the intestine. A variety of cell types can be involved in equine abdominal lymphoma, including large granular lymphocytes, B-cells, and epitheliotropic T-cells. Histopathologic differentiation of intestinal lymphoma from equine granulomatous enteritis is often difficult.

Mesothelioma

Mesothelioma arising in the peritoneum is rare and occurs in middle-aged to older horses, with a reported age range of 6 to 18 years.[42] Mesothelioma is associated with marked abdominal effusion, and neoplastic mesothelial cells are often present in cytologic preparations of abdominal fluid. Be aware that the differentiation of reactive and neoplastic mesothelial cells often requires the expertise of an experienced veterinary clinical pathologist. In some cases, histopathology may be required for confirmation of a diagnosis of mesothelioma. Widespread involvement of the abdominal cavity with nodular to villous thickening of the serosal and peritoneal surfaces is typical, and surgical excision is not possible.

Nonlymphomatous Gastrointestinal Tumors

A variety of cell types can give rise to tumors within the stomach or intestines. Those involving the mucosa often cause signs of colic or obstruction sooner than those arising in the wall. These tumors occur primarily in adult to aged horses.

Leiomyoma and Leiomyosarcoma: Benign and malignant smooth muscle tumors occur in the wall of the gastrointestinal tract in the horse and are most common in mature to aged horses.[19] Leiomyosarcoma is less common than leiomyoma. The small intestine is most commonly affected. Leiomyoma of the stomach or intestine may be an incidental finding at necropsy. Leiomyoma of the intestine, however, more often results in clinical signs of colic due to obstruction or intussusception. Leiomyosarcoma of the stomach can cause clinical signs of anorexia and weight loss, whereas intestinal leiomyosarcomas are associated with clinical signs of colic. Leiomyoma and leiomyosarcoma arise within the muscular wall and do not often involve the mucosa. Tumors are most often smooth, pink, firm, and fleshy, although ulceration and hemorrhage of larger tumors is possible. Leiomyoma is a discrete and well-differentiated tumor with histopathologic features characteristic of smooth muscle. Leiomyosarcoma is locally invasive and formed by a more pleomorphic population of spindle cells retaining some characteristics indicative of smooth muscle origin. A definitive diagnosis of poorly differentiated tumors may require immunohistochemistry. Metastasis of leiomyosarcoma appears to be very uncommon in the horse, and surgical excision of sections of intestine containing smooth muscle tumors can be curative.

Neural Tumors: In people and animals, it has become increasingly apparent that some mesenchymal tumors of the gastrointestinal wall previously diagnosed as leiomyoma or leiomyosarcoma actually consist of cells with neural differentiation. Such tumors may be exclusively of neural origin, or can contain an admixture of neural, smooth muscle, and fibroblastic cells. Origin from pluripotential cells within the gastrointestinal wall is proposed, and the term *gastrointestinal stromal tumor* has been used to encompass this heterogeneous group of tumors. Gastrointestinal tumors with neural differentiation appear to be particularly common in horses, and they can be multiple.[19,53] These tumors are most common in aged horses. Many cases of solitary tumors are identified as incidental findings during exploratory surgery or necropsy. Other cases have been associated with clinical signs of colic.[53] Tumors are typically smooth, raised, and often multinodular and arise from the serosal surface of affected intestine. These tumors do not metastasize, and surgical excision of affected portions of bowel can be curative.

Gastric Carcinoma and Adenocarcinoma: Squamous cell carcinoma arising in the nonglandular portion of the stomach is the most common epithelial tumor of the equine gastrointestinal tract (Fig. 13-9). This tumor is most common in middle-aged to older horses, with a mean reported age range of 8.6 to 14.6 years.[42] Quarter horse and draft related breeds appear to have an increased risk of developing gastric squamous cell carcinoma. Clinical signs are often nonspecific and include weight loss and episodic colic and anorexia. Choking, regurgitation, and resistance to passage of a nasogastric tube can be associated with tumors in the cardiac region.[1] Paraneoplastic hypercalcemia can occur. Gastroscopy reveals raised or plaque-like proliferative tissue that is often ulcerated and secondarily infected. Endoscopic biopsy will reveal characteristic invasive and atypical squamous epithelium. Gastric squamous cell carcinoma will often have spread within the abdomen, to the thorax, or both at the time of diagnosis. Only occasionally are neoplastic cells identified on cytologic evaluation of abdominal fluid, and finding such cells is almost certainly indicative of metastasis. Laparoscopy to evaluate for metastasis may be of value in cases in which surgical or medical therapy is contemplated.

Rarely, adenocarcinoma arises in the glandular stomach of horses. Diagnosis is based on histopathologic features indicative of glandular neoplasia, and behavior is similar to that described for squamous cell carcinoma.

Intestinal Adenocarcinoma: Adenocarcinoma of the small or large intestine of the horse is uncommon and typically occurs in horses older than 13 year of age.[54] Clinical signs of colic due to intestinal obstruction are most common. Hematochezia may be apparent. Evaluation of abdominal fluid does not typically reveal neoplastic cells. Segmental enlargement of affected bowel by fleshy tissue with extensive mucosal involve-ment and with frequent ulceration is typical. Osseous metaplasia is a peculiar change recognized to occur within intestinal adenocarcinomas of horses. Intra-abdominal and intrathoracic metastasis of intestinal adenocarcinoma is common,[42] although one case of colonic adenocarcinoma was apparently successfully treated by surgical resection.[55]

Rare Tumors and Tumor-Like Lesions: Carcinoid tumors composed of intestinal endocrine cells, and intestinal myxosarcoma histologically identical to myxosarcoma of the gingiva (see Tumors of the Head), are uncommon causes of colic in aged horses.[56,57] Non-neoplastic polyps can occur within the mucosa of the stomach or rectum.[42] Histopathologic evaluation is necessary to distinguish inflammatory polyps from polypoid neoplasia and to determine the nature of neoplastic processes. Surgical excision of gastrointestinal polyps is usually curative. Mesenteric hematoma and locally extensive small intestinal fibrosis occur in aged horses and can mimic neoplasia. Surgical excision of affected intestine can be curative.

Liver

The most common primary tumor of the equine liver is biliary carcinoma (cholangiocarcinoma). These tumors occur in aged horses and mules. Involvement of hepatic parenchyma results in alterations in hepatic enzymes as well as of bilirubin, and overt icterus can occur. In addition to intrahepatic metastasis, biliary carcinoma often undergoes widespread intra-abdominal metastasis resulting in abdominal effusion due to carcinomatosis (Fig. 13-10). Intrathoracic metastasis can also occur.

Lymphoma frequently involves the liver and can result in clinical and clinicopathologic evidence of

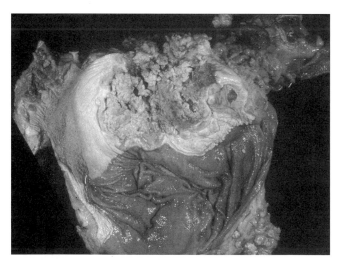

Figure 13-9 Irregular raised friable tissue indicative of squamous cell carcinoma in the gastric mucosa of a horse. (Courtesy of the Department of Biomedical Sciences, College of Veterinary Medicine, Cornell University.)

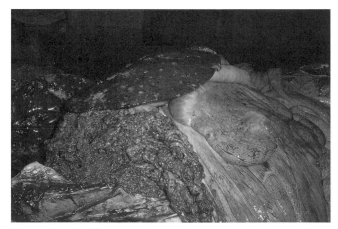

Figure 13-10 Biliary carcinoma in an aged mule resulting in multifocal pale nodular tumors within the liver. Widespread involvement of the abdominal serosa is characteristic of carcinomatosis.

hepatic disease but is rarely confined to this organ. Diffuse enlargement of the liver occurs due to leukemia (see Tumors of Bone Marrow). Hemangiosarcoma and gastrointestinal carcinoma and adenocarcinoma often metastasize to the liver.

Diagnosis of hepatic neoplasia relies on evaluation of cytologic and histopathologic specimens. In cases of carcinomatosis, neoplastic epithelial cells may be identified in samples of abdominal fluid.

Spleen

Tumors of the spleen are rare in horses and occur primarily in mature to aged horses. Lymphoma (Fig. 13-11) is the only tumor that occurs with any frequency. In most cases of lymphoma, splenic involvement is part of a widespread process. Diffuse enlargement of the spleen occurs due to leukemia (see Tumors of Bone Marrow). Disseminated hemangiosarcoma and metastatic melanoma can also involve the spleen. Diagnosis of splenic neoplasia relies on cytologic and histopathologic evaluation. In cases of hemangiosarcoma, histopathologic examination of multiple areas may be necessary to identify the characteristic neoplastic endothelial cells.

Pancreas

Pancreatic neoplasia is rare in horses and occurs in horses older than 10 years of age.[42] Tumors of the endocrine pancreas (islet cell tumor; insulinoma) can cause hypoglycemia due to excessive insulin production. Tumors of the exocrine pancreas (pancreatic adenocarcinoma) often result in marked weight loss. Diagnosis relies on histopathology. Metastasis of an islet cell tumor has not been reported, but widespread metastasis of pancreatic adenocarcinoma is possible.

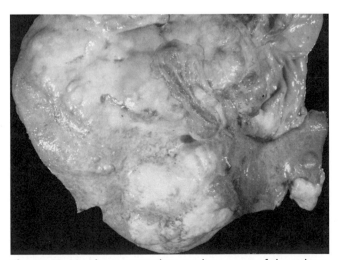

Figure 13-11 Almost complete replacement of the spleen by a soft, pale, fleshy mass characteristic of lymphoma. (Courtesy of the Department of Biomedical Sciences, College of Veterinary Medicine, Cornell University.)

Unusual Intra-abdominal Tumors

Mesenchymal tumors of smooth muscle cell, fibroblast, or myofibroblast origin are rare causes of localized intra-abdominal neoplasia within the omentum or mesentery of mature to aged horses.[42] Diagnosis relies on histopathologic evaluation of tumor samples. Surgical resection of these tumors, if possible, can be curative. Disseminated lymphangiosarcoma within the abdomen and thorax has been reported in a 10-year-old mare.[58] Diagnosis required histopathology and immunohistochemistry.

Tumors of the Urogenital System and Mammary Gland

Neoplasia of the equine urinary system and mammary gland is uncommon. Gonadal tumors, however, are relatively common, especially in mares. Tumors of the kidney and gonad occur in young horses as well as in older horses, whereas tumors of the urinary bladder and mammary gland are only seen in aged horses. Clinical signs are quite variable. Tumors of the urinary tract can result in hematuria, but clinical signs of renal carcinoma are often referable to sites of metastasis rather than to the primary tumor. Tumors of descended testes cause obvious enlargement of the affected testis, but tumors arising within retained testis can cause a variety of signs from none to colic and wasting. Ovarian tumors are often hormonally active and cause behavioral changes ranging from nymphomania to aggression. Hormonally active testicular tumors are uncommon. Equine mammary neoplasia is typically malignant and results in clinical signs similar to mastitis.

Kidney

Primary renal neoplasia is rare in the horse, with an incidence of approximately 0.11 percent to 0.15 percent. In horses, renal cell carcinoma is the most common primary tumor of the kidney, with a reported incidence of 0.055 percent.[59] Renal cell carcinoma has been seen in horses from 4 to 20 years of age and occurs with approximately equal frequency in horses younger than 10 years of age and in horses 10 years of age or older.[60] Renal cell carcinoma metastasizes readily and widely. Renal enlargement is evident on rectal palpation. Ascites due to intra-abdominal metastases resulting in carcinomatosis can occur. Cytologic evaluation of abdominal fluid in such cases may reveal neoplastic epithelial cells. Tumors are pale tan to white and are soft to firm due to variable associated sclerosis. Diagnosis depends on histologic evaluation. Confirmation of primary renal neoplasia in cases of carcinomatosis often requires a complete necropsy examination. The kidney can also be involved in widespread intra-abdominal lymphoma.

Urinary Bladder

Urinary bladder neoplasia in the horse invariably arises from mucosal epithelium, resulting in squamous cell carcinoma and transitional cell carcinoma. Masses are often palpable during rectal examination. Squamous cell carcinoma is the most common primary tumor of the urinary bladder in horses and is thought to arise either from foci of squamous epithelium normally present in the bladder mucosa of horses or from metaplastic change of transitional epithelium. Of six horses aged 13 to 23 years of age with primary urinary bladder tumors, four had squamous cell carcinoma, one had a transitional cell carcinoma, and one had a fibromatous polyp.[60] Neoplastic squamous or transitional epithelial cells may be evident in urinary sediment, but confirmation by histopathology is often needed. These tumors in the horse typically cause carcinomatosis due to transmural invasion and widespread abdominal metastasis rather than distant metastasis due to lymphatic invasion. Although surgical resection of epithelial tumors in early stages of development may be curative, recurrence and metastasis are common.

Gonads

Although not often described in the veterinary literature, equine gonadal neoplasia can be classified in the same way as gonadal neoplasia in humans. Tumors are either of germ cell or of gonadal stromal origin. Germ cell neoplasia is further subdivided into the nondifferentiating tumors seminoma and dysgerminoma, and the tumors of pluripotential cells. The least differentiated tumor of pluripotential germ cells is embryonal carcinoma. Differentiation of pluripotential cells along embryonic pathways results in teratoma and teratocarcinoma, tumors with somatic tissues. Differentiation along extraembryonic (placental) pathways results in tumors such as choriocarcinoma and yolk sac (endodermal sinus) tumor.[61] To date, gonadal germ cell tumors described in the horse include all but those with placental differentiation. Stromal tumors include granulosa cell tumors in mares, Sertoli cell and interstitial cell tumors in stallions, and mixed stromal tumors in both sexes.

Surgical excision of an enlarged testis or ovary is the treatment of choice, both diagnostically and therapeutically. Accurate histopathologic diagnosis can be difficult in small tissue samples. Histologic evaluation of multiple sections from equine testicular and ovarian tumors is often needed for accurate classification. Ideally, the entire gonad should be submitted (Fig. 13-12), although this will often require a large volume of formalin. Submission of the unfixed organ on ice is acceptable, provided the sample reaches the laboratory in a timely manner.

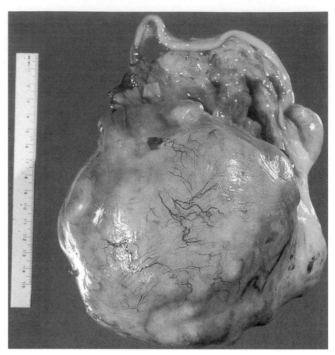

Figure 13-12 Irregular enlargement and replacement of the testis by a pale, multinodular tumor. The differential diagnoses for these findings are seminoma and embryonal carcinoma.

Testis: Equine testicular neoplasia is reported far less frequently than is ovarian neoplasia, but this is undoubtedly due to the early age that most male horses are castrated. The incidence of testicular neoplasia in horses is less than 1% of all equine neoplasms.[62] Clinical signs in descended testes are of a progressive nonpainful testicular enlargement. Involvement of the epididymis and spermatic cord is rare. Neoplasia within undescended testes can be an incidental finding or can result in signs of colic, especially if tumors are associated with torsion of the spermatic cord.[63] Progressive weight loss occurs in horses with metastases. Much of what we know about the behavior of testicular neoplasia in veterinary medicine is based on the dog, in which testicular neoplasia is common and is almost always benign. This is not the case in humans or in horses, especially as regards germ cell tumors. With the exception of teratoma, most equine testicular germ cell neoplasms are malignant and capable of widespread metastasis. The site of regional lymph node metastasis of testicular tumors will be the sublumbar lymph nodes, not the inguinal nodes, even in tumors arising in retained testes. Stromal tumors are most often benign. Use of chemotherapy and radiation therapy has drastically reduced the incidence of death due to malignant testicular neoplasia in men, but this is not the case in horses. As in humans, equine testicular neoplasia can arise in the young as well as in the aged.

Germ cell neoplasia reported in the equine testis includes seminoma, embryonal carcinoma, teratocarcinoma, and teratoma. Seminoma is the most common equine testicular neoplasm and is definitely the most likely tumor to arise in an aged stallion. Seminoma results in partial to complete replacement of testicular tissue by fleshy, soft to slightly firm, pale tan tissue that is often multilobular. Sheets of large round germ cells are seen on cytologic and histopathologic preparations. Almost all reports of seminoma in the horse describe widespread metastasis at the time of diagnosis or soon thereafter. Seminoma occurs within descended as well as cryptorchid testes. Teratoma is a benign tumor that is perhaps the most widely known equine testicular tumor. This is likely due to the innate appeal of these unusual tumors, as well as to the fact that teratoma is most common in young stallions and can be detected after routine castration. Teratoma is the most differentiated of the nonseminomatous germ cell neoplasms and is characterized by formation of an admixture of at least two embryonic tissues (endoderm, mesoderm, and ectoderm), forming recognizable tissue such as bone, cartilage, and hair. Teratocarcinoma is a rare malignant tumor of young horses in which a malignant tumor of undifferentiated germ cells (embryonal carcinoma) and neoplastic elements composed of differentiated somatic tissues are recognizable. Embryonal carcinoma is a rare malignant neoplasm of older horses composed of embryonal germ cells forming cords, nests, and acini.[61]

Of the non-germ cell testicular tumors in horses, interstitial cell tumor is the most common. Interstitial (Leydig) cell tumors occur most often in retained testes[64] but can occur in descended testes.[62] In one study, the mean age of affected horses was 8.1 years, with a range of 3 to 20 years.[64] Tumors are nodular to multinodular, soft, and often hemorrhagic and are composed of closely packed large round to polygonal cells with abundant eosinophilic cytoplasm. These tumors are benign and are cured by excision of the affected testis. Sertoli cell tumor is a rare neoplasm in aged horses characterized by nests of columnar cells mimicking seminiferous tubules, with prominent fibrous stroma. Sertoli cell tumors can be either malignant or benign. Mixed germinal and stromal tumors occur rarely in aged horses. Testicular involvement by lymphoma can also result in testicular swelling, and characteristic sheets of neoplastic lymphocytes are seen on cytologic and histopathologic evaluation.

Ovary: Ovarian germ cell neoplasia (dysgerminoma, teratoma, and teratocarcinoma) is rare in the horse and occurs most often in young mares. Dysgerminoma and teratocarcinoma are often associated with widespread intra-abdominal metastases at the time of diagnosis.

Teratoma is usually a benign neoplasm, but epithelial elements of ovarian teratomas can give rise to adenocarcinoma and widespread intra-abdominal metastasis. Cytologic evaluation of abdominal fluid in cases of metastatic ovarian tumors may or may not reveal neoplastic cells. Cytologic and histopathologic features of germ cell neoplasia in the mare are virtually identical to those of corresponding testicular germ cell tumors.

Stromal tumors, including granulosa cell tumor and granulosa-thecal cell tumor, are by far the most common ovarian tumor in the mare. Although these tumors can occur in young mares, most cases are in adult to aged mares. The presence of these tumors is suspected when there are anomalies of behavior or of the estrus cycle and can be confirmed by rectal palpation and/or by determination of blood levels of hormones, including inhibin, estrogens, and androgens. On occasion, ovarian tumors result in intestinal obstruction and signs of colic. Tumors are typically large, replacing the entire ovary, and are often multicystic with areas of hemorrhage (Fig. 13-13). Granulosa cells admixed with variable amounts and types of stroma are characteristic histopathologic features. Surgical excision is generally curative.

Mammary Gland

Mammary neoplasia is uncommon in the mare, with a reported incidence of between 0.11% and 1.99% of horses examined at slaughter.[65] Mammary neoplasia occurs in aged mares and is invariably malignant.

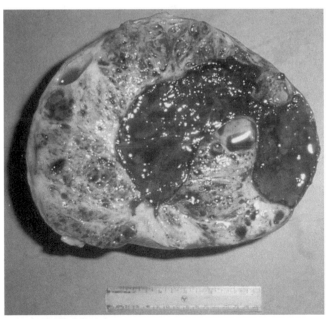

Figure 13-13 Enlargement and replacement of ovarian tissue by a multicystic tumor with zones of hemorrhage characteristic of granulosa cell tumor. (Photograph by Dr. Rob Bildfell.)

Typically, only one gland is affected. Clinical signs often mimic mastitis, with painful enlargement of the affected gland by firm white to tan tissue and a discolored secretion that can be secondarily infected by various bacteria.

Carcinoma and adenocarcinoma are the most common mammary tumors in the mare. The age of affected horses has ranged from 12 to 21 years of age.[66] Examination of biopsy or cytology samples will reveal atypical epithelial cells indicative of neoplasia. Both vascular and lymphatic spread is possible, resulting in involvement of regional as well as distant lymph nodes, and of pleura and lungs as well as abdominal organs. Surgical excision of the entire affected mammary gland can be performed, although subsequent metastatic disease typically results in eventual death or euthanasia.[66]

In adult gray mares, multicentric or metastatic melanoma can involve the mammary gland. Melanin pigment in mammary secretory material or fluid obtained by aspiration is diagnostic. Infiltration by multicentric lymphoma can also cause mammary gland enlargement. Cytologic evaluation of aspirates or needle biopsies of the affected area will reveal neoplastic lymphocytes.

Tumors of Bone Marrow

Leukemia and multiple myeloma are primary tumors of bone marrow. Both are uncommon in the horse. These tumors can occur in horses of all ages, including horses 1 to 2 years of age, but are most common in aged horses. Diagnosis is based on evaluation of peripheral blood and of bone marrow. Immunophenotyping is often necessary to determine the cell of origin. A leukemic phase can occur in late stages of solid tissue lymphoma, and extramedullary disseminated plasma cell neoplasia occurs in the horse, but this section focuses only on those tumors that arise in bone marrow.

Leukemia

Leukemia can be of lymphoid, myeloid, monocytic, or erythroid cells. Although the term *leukemia* refers to white cells within the blood, marrow infiltration by leukemic cells can result in pancytopenia[68] or a normal number of circulating white blood cells, as well as leukocytosis. The term "subleukemic" is applied to leukemia in which the peripheral white blood cell count is normal. As in humans, leukemia in the horse is classified as acute or chronic based on the stage of differentiation of the neoplastic cells. Acute leukemia is a tumor of immature or blast cells that typically has a rapidly progressive course. Acute leukemia occurs in individuals of all ages, but is more common in the young. Chronic leukemia is of more mature leukocytes, typically occurs in aged individuals, and has a more insidious and prolonged course.

Common clinical signs of leukemia in the horse include chronic weight loss, fever of unknown origin, peripheral lymphadenopathy, ventral edema, depression, and exercise intolerance. Anorexia may or may not be apparent. Marked hepatomegaly and splenomegaly due to leukemic infiltrates are typical. Anemia, thrombocytopenia, and hyperproteinemia are common. Persistent lymphocytosis is common in horses with chronic lymphocytic leukemia. Serum electrophoresis of cases of lymphoid leukemia often reveals abnormal globulin fractions.[69]

Neoplastic cells may or may not be seen on peripheral blood smears. It is vital that blood from suspect horses be evaluated by an experienced veterinary clinical pathologist. Automated cell counters often mistake circulating neoplastic cells for normal leukocytes, and those unfamiliar with the appearance of atypical leukocytes in the horse can overlook the presence of circulating leukemic cells. In many cases, examination of aspirates and core biopsies of sternal bone marrow is needed for diagnosis. Bone marrow examination is essential in cases in which circulating neoplastic cells are not present.[68] The pattern of leukemic infiltration of lymph nodes is different from the pattern of nodal solid tissue lymphoma, but it may take immunohistochemical procedures and a veterinary pathologist with a special interest in lymphoproliferative disorders to detect this pattern.

To date there are no reports of successful chemotherapeutic treatment of equine leukemia, although newer therapeutic regimens are being developed and may prove to be of value.

Multiple Myeloma

Multiple myeloma is a multicentric tumor of plasma cells. It is uncommon in the horse, occurring in horses from 3 months to 22 years of age, with a median age of 11 years.[67] The most common clinical signs are weight loss, anorexia, fever, and limb edema. Less common signs include lameness, epistaxis, and lymphadenopathy. Macrocytic anemia and hyperproteinemia due to hypergammaglobulinemia are characteristic. Electrophoresis of serum will reveal a monoclonal globulin spike. Proteinuria due to passage of Bence-Jones protein, a characteristic feature of multiple myeloma in humans, is rare in the horse. An increased number of plasma cells in bone marrow is diagnostic, but multiple bone marrow core biopsies as well as aspirates may be necessary to detect infiltrating cells. Pathologic evaluation of peripheral lymph nodes in cases with lymphadenopathy may be of value. Radiologic studies often reveal bone lesions, varying from punctuate zones of lysis to sclerosis or diffuse osteoporosis.

Survival of horses with multiple myeloma is typically less than 6 months, although survival up to 2 years after diagnosis has been reported.[67] To date, there are no reports of successful treatment of equine multiple myeloma. But, as with lymphoma and leukemia, newer chemotherapeutic regimens may prove to be useful.

Tumors and Tumor-Like Lesions of the Nervous System

Neoplasia affecting the brain, spinal cord, and peripheral nerves is quite uncommon in the horse but should be included in the differential diagnosis in cases of neurologic disease in horses of all ages. Clinical signs are generally progressive and will be referable to the area or areas affected. A careful neurologic examination and determination of the neuroanatomic basis of the clinical signs is imperative. Evaluation of cerebrospinal fluid is an invaluable ancillary test to aid in the diagnosis of central nervous system neoplasia. Ultrasonography and computed tomography allow for imaging of intracranial lesions. Neoplasia involving peripheral nerves will require nerve biopsy and histopathologic evaluation for diagnosis.

Brain and Spinal Cord

Primary tumors of the nervous system parenchyma are exceedingly rare in the horse. The vast majority of tumors arise in the meninges, ependymal lining cells, and choroid plexus. In some cases, neoplastic cells are identified in cerebrospinal fluid. In other cases, definitive diagnosis can only be made after necropsy and histopathologic examination of tumor tissue.

Ependymoma and Choroid Plexus Papilloma: Ependymoma is a tumor that arises in the lining cells of the ventricles of the brain. Tumors involving the third and fourth ventricles are most common in the horse. Although these tumors can arise in young horses, most are in aged animals. Clinical signs are of progressive tetraparesis. Ependymoma is often associated with hemorrhage into the cerebrospinal fluid, which will often be apparent on analysis of cerebrospinal fluid.[70] Ependymoma in the third ventricle can cause compression of the hypothalamus and persistent hypernatremia.[71]

Choroid plexus papilloma is a very rare tumor in the horse. One reported case was in a 5-year-old mare and involved the choroid plexus of the third ventricle. Clinical signs were progressive tetraparesis, depression, and circling to one side.[72]

Lymphoma: Involvement of the central nervous system by lymphoma can occur as part of a multicentric lymphoma or due to primary meningeal lymphoma. Central nervous system lymphoma occurs in horses from 20 months to 15 years of age. Most cases are of discrete extradural masses causing compression of the thoracic spinal cord, although diffuse meningeal lymphoma causing thickening of the meninges of the spinal cord has been reported.[73] Neoplastic lymphocytes are often, but not always, found in cerebrospinal fluid.

Metastatic Neoplasia: Various types of metastatic neoplasms are occasionally seen causing central nervous system dysfunction in the horse. The most common is melanoma in aging gray horses. Metastatic melanoma most often affects the spinal canal, causing progressive ataxia. Melanin-containing cells may or may not be seen in cerebrospinal fluid.

Cholesterol Granuloma (Cholesterinemic Granuloma; Cholesteatoma): Cholesterol granuloma is a non-neoplastic mass lesion that occurs within the choroid plexus of the lateral ventricle. These lesions are quite common, occurring in up to 20% of aged horses, and in most instances are found as incidental lesions at necropsy. Repeated hemorrhage into the choroid plexus has been proposed as a cause. Cholesterol granulomas can be unilateral or bilateral. If large enough, these masses will cause compression of the cerebrum and clinical signs of profound depression. Although the gait may be stiff, ataxia is uncommon. Cerebrospinal fluid is often xanthochromic, indicative of chronic hemorrhage, with an increased protein level. Scintigraphy can detect these intracranial lesions.[74] On gross examination, these lesions are glistening and granular in appearance, with variable color from dark tan to brown (Fig. 13-14). Characteristic histopathologic features are organized

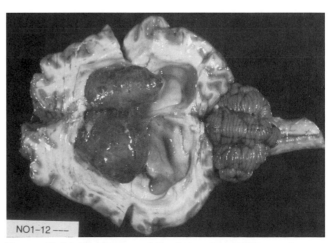

Figure 13-14 Distension of the lateral ventricles and thinning of the cerebral cortex by bilateral cholesterol granulomas. (Photograph by Dr. Alexander de Lahunta.)

granulomatous inflammation admixed with hemorrhage and prominent cholesterol crystals.

Peripheral Nerve

Equine lymphoma can be neurotropic, causing enlargement and dysfunction of one or more peripheral nerves. Clinical signs include localized denervation atrophy of skeletal muscle and lower motor neuron dysfunction. Cranial nerves seem to be particularly prone to this form of lymphoma. Peripheral nerve infiltration by lymphoma must be distinguished from granulomatous inflammation due to polyneuritis equi, and biopsy of affected nerves is diagnostic. Tumors arising in visceral nerves have been described in the section on tumors of the gastrointestinal tract, and dermal schwannomas are described in the section on tumors of the skin, subcutis, and skeletal muscle.

REFERENCES

1. Cotchin E: A general survey of tumours in the horse. Equine Vet J 9:16, 1977.
2. Kerr KM, Alden CL: Equine neoplasia, a ten year survey. Proc Ann Meet Am Assoc Vet Lab Diag 17:183, 1974.
3. Valentine BA: Equine melanocytic tumors: A retrospective study of 53 horses (1988–1991). J Vet Intern Med 9:291, 1995.
4. MacGillivray KC, Sweeney RW, Del Piero F: Metastatic melanomas in horses. J Vet Intern Med 16:452, 2002.
5. Goetz TE, Ogilvie GK, Keegan KG: Cimetidine for treatment of melanomas in three horses. J Am Vet Med Assoc 196:449, 1990.
6. Junge RE, Sundberg JP, Lancaster WD: Papillomas and squamous cell carcinomas of horses. J Am Vet Med Assoc 185:656, 1984.
7. Théon AP, Pascoe JR, Galuppo LD, et al: Comparison of perioperative versus postoperative intratumoral administration of cisplatin for treatment of cutaneous sarcoids and squamous cell carcinomas in horses. J Am Vet Med Assoc 215:1655, 1999.
8. Gerard MP, Healy LN, Bowman KF, et al: Cutaneous lymphoma with extensive periarticular involvement in a horse. J Am Vet Med Assoc 213:391, 1998.
9. Finley MR, Rebhun WC, Dee A, et al: Paraneoplastic pruritus and alopecia in a horse with diffuse lymphoma. Am J Vet Med Assoc 213:102, 1998.
10. Platt H: Observations on the pathology of non–alimentary lymphomas in the horse. J Comp Pathol 98:177, 1988.
11. Henson KL, Alleman AR, Cutler TJ, et al: Regression of subcutaneous lymphoma following removal of an ovarian granuloma-theca cell tumor in horse. J Am Vet Med Assoc 212:1419, 1998.
12. McEntee MF: Equine cutaneous mastocytoma: Morphology, biological behavior and evolution of the lesion. J Comp Pathol 104:171, 1991.
13. Samii VF, O'Brien TR, Stannard AA: Radiographic features of mastocytosis in the equine limb. Equine Vet J 29:63, 1997.
14. Southwood LL, Schott HC II, Henry CJ, et al: Disseminated hemangiosarcoma in the horse: 35 cases. J Vet Intern Med 14:105, 2000.
15. Williams MA, Dowling PM, Angarano DW, et al: Paraneoplastic bullous stomatitis in a horse, J Am Vet Med Assoc 207:331, 1995.
16. Schuh JCL, Valentine BA: Equine basal cell tumors. Vet Pathol 24:44, 1987.
17. Slovis NM, McEntee MC, Fairley RA, et al: Equine basal cell tumors: 6 cases (1985–1999). J Vet Intern Med 15:43, 2001.
18. Render JA, Harrington DD, Wells RE, et al: Giant cell tumor of soft parts in six horses. J Am Vet Med Assoc 183:790, 1983.
19. Cooper BJ, Valentine BA: Tumors of muscle. In Meuten DJ, editor: Tumors in Domestic Animals, 4th ed. Ames, IA, Iowa State Press, 2002.
20. Held JP, Patton CS, Shires M: Solitary osteochondroma of the radius in three horses. J Am Vet Med Assoc 193:563, 1988.
21. Bertone AL, Powers BE, Turner AS: Chondrosarcoma in the radius of a horse. J Am Vet Med Assoc 185:534, 1984.
22. Nelson AM, Baker DC: Pedal osteosarcoma in a donkey. Vet Pathol 35:407, 1998.
23. Ritmeester AM, Denicola DB, Blevins WE, et al: Primary intraosseous mast cell tumour of the third phalanx in a Quarter horse. Equine Vet J 29:151, 1997.
24. Jorgensen JS, Geoly FJ, Berry CR, et al: Lameness and pleural effusion associated with an aggressive fibrosarcoma in a horse. J Am Vet Med Assoc 210:1328, 1997.
25. Durando MM, MacKay RJ, Staller GS, et al: Septic cholangiohepatitis and cholangiocarcinoma in a horse. J Am Vet Med Assoc 206:1018, 1995.
26. Lloyd KCK, Peterson PR, Wheat JD, et al: Keratomas in horses: Seven cases (1975–1986). J Am Vet Med Assoc 193:967, 1988.
27. Dugan SJ, Roberts SM, Curtis CR, et al: Prognostic factors and survival of horses with ocular/adnexal squamous cell carcinoma: 147 cases. J Am Vet Med Assoc 198:298, 1991.
28. Bacon CL, Davidson HJ, Yvorchuk K, et al: Bilateral Horner's syndrome secondary to metastatic squamous cell carcinoma in a horse. Equine Vet J 28:500, 1996.
29. Rebhun WC, Del Piero F: Ocular lesions in horses with lymphosarcoma: 21 cases (1977–1997). J Am Vet Med Assoc 212:852, 1998.
30. Moore PF, Hacker DV, Buyukmihci NC: Ocular angiosarcoma in the horse: Morphological and immunohistochemical studies. Vet Pathol 23:240, 1986.
31. Basher AWP, Severin GA, Chavkin MJ, et al: Orbital neuroendocrine tumors in three horses. J Am Vet Med Assoc 210:668, 1997.
32. Bistner S, Campbell RJ, Shaw D, et al: Neuroepithelial tumor of the optic nerve in a horse. Cornell Vet 73:30, 1983.
33. Rosol TJ, Nagode LA, Robertson JT, et al: Humoral hypercalcemia of malignancy associated with ameloblastoma in a horse. J Am Vet Med Assoc 204:1930, 1994.
34. Camus AC, Burba DJ, Valdes MA, et al: Intraosseous epidermoid cyst in a horse. J Am Vet Med Assoc 209:632, 1996.
35. Schuh JCL: Squamous cell carcinoma of the oral, pharyngeal and nasal mucosa in the horse. Vet Pathol 23:205, 1986.
36. Jones DL: Squamous cell carcinoma of the larynx and pharynx in horses. Cornell Vet 84:15, 1994.
37. Adams R, Calderwood-Mays MB, Peyton LC: Malignant lymphoma in three horses with ulcerative pharyngitis. J Am Vet Med Assoc 193:674, 1988.
38. Weaver MP, Dobson JM, Lane JG: Treatment of intranasal lymphoma in a horse by radiotherapy. Equine Vet J 28:245, 1996.
39. Specht TE, Colahan PT, Nixon AJ, et al: Ethmoidal hematoma in nine horses. J Am Vet Med Assoc 197:613, 1990.
40. Schumacher J, Yarbrough T, Pascoe J, et al: Transendoscopic chemical ablation of progressive ethmoidal hematomas in standing horses. Vet Surg 27:175, 1998.
41. Fintl C, Dixon PM: A review of five cases of parotid melanoma in the horse. Equine Vet Educ 13:17, 2001.
42. East LM, Savage CJ: Abdominal neoplasia (excluding urogenital tract). Vet Clin North Am Equine Pract 14:475, 1998.
43. Sweeney CR, Stebbins KE, Schelling CG, et al: Hypertrophic osteopathy in a pony with a pituitary adenoma. J Am Vet Med Assoc 195:103, 1989.
44. Sweeney CR, Gillette DM: Thoracic neoplasia in equids: 35 cases (1967–1987). J Am Vet Med Assoc 195:374, 1989.
45. Mair TS, Brown PJ: Clinical and pathologic features of thoracic neoplasia in the horse. Equine Vet J 25:220, 1993.
46. Ohnesorge B, Gehlen H, Wohlsein P: Transendoscopic electrosurgery of an equine pulmonary granular cell tumor. Vet Surg 21:375, 2002.
47. Scarratt WK, Crisman MV, Sponenberg DP, et al: Pulmonary granular cell tumour in 2 horses. Equine Vet J 25:244, 1993.
48. Kelley LC, Hill JE, Hafner S, et al: Spontaneous equine pulmonary granular cell tumors: Morphologic, histochemical and immunohistochemical characterization. Vet Pathol 32:101, 1995.
49. Facemire PR, Chilcoat CD, Sojka JE, et al: Treatment of granular cell tumor via complete right lung resection in a horse. J Am Vet Med Assoc 217:1522, 2000.

50. Blikslager AT, Bowman KF, Haven ML, et al: Pedunculated lipomas as a cause of intestinal obstruction in horses: 17 cases (1983–1990). J Am Vet Med Assoc 201:1249, 1992.

51. Edwards GB, Proudman CJ: An analysis of 75 cases of intestinal obstruction caused by pedunculated lipomas. Equine Vet J 26:18, 1994.

52. Freeman DE, Schaeffer DJ: Age distributions of horses with strangulation of the small intestine by a lipoma or in the epiploic foramen: 46 cases (1994–2000). J Am Vet Med Assoc 219:87, 2001.

53. Del Piero F, Summers BA, Cummings FJ, et al: Gastrointestinal stromal tumors in equids. Vet Pathol 38:689, 2001.

54. Rottman JB, Roberts MC, Cullen JM: Colonic adenocarcinoma with osseous metaplasia in a horse. J Am Vet Med Assoc 198:657, 1991.

55. Roy M-F, Parente EJ, Donaldson MT, et al: Successful treatment of a colonic adenocarcinoma in a horse. Equine Vet J 34:102, 2002.

56. Orsini JA, Orsini PG, Sepesy L, et al: Intestinal carcinoid in a mare: An etiologic consideration for chronic colic in horses. J Am Vet Med Assoc 193:87, 1988.

57. Edens LM, Taylor DD, Murray MJ, et al: Intestinal myxosarcoma in a Thoroughbred mare. Cornell Vet 82:163, 1992.

58. Sanchez B, Nieto A, Ruiz de Leon A, et al: Metastatic lymphangiosarcoma in a horse. Vet Pathol 39:266, 2002.

59. Haschek WM, King JM, Tennant BC: Primary renal cell carcinoma in two horses. J Am Vet Med Assoc 179:992, 1981.

60. Traub-Dargatz JL: Urinary tract neoplasia. Vet Clin North Am Equine Pract 14:495, 1998.

61. Valentine BA, Weistock D: Metastatic testicular embryonal carcinoma in a horse. Vet Pathol 23:92, 1986.

62. May KA, Moll HD, Duncan RB, et al: Unilateral Leydig cell tumour resulting in acute colic and scrotal swelling in a stallion with descended testes. Equine Vet J 31:343, 1999.

63. Hunt RJ, Hay W, Collatos C, et al: Testicular seminoma associated with torsion of the spermatic cord in two cryptorchid stallions. J Am Vet Med Assoc 197:1484, 1990.

64. Gelberg HB, McEntee K: Equine testicular interstitial cell tumors. Vet Pathol 24:231, 1987.

65. Foreman JH, Weidner JP, Parry BW, et al: Pleural effusion secondary to thoracic metastatic mammary adenocarcinoma in a mare. J Am Vet Med Assoc 197:1193, 1990.

66. Seahorn TL, Hall G, Brumbaugh GW, et al: Mammary adenocarcinoma in four mares. J Am Vet Med Assoc 200:1675, 1992.

67. Edwards DF, Parker JW, Wilkinson JE, et al: Plasma cell myeloma in the horse: A case report and literature review. J Vet Intern Med 7:169, 1993.

68. Lester GD, Alleman AR, Raskin RE, et al: Pancytopenia secondary to lymphoid leukemia in three horses. J Vet Intern Med 7:360, 1993.

69. Dascanio JJ, Zhang CH, Antczak DF, et al: Differentiation of chronic lymphocytic leukemia in the horse: a report of two cases. J Vet Intern Med 6:225, 1992.

70. Huxtable CR, de Lahunta A, Summers BA, et al: Marginal siderosis and degenerative myelopathy: a manifestation of chronic subarachnoid hemorrhage in a horse with a myxopapillary ependymoma. Vet Pathol 37:483, 2000.

71. Heath SE, Peter AT, Janovitz EB, et al: Ependymoma of the neurohypophysis and hypernatremia in a horse. J Am Vet Med Assoc 207:738, 1995.

72. Pirie RS, Mayhew IG, Clarke CJ, et al: Ultrasonographic confirmation of a space-occupying lesion in the brain of a horse: choroid plexus papilloma. Equine Vet J 30:445, 1998.

73. Lester GD, MacKay RJ, Smith-Meyer B: Primary meningeal lymphoma in a horse. J Am Vet Med Assoc 201:1219, 1992.

74. Jackson CA, de Lahunta A, Dykes NL, et al: Neurological manifestation of cholesterinic granulomas in three horses. Vet Rec 135:228, 1994.

Nutrition of the Geriatric Horse

Sarah L. Ralston

Many horses older than 20 years are able to maintain good to excellent body condition and health on normal maintenance rations.[1] However, weight loss is not uncommon in old horses, especially in severe weather conditions, qualifying them as geriatrics in need of special care considerations. Causes of the inability to maintain good body condition in older horses include irreparable dental abnormalities (tooth loss, wave mouth), reduced digestion or absorption of nutrients, and pituitary dysfunction. If renal or hepatic function is also reduced, tolerance of excess dietary protein, calcium, and edible oil may be adversely affected. Chronic pain associated with arthritic changes may exacerbate the problem by decreasing appetite.

Evaluation

When confronted with a failing older horse, the first step should be to thoroughly evaluate what the horse is being fed, determine whether there have been any recent changes in diet or environment, and check the schedule of dental care and anthelminthic administration. Changing the ration to a better quality feed or hay, correcting severe dental abnormalities, and administering an anthelminthic will often solve the problem. Changes in environment can be particularly stressful to aged horses. Competition from new herd mates or loss of a herd companion can result in reduced intake and weight loss and should be taken into consideration. Old horses are more sensitive to extremes of weather than are younger horses, regardless of body condition or pituitary/thyroid func-

tion.[2] Geriatric horses should have adequate shelter, although confinement to a stall can exacerbate orthopedic problems and stiffness.

The older horse should be given a thorough dental examination (see Chapter 5). Correctable dental abnormalities (e.g., sharp points, hooks, broken or infected molars) should be addressed, but since most of these horses do not have much tooth growth left, overcorrection or aggressive floating should be avoided if possible.[3] The angle of the occlusal surface of the molars should be between 72 to 80 degrees relative to the lateral surface of the tooth for optimal grinding.[4] If dental abnormalities are not correctable, dietary changes may be necessary to optimize digestion and absorption of nutrients.

Before instituting dietary changes, however, blood should be drawn for complete blood chemistry assessment and a blood cell count to rule out medical causes of weight loss such as chronic infection, neoplasia, renal dysfunction, or hepatic failure (see Chapters 7, 13, and 21). The standard indices for renal and hepatic function can be applied to the geriatric horse.[2,5] Chronic laminitis or infections, hyperglycemia or hyperinsulinemia after a glucose challenge, polyuria/polydipsia, and hirsutism are suggestive of pituitary dysfunction (equine Cushing's disease), which is extremely common in geriatric horses.[2,6,7] If these signs are present, the horse should be tested. A modified dexamethasone suppression test is the single most sensitive and specific test for pituitary dysfunction[6] (see Chapter 7 for details). However, a simple screening test for hyperglycemia/hyperinsulinemia can be employed to assess the need for the modified dexamethasone suppression test or other testing. A blood sample can be obtained for glucose and insulin analysis before and then 1 to 2 hours after feeding the horse 3 pounds of concentrate, preferably a sweet grain mix (S.L. Ralston, unpublished data, 1989-1999). If the values reported for the two samples differ by more than 100 mg/dL for glucose or by more than 200 IU/mL for insulin, these results are strongly suggestive of pituitary dysfunction (S.L. Ralston, unpublished data, 1989-1999), and further tests should be conducted to verify the problem. Obesity alone can cause the same degree of insulin resistance as thyroid dysfunction or peripheral resistance (see Chapter 6).

Feeding Older Horses in Poor Body Condition

If no obvious medical problems are found other than pituitary dysfunction or poor dentition, the horse may benefit from a dietary change.[1] Reduced digestion of fiber, protein, and phosphorus was reported in horses older than 20 years of age in the 1980s.[8,9] Because the horses used in the study were born well before effective anthelminthic drugs were in common use and the digestive profile was identical to that found in horses that had undergone complete resection of the large colons, it is hypothesized that chronic parasitic scarring of the large intestine may be responsible for some of the apparent malabsorption/maldigestion observed in the earlier study.[8,9] The reduction in fiber digestion may also be attributable to the abnormal dentition.[3,4]

In these cases, one should slowly switch the horse to a ration formulated specifically for geriatric horses. Most major feed companies now offer "geriatric" feeds (which usually have the word "Senior" or "Vintage" in the product name) that contain 12 to 16 percent protein, less than 1.0 percent calcium, and 0.45 to 0.6 percent phosphorus and may contain added water-soluble vitamins. Most are designed to be "complete" feeds and contain at least 12 percent crude fiber. These feeds are usually either "predigested" or extruded to increase digestibility for the geriatric horse. If the horse has demonstrated insulin resistance or pituitary dysfunction, a product should be selected that has little or no added molasses. All changes should be done over the course of 4 to 5 days, gradually switching the old ration to the new product. No more than 0.5 percent of the horse's ideal body weight should be offered per feeding in the form of concentrates. If the new concentrate product is designed as a "complete" feed, up to 2.5 percent of the horse's ideal body weight could be offered daily, divided in five separate feedings. This, however, is often impractical and also may cause the horse to go "off feed." If it takes that much feed to maintain the horse, one should look for a higher caloric density product or add other feeds such as beet pulp or hay cubes or high-calorie supplements, such as edible oils or rice bran products. Long stem hay can still be offered and is recommended as long as choke is not a problem. Hay cubes can be used as a forage source if the horse has a problem chewing long stem hay. The hay cubes should be a mixture of grass hay or the whole corn plant and alfalfa. Soaked beet pulp or hay cubes (up to 0.5% body weight before adding the water) may be added to each feeding.

Cautions

Calcium intakes in excess of need result in high urinary calcium excretion in horses (SL Ralston, unpublished data, 1989-1999). In the author's experience, there is an unusually high incidence of renal and bladder calculi in otherwise clinically normal older horses fed straight alfalfa. Therefore, alfalfa and beet pulp, both relatively high in calcium, should be used with caution in failing older horses. Sweet feeds (>3% molasses) may exacerbate glucose intolerance and also should be used with caution in horses with pituitary dysfunction or hyperinsulinemia. Hay cubes and pelleted or extruded geriatric feeds can be soaked in water to make slurries if choke or impactions are a problem.

Supplements

Vegetable oil (1-2 cups per day) can be added to the ration for extra calories but must be introduced slowly. Aged horses were documented to have lower plasma ascorbic acid than did younger, healthy horses,[2] the cause of which has yet to be determined. However, vitamin C supplementation (10 g twice a day) increased antibody response to vaccines in aged horses, especially those with pituitary dysfunction (SL Ralston, unpublished data, 1989-1999) and may help old horses with chronic infections.

Other Considerations and Treatments

If chronic pain due to arthritis appears to be a contributing factor to the weight loss due to inappetence, the horse can be administered amounts of anti-inflammatory agents or glucosamine/chondroitin sulfate compounds. Nontraditional therapies such as acupuncture have also been effective in some cases. Confinement appears to exacerbate the stiffness and pain (SL Ralston, unpublished data, 1989-1999), so the horses should be turned out as much as possible.

If pituitary dysfunction is present, consideration should be given to treating the horse with either cyproheptadine or pergolide (see Chapters 6 and 12) in addition to the dietary modifications discussed above.

If renal or hepatic dysfunction is present, lower concentrations of protein (8%-10%) and higher concentrations of carbohydrate should be fed (S.L. Ralston, unpublished data, 1989-1999). Grass hay (chopped or cubed), corn, and barley are the feeds of choice. Salt should always be available free-choice. Beet pulp can be used as a roughage source for horses with hepatic disease but should be avoided in horses with renal disease because of its higher calcium content. Vegetable oil can be used as an additional calorie source for horses with renal disease but not for horses with evidence of hepatic dysfunction due to the danger of hyperlipidemia. Digestive aids such as yeast cultures may be of benefit.

Summary

Just because a horse is old does not mean it has to be thin and in poor health. With proper attention to dentition, ration, and veterinary care, horses can maintain excellent body condition and health well past 30 years of age.

REFERENCES

1. Ralston SL, Breuer LH: Field evaluation of a feed formulated for geriatric horses. J Equine Vet Sci 16:334, 1996.
2. Ralston SL, Nockels CF, Squires EL: Differences in diagnostic test results and hematologic data between aged and young horses. Am J Vet Res 49.1387, 1988.
3. Scrutchfield WL, Schumacher J, Martin MT: Correction of abnormalities of the cheek teeth. Proc ΛΛEP 42:11, 1996.
4. Ralston SL, Foster DL, Divers T, Hintz HF: Effect of dental correction on feed digestibility in horses. Equine Vet J 33:390, 2001.
5. McFarlane D, Sellon DC, Gaffney D, et al: Hematologic and serum biochemical variables and plasma corticotrophin concentrations in aged horses. Am J Vet Res 59:1247, 1998.
6. Dybdal NO, Hargreaves KM, Madigan JE, et al: Diagnostic testing for pituitary pars intermedia dysfunction in horses. JAVMA 204:627, 1994.
7. Beech J: Pituitary tumors. In Robinson NE, editor: Current Therapy in Equine Medicine 2. Philadelphia, WB Saunders, 1987, pp 182–185.
8. Ralston SL: Digestive alterations in aged horses. J Equine Vet Sci 9:203, 1989.
9. Ralston SL, Malinowski KM, Christensen R, Hafs H: Digestion in the aged horse re-visited. J Equine Vet Sci 21:310, 2001.

CHAPTER 15

Eye Disease in Geriatric Horses

Keith J. Chandler,

Andrew G. Matthews

Little is known about senile ophthalmic changes in equine animals, although in humans certain ophthalmic pathologic conditions become more common with increasing age, including vitreous degeneration (liquefaction), asteroid hyalosis, synchysis scintillans, senile retinal hyperpigmentation, and chorioretinal degeneration (cobblestone degeneration).[1] Among horses and ponies older than 15 years of age, more than 80 percent have eye lesions, although these lesions are not all age-related.[2] There are several equine ocular conditions, however, that are reportedly more common with advancing age, and these include senile retinopathy,[3] proliferative optic neuropathy,[4,5] and vitreal degeneration.[6]

In a study on the health of horses in the United Kingdom, only 1 percent of horse owners reported that their animals suffered from ocular disorders.[7] This may indicate that elderly animals are coping well with poor sight. The fact that so many elderly animals have ophthalmic lesions suggests that the lesions, and the potential visual disturbance, are not significant to the survival of aging domesticated horses. In wild horses, there are a number of limiting factors to longevity, including dental disease, but it would not be unreasonable to assume that deterioration in sight may also be a limiting factor.

There are no published data on the prevalence of ocular pathologic conditions in younger horses, so it is difficult to compare the prevalence in geriatric equine animals with the remainder of the equine population. Comparing lesions in old and young animals gives a cross-sectional indication of aging changes within the eye, but this method does not provide a direct measurement of senescence in individuals, since differences between age groups may be due to age-cohort effects. However, to qualify whether the lesions are true ageing changes, it would be necessary to repeatedly examine the same individual as it becomes older. These types of longitudinal studies in which the animals are drawn from a similar birth cohort are not usual in veterinary medicine because they are very time-consuming and costly.

Cornea and Ocular Surface

The ocular surfaces are continuously challenged, both by minor physical insults and by overgrowth of potential microbial pathogens, including bacteria and fungi, which make up the normal commensal population of the external eye. The health of the ocular surfaces, including the cornea, in the face of such challenge is to a large extent dependent on the ocular surface defense mechanisms. Most superficially, these include the physical and biochemical integrity of the tear film. The tear film mucin lysozyme, possibly the most potent of the tear film bacteriolytic agents, has been shown to decrease with age in humans. A nonspecific, innate immunity is present on the ocular surface. Innate immunity has no immunologic memory and comprises both phagocytic cells such as natural killer cells and leukocytes and serum-derived macromolecules such as defensins, complement components, and creative protein. These latter cells enter the tear film via increased capillary permeability after surface insult. In laboratory animals, the recruitment and phagocytic activity of polymorphonuclear leukocytes on the ocular surface is significantly reduced with age. Similarly, specific surface immunity driven by T cells and based on cell-mediated immunity is believed to become impaired in aging animals.

The result of age-based compromise of ocular surface defense mechanisms is seen in the increased risk of microbial disease, in particular keratomycosis, in older horses. In addition, these diseases may be more difficult to treat in older animals and, in general, carry a more guarded prognosis. Other clinical considerations arising from this include the imperative to select bacteriocidal over bacteriostatic antibiotics in treating bacterial ulceration in older animals, and in electing to use topical corticosteroids only with considerable circumspection.

Age is only one of a number of risk factors in microbial disease of the ocular surface, in particular of the cornea. Others include geographic and seasonal variation in the prevalence of potential keratopathogens among the microflora of the external eye, the liability to minor injury of the corneal surface, and the protracted or inappropriate use of topical antibiotics and corticosteroids.

Retina

The incidence of so-called senile retinopathy, a form of retinal degeneration, has been shown to increase with age (Fig. 15-1).[2] The retinopathy is characterized ophthalmoscopically by a generalized depigmentation and linear or branching hyperpigmentation in the non-tapetal fundus and, in some cases, by attenuation of the peripapillary retinal blood vessels (Figs. 15-2 and 15-3). In advanced cases, there may be hyper-reflectivity in the non-tapetal fundus. Histologically, this condition is characterized by disruption of the of the retinal pigment epithelium, loss of photoreceptors, and cystic degenera-

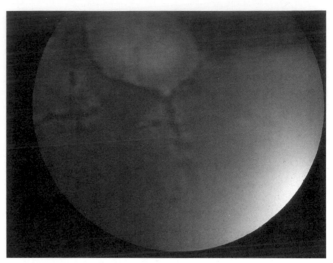

Figure 15-2 Senile retinopathy.

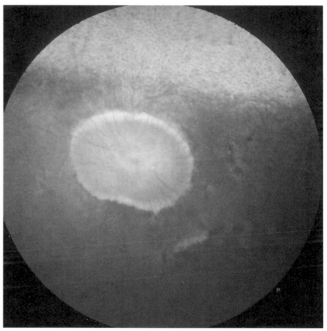

Figure 15-3 Senile retinopathy. Note the blood vessel attenuation.

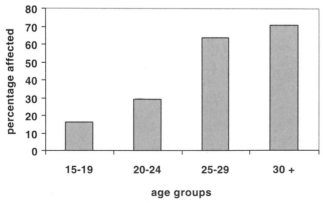

Figure 15-1 The prevalence of senile retinopathy in each age group of geriatric equine animals. Senile retinopathy is significantly more prevalent in older age groups ($P = .0007$).

tion of the inner layers of the neurosensory retina,[3] causing functional injury to the neurosensory retina and inevitably resulting in some degree of visual disruption.[5] The extent of any visual disability in affected horses is notoriously difficult to assess. Ophthalmoscopy has limitations, and electroretinography and visually evoked responses are not particularly accurate or practical.[5,8] Horses have the largest globe among domestic animals,[9] but the visual field of the direct ophthalmoscope corresponds to approximately 2 percent of the visually receptive fundus, permitting examination of only 15 percent to 20 percent of the retina through a maximally dilated pupil. As a result, lesions that appear large on ophthalmoscopic examination may represent only a small and possibly inconsequential defect.[5] However, there is little doubt that senile retinopathy does affect vision, particularly under poor lighting conditions. The visually attributable behavioral changes noted by the owners of affected animals include avoiding standing inside darkened stables and clumsiness in failing light. The photoreceptor and ganglion cell geography of the rod-rich equine retina permits a high degree of sensitivity to movement and changes in luminosity in dim light, but at the expense of visual acuity and point discrimination,[10] which may partly explain why disruption in photopic vision is commonly the first indication of visual disability. However, many geriatric animals are no longer working at a competitive level, and reduced or impaired vision may be less important. Retired animals are often managed in such a way that owners may miss cues to disturbances in vision; these animals are often kept in familiar surroundings and on a regular daily routine.

Other fundic lesions, such as focal chorioretinopathy (Fig. 15-4), affect up to 10 percent of the equine population in the United Kingdom.[11] Focal chorioretinopathy is found commonly in older horses, but it is likely that the initial inflammatory insult occurred some time before, most probably as a result of equine herpes virus infection. The resultant chorioretinal pathologic condition is present for the rest of the animal's life.

Optic Nerve

Optic nerve disease is more common in older horses. Optic atrophy is the end stage of ischemic injury to the nerve and in animals of any age can result from head trauma, optic neuritis, and, rarely, septic embolism. In older animals, optic atrophy may be associated with local perineural or infiltrative pathologic conditions such as orbital space-occupying lesions, tumors of the diencephalon, midbrain, meninges, or the optic nerve itself, and from sphenopalatine sinusitis. Affected eyes are invariably blind and may appear ophthalmoscopically normal in the early stages of the disease. Subsequently, the optic disc becomes pale and may have a granular appearance as the lamina cribrosa of the sclera foramen is exposed. There is profound attenuation of the retinal vasculature, and ischemic retinopathy may be evident. The condition may be found coincidentally with senile retinopathy.

Proliferative optic neuropathy is also reported to be more common in older horses; however, it is likely to be present in less than 2 percent of geriatric eyes.[2] This is a discrete, nonprogressive, whitish-pink lobular lesion located at the edge of the optic disc (Fig. 15-5) that does not appear to affect vision.[5,12] Histologically, the lesion

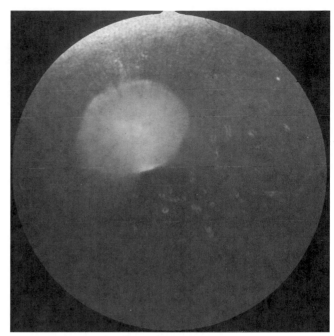
Figure 15-4 Focal chorioretinopathy.

typically consists of extruded glial tissue with lipid-filled cytoplasm vesicles, and in one case has been described as a schwannoma.

Vitreous

The vitreous occupies the greater part of the ocular volume and has a number of functions, including metabolic support of the neuroretina, maintenance of the spatial and geographic integrity of the neuroretina, removal of

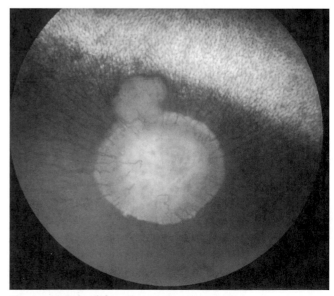
Figure 15-5 Proliferative optic neuropathy.

metabolic waste, and the unhindered transmission of light to the retina.

In humans, the consistency and optical clarity of the vitreous changes throughout life, and with increasing age liquefaction (syneresis) and collapse of the vitreal body occurs.[13] In horses, the uniformly low-density vitreal hydrogel probably does not undergo true age-related liquefaction until extreme old age. However, progressive dilution of the hydrogel throughout life appears to convey the clinical impression of liquefaction from a relatively early age, usually evident in the movement of intravitreal "floaters" with ocular saccades. Pathologic liquefaction arising from posterior segment inflammatory disease may also commonly contribute to the apparent vitreal liquefaction in relatively young horses. The cumulative effect of apparent liquefaction and the appearance of inflammatory or other cellular debris is referred to as *vitreal degeneration* and begins to affect horses from the age of 6 years.[6] Inflammatory debris in the vitreous can result from diseases such as equine recurrent uveitis. Vitreal degeneration may affect up to half of all equine animals older than 15 years of age,[2] and these vitreal changes may be even more common in areas where there is a high prevalence of recurrent uveitis, such as in continental Europe, where uveitis affects up to 15 percent of that equine population.[14]

Vitreous degeneration is best visualized using direct ophthalmoscopy or slit-lamp biomicroscopy. Typically, there is clouding or discoloration of the vitreous gel, and particulate, membranous, or cellular debris may be suspended within the vitreal body. These changes are rarely severe enough to adversely affect vision, but in some cases direct ophthalmoscopic examination of retinal detail may be markedly hindered.

Synchysis scintillans, or cholesterosis bulbi (Fig. 15-6), is a rare condition in horses and is reportedly more common in older animals. It manifests as highly refractile, golden particles floating freely within the vitreous. These particles are made up of cholesterol crystals and usually reflect previous hemorrhage within the vitreous, which in most instances is likely to be secondary to head trauma.

Asteroid hyalosis (Fig. 15-7) is a very rare finding in old horses. It appears as relatively large whitish or refractile particles enmeshed in the vitreous gel structure. The particles probably consist of lipid-mineral complexes and typically remain suspended in the vitreous body, although some movement is provoked by ocular saccades. Their origin is unknown.

Lens

Cataracts are the loss of optical homogeneity of the lens, and they are common in older horses.[15,16] As horses and ponies age, there is increased risk of cataract development

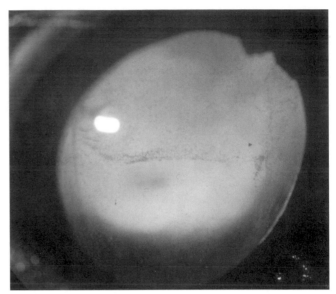

Figure 15-6 Synchysis scintillans in a 38-year-old pony.

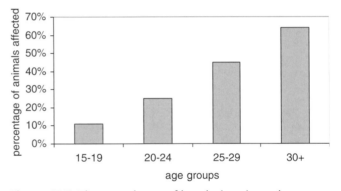

Figure 15-7 The prevalence of lens lesions in each age group of geriatric equine animals. The prevalence of lens lesions is significantly higher in older age groups ($P = .0048$).

(Fig. 15-8). Senile cataracts are age-dependant opacities found commonly in animals older than 18 years. It is unclear how senile cataracts develop in the horse. They may represent true senescence of the lens but in most cases are more likely to be associated with an age-determined susceptibility of the lens to autocrine or oxidative injury associated with subclinical intraocular pathologic conditions. Senile cataracts typically involve the posterior nuclear suture lines and anterior or posterior cortex (Fig. 15-9). Complete and occasionally hypermature cataracts occur in some animals, with the animal losing the pupillary light response in advanced cases.

Posterior capsular cataract is found in association with posterior uveitis and, on occasion, with vitreal degeneration. This type of cataract becomes increas-

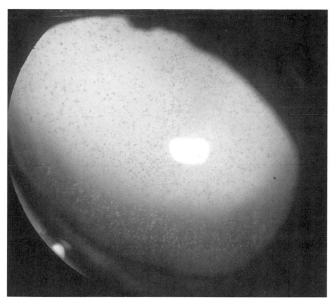

Figure 15-8 Unilateral asteroid hyalosis.

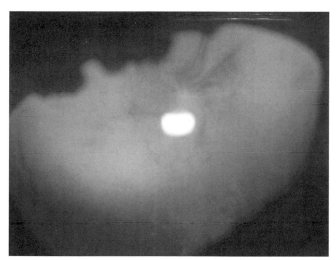

Figure 15-9 Senile cataract with posterior suture condensations.

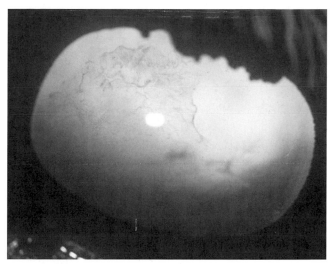

Figure 15-10 Posterior capsular cataract with incidental anterior cataract.

Glaucoma

Glaucoma is relatively uncommon in horses and ponies. Animals older than 15 years are at an increased risk, however, particularly if they have been previously or are currently affected by anterior segment inflammatory disease, including equine recurrent uveitis (Figs. 15-11 and 15-12).[17] Appaloosas are at particular risk from the disease. Clinical signs in the early stages of equine glaucoma are often subtle, and ocular pain may not be apparent. Corneal opacity is a common and early presenting sign, either as diffuse "ground glass" opacity or as branching striate opacities arising from dehiscences in Descemet's membrane caused by elevations in intraocular pressure. As the condition progresses, other signs, including cataract and posterior synechiae, may become apparent. Diagnosis is based on clinical signs and tonometric measurement of intraocular pressure. However, intraocular pressure rises may be transient, and some glaucomatous eyes may be normotonic at the time of examination. Treatment of the condition is directed at reducing intraocular pressure using topical carbonic-anhydrase inhibitors such as dorzolamide and topical beta blockers such as timolol maleate. In addition, some horses will respond to treatment of underlying uveitis with topical corticosteroids and systemic anti-inflammatory medication. Topical prostaglandins, as used in the management of some human glaucomas, are contraindicated in the horse. All glaucoma cases in the horse are difficult to manage medically over the long term, and surgical options including cyclodestruction or enucleation should be considered.

Ocular Neoplasia

Squamous cell carcinoma is the most common tumor of the eye, and there is an increased prevalence with age: an

ingly common with age and appears as an irregular diffuse opacity of the posterior lens (Fig. 15-10). This type of cataract may be progressive and can hinder ophthalmoscopic examination of the posterior segment.

Nuclear sclerosis has not been definitively described in equines. In extreme old age, however, horse lenses commonly show an enhanced nuclear delineation, which may be associated with senile cataracts and, rarely, brunescence of the lens. Vision is unlikely to be affected by these types of lens changes.

Aged animals with senile cataracts are likely to be a poor surgical risk and are not suitable candidates for lensectomy.

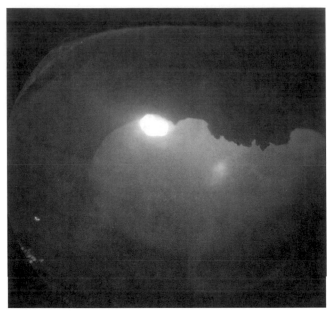

Figure 15-11 Uveitic glaucoma, note incidental anterior capsular cataract.

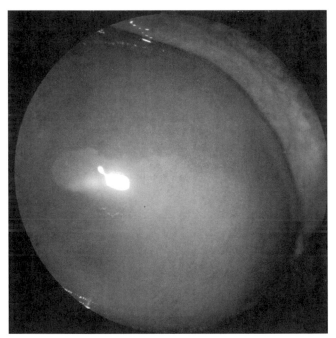

Figure 15-12 Acute uveitic glaucoma.

11-year-old horse is 2.4 times more likely to develop squamous cell carcinoma than a 2-year-old.[18] With advancing age comes long-term exposure to carcinogens, in this case ultraviolet light. However, there may be age-related biochemical or immunologic factors that influence the risk of development of these neoplasms.

Squamous cell carcinoma primarily affects the limbal conjunctiva and the third eyelid. Some cases are quite subtle and manifest as a persistent nonresponsive conjunctivitis, although closer inspection may reveal roughening of the surface of the conjunctiva by tumor formation. Diagnosis is based on history and, ultimately, biopsy results. Excision or radiotherapy is effective, and the prognosis is favorable if the tumor is removed at an early stage. Metastasis is uncommon.

Melanomas are usually found in older gray horses, although they rarely cause more than local affects such as protrusion of the third eyelid. Periorbital sarcoids tend to affect young adult horses and do not commonly appear for the first time in geriatric animals.

REFERENCES

1. Naumann GOH, Apple DJ: Pathology of the Eye. New York, Springer-Verlag, 1986.
2. Chandler KJ, Billson FM, Mellor DJ: Ophthalmic lesions in 83 geriatric horses and ponies. Vet Rec 153:319, 2003.
3. Barnett KC: The ocular fundus of the horse. Equine Vet J 4:17, 1971.
4. Rebhun WC: Equine retinal lesions and retinal detachments. Equine Vet J Suppl 2:86, 1983.
5. Matthews AG, Crispin SM, Parker J: The equine fundus III: Pathological variants. Equine Vet J Suppl 10:55, 1990.
6. Gellat KN: Equine ophthalmology. In Essentials of Veterinary Ophthalmology. Philadelphia: Lippincott, Williams & Wilkins, 2000, pp 337–377.
7. Mellor DJ, Love S, Walker R, et al: Sentinel practice-based survey of the management and health of horses in northern Britain. Vet Rec 149:417, 2001.
8. Crispin SM, Matthews AG, Parker J: The equine fundus I: Examination, embryology, structure and function. Equine Vet J Suppl 10:42, 1990.
9. Davidson MG: Equine ophthalmology. In Gellat KN, editor: Veterinary Ophthalmology. Philadelphia: Lea & Febiger, 1991, pp 576–611.
10. Ehrenhofer MCA, Deeg CA, Reese S, et al: Normal structure and age-related changes in the equine retina. Vet Ophthalmol 5:39, 2002.
11. Slater JD, Ellis MA, Froesch N, et al: Herpesvirus chorioretinal lesions. In Proceedings of the 40th British Equine Veterinary Association Congress, 2001, pp 169–170.
12. Rebhun WC: Equine retinal lesions and retinal detachments. Equine Vet J Suppl 2:86, 1983.
13. Sebag J: The vitreous. In Hart WM, editors: Alders Physiology of the Eye, 9th edition. London, Butterworth, 1992, pp 268–348.
14. Deeg C: Equine recurrent uveitis: An inflammatory disease mediated by organ-specific autoimmunity. In Proceedings of the 40th British Equine Veterinary Association Congress, 2001, pp 167–168.
15. Matthews AG: Lens opacities in the horse: a clinical classification. Vet Ophthalmol 3:65, 2000.
16. Matthews AG: Classification, diagnosis and prognosis of equine cataracts. In Proceedings of the 40th British Equine Veterinary Association Congress, 2001, pp 173–175.
17. Miller TR, Brooks DE, Smith PJ, et al: Equine glaucoma: clinical findings and response to treatment in 14 horses. Vet Comp Ophthalmol 5:170, 1995.
18. Dugan SJ, Curtis CR, Roberts SM, et al: Epidemiological study of ocular/adnexal squamous cell carcinoma in horses. J Am Vet Med Assoc 198:251, 1991.

CHAPTER 16

Respiratory Disease in the Geriatric Equine Patient

Elizabeth Davis,

Bonnie R. Rush

Recurrent Airway Obstruction

Geriatric horses have the potential to suffer from a variety of age-associated health issues. The body systems most commonly affected include the musculoskeletal, endocrine, gastrointestinal, and respiratory systems. Although a variety of conditions can result in pulmonary disease in geriatric equines, by far the most common disorder is heaves. This condition is more descriptively termed *recurrent airway obstruction* (RAO), and as the name implies it is a recurrent inflammatory condition of the equine pulmonary system. When the diagnosis of heaves is made in a geriatric patient, the condition is more likely to be advanced. Recurrent airway obstruction is a relatively drug-responsive disease in middle-aged horses, but when diagnosed later in life, horses are more likely to have permanent pulmonary remodeling and fibrosis that is less amenable to drug therapy.

Recurrent obstruction of the lower airways is characterized by bronchospasm, excessive mucous production, and pathologic changes of the bronchiolar walls that result in terminal airway obstruction.[1,2] Since the total cross-sectional area of the small airways is notably large, clinical signs develop at rest only after obstructive disease is generalized, involving the majority of the small airways. There is no recognized breed or gender predisposition, and disease incidence correlates linearly with age.[3] Previous studies have demonstrated a hereditary basis of disease, and specific lines appear predisposed to the development of RAO.[4] These data are supported by the fact that human asthma is highly heritable in young children, even though the mode of inheritance does not follow a classic mendelian inheritance pattern.

Equine heaves causes a reproducible series of clinical signs in affected horses, regardless of age. Disease exacerbation is often seasonal and tends to be more intense when horses are housed indoors and exposed to specific allergens or airway irritants such as organic dust, poor-quality hay, ammonia fumes, fungal spores, and other stimuli.[4] In contrast, summer-pasture associated obstructive pulmonary disease is a syndrome similar to heaves, except that the clinical signs are triggered by exposure to late summer pollens at pasture in the southeastern United States.[7,14,22,23] The primary differences between heaves and summer-associated disease involve the local climate with exposure to specific aeroallergens that induce clinical signs of airway obstruction. The clinical signs and medical therapy of summer-pasture associated obstructive pulmonary disease are identical to heaves.

The most common presenting symptom for horses with RAO is chronic cough. Exercise intolerance, respiratory distress, mucopurulent nasal discharge, abnormal pulmonary sounds, and an enlarged field of percussion are additional abnormalities that may be noted during physical examination. Diagnostic challenges are encountered when clinical signs are mild, exhibited by an occasional cough, exercise intolerance, or minimal abdominal effort. A rebreathing procedure enhances pulmonary sounds on auscultation and may aid in clinical diagnosis. Horses suffering from mild heaves will require ancillary diagnostic testing. Blood gas analysis at rest and 5 minutes after exercise may provide supportive evidence for the presence of low-grade RAO, indicating pulmonary gas exchange impairment. This is particularly important if the PaO_2 values at rest are low (normal values at sea level are 100 ± 5 mm Hg or 13.3 ± 0.7 kPa).[2] When pulmonary function testing is performed in RAO-affected horses, the most reproducible change is increased pulmonary resistance, which is more apparent in moderate to severely affected horses. Histamine challenge can identify horses with low-grade disease by determining hyperresponsive bronchoconstriction. Histologic evaluation of pulmonary tissue obtained from heaves-affected horses is characterized by evidence of persistent pulmonary inflammation during disease remission. These findings indicate that although clinical signs of disease are reversible, pulmonary parenchymal changes are permanent.

Goals of therapy for heaves-affected horses are (1) reduction in airway inflammation, (2) elimination of bronchoconstriction, and (3) enhancement of mucociliary clearance mechanisms. Environmental modification to reduce allergic exposure is the most important treatment principle. Combination therapy with corticosteroids and bronchodilator therapy is a commonly employed treatment strategy for RAO-affected patients.

Pathophysiology

Although incompletely understood, pulmonary structural changes and pulmonary inflammation are not consistently correlated in heaves-affected horses (Box 16-1). In an effort to characterize equine RAO, research has focused on the role of submucosal inflammatory changes in combination with epithelial components as a function of disease progression. The hypothesis suggests a correlation involving these anatomic regions and is based on the pathophysiology of human asthma, in which the primary role of the submucosa in the pathophysiology is well documented.[2]

Box 16-1

Pathologic Changes of Recurrent Airway Obstruction

Mucous production and bronchoconstriction are consistent, clinically recognizable features of RAO.

Luminal neutrophilic infiltrates resulting from increased interleukin-8 expression.

Irreversibility of disease is associated with submucosal hyperplasia, fibrosis, and peribronchiolar mineralization. These changes are more likely to be identified in geriatric equine patients suffering from long-standing disease.

Early in the course of disease, acute exposure to a challenge (allergen) environment results in destruction of surface cilia and loss of epithelial cells, resulting in submucosal and intercellular edema. Acute bronchiolar disease typically results in degeneration, necrosis, and Clara cell exfoliation. With chronicity, structural changes are characterized by regions of proliferating progenitor type cells centralized around irregular hyperplastic foci. Histologic changes of the mucosal lining are typically observed in the peripheral bronchioles located in the caudodorsal pulmonary fields.[2] Severe obstructive disease is associated with multifocal mucous cell metaplasia in the smaller peripheral airways of affected horses. Excessive mucin production results in peripheral bronchiolar obstruction with viscous-appearing mucin, visible on histopathologic examination. Severe disease involves the development of mineralized peribronchiolar plaques in combination with significant mucous accumulation. Changes that are observed in horses with severe, long-standing disease explain the irreversibility of this disease in geriatric horses.

The inflammation of heaves is characterized by influx of luminal neutrophils,[5] whereas submucosal infiltrates are composed of lymphocytes, mast cells, plasma cells, and occasionally eosinophils. When inflammation is severe, organization of lymphoid follicles in the submucosa has been observed. Peribronchial lymphocytes are immunoglobulin-producing B-lymphocytes and CD4+ T-lymphocytes. The CD4+ T-lymphocytes follow the TH_2 phenotype, characterized by the release of interleukins 4, 8, and 13, contributing to IgE antibody production and neutrophil recruitment.[5,6] These findings are similar to those of human asthma with the absence of interleukin-5 expression in heaves-affected horses. Increased interleukin-5 in human asthmatics results in classic eosinophil-dominated type I hypersensitivity. Analysis of bronchoalveolar lavage cells and peripheral blood mononuclear cells of horses affected with summer-pasture associated obstructive pulmonary disease, during episodes of disease, has demonstrated increased interleukin-4 mRNA production.[7,8] These findings support the histopathologic findings of neutrophilic infiltrates and the absence of eosinophils in the lower airways of heaves-affected horses. Interleukin-4 induced production of IgE antibodies directed against specific aeroallergens likely plays a pivotal role in the pathology of heaves.[12]

Another proximal mediator of disease is the nuclear transcription factor nuclear factor-κB (NF-κB), which is partially regulated through the binding of inhibitor-κB (I-κB). Upon stimulation (i.e., inflammation), dissociation of I-κB from NF-κB occurs in the cytoplasm of affected cells. This dissociation allows for translocation of NF-κB into the nucleus, where it binds to its binding site in the promoter region of DNA. This binding initiates the process of gene transcription and ultimately protein synthesis for inflammatory proteins, such as cellular cytokines. When present as a homodimer of p65 subunits, this transcription factor is recognized to specifically upregulate the synthesis of interleukin-8.[9,10] It is this pathway that is constitutively active in heaves-affected horses and is believed to play a major role in neutrophilic chemotaxis demonstrated by RAO patients[2].

Clinical Signs

Early manifestations of disease may be subclinical, with affected horses appearing bright, alert, and afebrile. Occasional coughing at the initiation of exercise or while eating may be the first abnormalities detected. Typically, the frequency and intensity of coughing episodes increases and develops into paroxysmal periods of nonproductive cough. Nasal discharge commonly accompanies episodes of respiratory distress. With disease exacerbation, episodes of tachypnea, nostril flare, and double expiratory effort occur. Significant weight loss and the presence of a "heave line" will accompany disease progression, particularly in untreated geriatric horses. The heave line represents hypertrophy of the external abdominal oblique muscles that have been recruited to aid in expiration of air trapped in terminal airways. The recurrent nature of the disease is variable, and episodes may last days to weeks.

Thoracic auscultation of horses with mild RAO may not identify abnormalities at rest, but a rebreathing procedure or examination after exercise may reveal expiratory wheezes in the pulmonary periphery.[11] A tracheal rattle due to excessive mucous production and wheezes throughout all lung fields are observed in horses with advanced disease. Air trapping in peripheral lung fields will result in hyper-resonance of ventral and caudal lung fields; these changes account for the increased size of pulmonary fields.

Box 16-2 lists the clinical signs of recurrent airway obstruction.

Diagnosis

When heaves-affected horses present with advanced disease, the diagnosis is straightforward, primarily based on clinical signs. It is important for the clinician to rule out primary or secondary bacterial pneumonia, which may contribute to pulmonary dysfunction. Recurrent airway obstruction will not influence hemogram results; therefore, a normal complete blood cell count rules out complicating infectious disease. Geriatric patients with concurrent pituitary pars intermedia dysfunction (PPID) may demonstrate evidence of a stress leukogram and hyperglycemia. Fibrinogen concentration should be within normal limits in horses with uncomplicated heaves.

Box 16-2

Clinical Signs of Recurrent Airway Obstruction

Occasional coughing progressing to paroxysmal attacks associated with eating or exercise.

Nasal discharge associated with episodes of dyspnea. Episodes of dyspnea are progressive in nature, rendering the untreated geriatric patient severely compromised for pulmonary functional reserve.

Chronic disease is accompanied by development of a "heave line" due to profound air trapping in the lower airways and hypertrophy of the external abdominal oblique muscle.

In horses with less severe disease, bronchoalveolar lavage is a valuable diagnostic tool to obtain samples for cytologic examination of the lower airways (Fig. 16-1). Transtracheal aspirate samples are less useful for diagnosis of RAO, because small airway secretions obtained using this method are contaminated by tracheal secretions. Classic cytologic changes associated with RAO include pulmonary neutrophilia (15%-85% of total bronchoalveolar lavage cells) and Curschmann's spirals, composed of inspissated mucous casts of small bronchioli. Although pulmonary neutrophilia will exist in all affected patients, good correlation does not always exist between severity of bronchoalveolar lavage (percentage of neutrophils) changes and clinical severity of disease.[12,13]

Additional diagnostic testing may include endoscopy, arterial blood gas analysis, and pulmonary function testing. Endoscopic examination during airway obstruction will reveal tracheal hyperemia, mucoid exudate, and increased sensitivity to cough. Radiographic evaluation reveals a mild to moderate interstitial pattern with a pronounced peribronchiolar radiodensity.[11,14] Arterial blood gas analysis is an easy and efficient method of assessing gas exchange in severely affected horses. Horses suffering from moderate heaves may have a PaO_2 less than 80 mm Hg at rest, whereas horses in severe distress may have a PaO_2 of 50 mm Hg.[2] Pulmonary function can be assessed by estimating fluctuations in pleural pressure as measured through intrathoracic esophageal pressures. The measurement is performed using a commercially available esophageal catheter linked to a portable physiologic recorder. This technique is limited in its usefulness because significant changes in intrathoracic esophageal pressures are detected only when obvious clinical signs of respiratory disease are present. However, bronchoprovocation challenge with histamine will reveal airway hypersensitivity in mildly affected horses or horses in disease remission and subsequently may aid in determining the diagnosis in mildly affected patients.

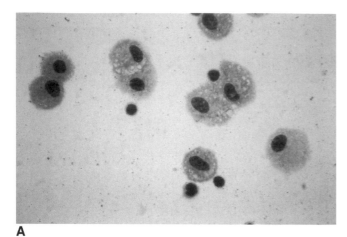

A

B

Figure 16-1 A, Normal cytologic results from a bronchoalveolar lavage sample obtained from a healthy horse. Mature macrophages (foamy cytoplasm) and dark-staining lymphocytes make up the predominant cell types. B, Sample obtained from a horse suffering from recurrent airway obstruction. Note the predominance of neutrophils (N <15%) that make up the majority of the leukocyte population on bronchoalveolar lavage cytologic examination.

Lung biopsy is a more invasive technique that is useful for yielding prognostic information. There is good correlation between parenchymal change and severity of disease. This procedure can be performed with ultrasound guidance or blind sampling at the seventh or eighth intercostal space, approximately 8 cm above the humeroradial joint. Hemorrhage is a potential life-threatening complication; therefore, lung biopsy is not recommended for routine diagnosis of RAO. Bronchoscopy has been attempted for biopsy samples, but these findings correlate poorly with transcutaneous thoracic biopsy results. A newer biopsy technique involves the use of thoroscopy, allowing for excellent visualization and monitoring for appropriate hemostasis.[16] A major advantage of biopsy sampling is to determine prognostic information for severely affected patients.

Equine recurrent airway obstruction is recognized to be a reversible, episodic condition. The previous nomenclature, chronic obstructive pulmonary disease, correlates to progressive and irreversible disease in humans, often associated with smoking, and is inappropriate to describe this syndrome in horses. On the other hand, the reversible nature of RAO allows these horses to continue to be functional with appropriate environmental and therapeutic management. Subsequently, identification of the level of reversibility may have a direct impact on the prognosis of horses suffering from RAO. Previous reports have suggested that this reversibility can be documented based on individual response to the parasympatholytic agent atropine (5 mg/kg IV, once). Potential complications of paralytic ileus and colic preclude widespread use of this agent in the diagnosis of RAO. Response to β_2-adrenergic agonist therapy (albuterol, 310 mg) in combination with pulmonary function testing before and after bronchodilation can provide the clinician with valuable information about the reversibility of the airway obstruction.[2]

Box 16-3 demonstrates diagnosis of recurrent airway obstruction.

Treatment

The primary goal of treatment for RAO-affected horses is prevention of exposure to allergens (organic dusts and molds), in combination with provision of symptomatic

---

Box 16-3

Diagnosis of Recurrent Airway Obstruction

1. Clinical signs in severely affected horses:
   a. Complete blood cell count with fibrinogen concentration in these individuals is important to rule out primary or secondary bacterial infection.
   b. Evaluation of hormonal testing may be indicated if PPID appears to be present in geriatric patients.
2. Mild to moderate disease:
   a. Endoscopy of the upper airway and trachea characterized by mucosal hyperemia and mucous exudates.
   b. Bronchoalveolar lavage cytologic examination characterized by neutrophilia (>15 % polymorphonuclear leukocytes), often in combination with Curschmann's spirals.
3. Bronchoprovocation with histamine may be necessary for diagnosis in mildly affected individuals.
4. Thoracic radiographs may be useful for staging chronic disease. A poor prognosis is associated with significant interstitial pattern and peribronchiolar mineralization.

relief with bronchodilators and anti-inflammatory therapy via corticosteroids.

Environmental Management

Reduced exposure to dust and molds is the cornerstone to successful management of horses suffering from RAO. Appropriate drug therapy will be incompletely effective if environmental management is not implemented. Reversal of clinical signs resulting from environmental change alone may take 3 to 4 weeks. A direct correlation has been observed between the severity of disease and the duration of remission of disease. For example, horses that are maintained in an outdoor environment and fed good-quality hay usually remain free from clinical signs of disease for extended periods of time. Therefore, owners should be encouraged to maintain an RAO-affected horse outdoors in a cold climate. Even in harsh winters, horses that are provided shelter, good-quality hay, and water are unlikely to experience clinical episodes of obstructive disease.

Horses that require indoor housing should be managed in a clean, controlled environment. The principles for maintaining the environment include (1) reduced allergen load in the surroundings, (2) modification of allergen exposure (wet hay, hay cubes, or pellets), and (3) enhanced environmental clearance of dust and molds with good ventilation systems. When comparing bedding materials, organic dust concentrations are 35-fold higher in the breathing zone for horses bedded on straw and fed dry hay when compared with shavings and pelleted feed. Alternatively, grass silage feeding is effective for reducing the allergen load for horses bedded on shavings. Hay that is offered wet will not adequately reduce allergen load for most heaves-affected horses. The most effective method of controlling allergen exposure is to limit source exposure in horses maintained in confinement.

As previously stated, the ideal environment for heaves-affected horses is pasture turnout, where exposure to respirable aeroallergens and endotoxin is minimized. Horses in remission, based on pulmonary function and clinical scores, will maintain low-grade pulmonary inflammation in a low-dust, controlled environment. These horses in apparent remission have persistent pulmonary neutrophilia, increased alveolar clearance rates, and hypersensitivity to bronchoprovocation challenge, suggesting that an outdoor environment is superior to controlled indoor housing. Geriatric horses maintained outdoors will have increased caloric needs, particularly during periods of harsh weather conditions. As RAO-affected horses age, they have increasing difficulty maintaining an appropriate body condition score. Poor body condition is a significant problem in older horses living outdoors, especially for those that compete with young horses for feed. Palatable, soft pelleted feed designed for geriatric horses will increase feed efficiency. Body condition will also be negatively affected by PPID, highlighting the need to appropriately manage endocrine function in older horses with heaves.

Anti-inflammatory Therapy

The cornerstone of therapy to induce remission of clinical signs in horses suffering from recurrent airway obstruction is reduced inflammation. It is well recognized that the inflammatory cytokines released by activated T-lymphocytes increase the pulmonary concentration of interleukin-4 and interleukin-8. Pulmonary neutrophilia resulting from increased interleukin-8 levels maintains a heightened level of immune reactivity, contributing to enhanced mucous production, bronchospasm, and coughing. Corticosteroids act as direct inhibitors of this inflammatory cascade, resulting in improved clinical signs. The combination of corticosteroids with bronchodilator therapy is most effective for inducing disease remission. However, geriatric horses with chronic heaves are less likely to demonstrate complete disease remission, despite appropriate environmental and pharmacologic management. When selecting long-acting potent systemic corticosteroids, the clinician must consider that this class of drug is more likely to produce detrimental effects such as laminitis and immune suppression. Therefore, therapeutic recommendations for glucocorticoids include administering the lowest effective dose and avoiding prolonged administration. In many cases, a course of therapy for approximately 2 weeks is sufficient to induce clinical remission.

Systemic administration of potent corticosteroids improves clinical signs, reduces airway inflammation, and improves pulmonary function in horses with recurrent airway obstruction. An additional benefit of glucocorticoid therapy is reduced β-adrenergic receptor downregulation, resulting in prolonged beneficial effects of bronchodilator therapy. Triamcinolone acetonide (0.09 mg/kg intramuscularly) as a single dose relieves lower airway obstruction for up to 4 weeks. Unfortunately, this therapy results in adrenal suppression for approximately 4 weeks, characterized by low resting serum cortisol. Dexamethasone (0.02-0.05 mg/kg IV q 24 hours) reduces airway obstruction and inflammation within 3 to 7 days while providing clinical benefit evident for up to 7 days. Administration of dexamethasone also produces adrenal suppression; however, this effect is relatively short-lived, lasting approximately 3 days after discontinuation of treatment.[17] Oral prednisolone (1 mg/kg PO daily) does not rapidly improve clinical signs of airway obstruction; this therapy may improve pulmonary inflammation in horses with RAO if administered for more than 1 week of therapy. Nonsteroidal anti-inflammatory drugs and anti-histamines appear to be ineffective for the treatment of inflammation associated with heaves.

Aerosolized corticosteroids are effective in horses with mild to moderate airway obstruction. Aerosolized drugs provide the benefit of drug delivery directly to the respiratory tract but represent a more substantial financial investment and may be reserved for valuable or performance horses. There are three aerosolized corticosteroid preparations available in metered-dose inhaler preparations: beclomethasone dipropionate, fluticasone propionate, and flunisolide. These medications can be administered via the Equine AeroMask or the Equine Haler. The relative potency of these surface-acting corticosteroids are fluticasone > beclomethasone > flunisolide = triamcinolone. When considering dexamethasone as a standard of 1, flunisolide = 1.9; triamcinolone = 2.0; beclomethasone = 13.5; and fluticasone = 18.0.

When comparing the commercially available corticosteroid products, fluticasone is the most potent and the most expensive. Fluticasone is highly lipophilic, resulting in the longest pulmonary residence time. Since fluticasone has extremely low oral bioavailability (<2%) and extensive first-pass metabolism (99%), fluticasone has the advantage of being the least likely to result in adverse systemic side effects while providing the most favorable therapeutic index of the commercially available aerosolized corticosteroids. Horses suffering from recurrent airway obstruction receiving fluticasone (2000 µg bid, AeroMask) demonstrate reduced pulmonary neutrophilia, improved pulmonary function assessment, and reduced responsiveness to histamine challenge during episodes of airway obstruction. When normal horses are evaluated after administration of fluticasone, serum cortisol levels are reduced by 40 percent after 1 day of therapy and by 65 percent after 1 week of treatment. Serum cortisol concentrations return to pretreatment levels approximately 24 to 48 hours after discontinuation of drug therapy. Despite the fact that human asthma patients remain on inhaled corticosteroids for extended periods of time without the detriment of adrenosuppression, horses have increased sensitivity to the adrenosuppressive effects of inhaled corticosteroids.

Inhaled corticosteroids are a valuable therapeutic option for treatment of heaves-affected horses. Beclomethasone (3750 µg bid, Equine Aeromask, Canadian Monaghan, London, Ontario, Canada) reduces pulmonary inflammation, improves pulmonary function, and improves ventilation imaging of horses suffering from recurrent airway obstruction. In contrast to rescue bronchodilator therapy, no immediate drug effect is observed with aerosolized corticosteroids. Administration of beclomethasone (3500 µg bid) using the AeroMask improves parameters of pulmonary function and arterial oxygen tension approximately 3 to 4 days after initiation of therapy.[18] Among the variety of available inhaled corticosteroid preparations, fluticasone (2000 µg bid) is the most potent, with the advantage of minimal adrenosuppressive effects.[6] Reduced pulmonary neutrophilia, improved pulmonary function, and reduced airway hyperresponsiveness are observed after fluticasone administration. Although inhaled corticosteroids are particularly useful for resolution of airway obstruction, unless environmental modification is implemented, clinical signs of obstructive disease will return within 2 to 4 days after discontinuation of therapy. Subsequently, it can be concluded that if environmental management is not addressed, clinical resolution will not be maintained when beclomethasone treatment is used.

Bronchodilator Therapy

Pulmonary bronchoconstriction associated with RAO requires specific therapy for immediate relief of smooth muscle contraction in the lower airways. Symptomatic bronchodilator therapy will improve clinical signs; however, lower airway inflammation is not altered by bronchodilator administration. Bronchodilator therapy is primarily indicated for symptomatic relief of bronchoconstriction.[2] The rapid onset of action of aerosolized bronchodilator treatment consistently provides immediate relief of bronchoconstriction. The most effective agents available for bronchodilation are β_2-adrenergic agonists and parasympatholytic agents. Methylxanthines are less reliable and have a narrow therapeutic index. Clinical improvement associated with bronchodilator treatment is characterized by reduced pulmonary resistance, increased pulmonary compliance, and decreased maximal change in pleural pressure.[2] Bronchodilator therapy is likely valuable in horses that appear to be in remission. Heaves-affected horses stabled in a dust-free environment demonstrate a positive response to bronchodilator therapy. These results illustrate the point that environmental management alone does not abolish the dominating bronchoconstrictive component of heaves; therefore, pharmacologic management, particularly prior to exercise, is beneficial to these patients, even when housed in an appropriate environment.[2]

Bronchoconstriction results from a variety of physiologic changes that occur in response to pulmonary hypersensitivity, including smooth muscle contraction, smooth muscle hypertrophy, and mucosal thickness leading to airway narrowing and subsequent air trapping. Pulmonary remodeling in heaves-affected horses includes mucous cell hyperplasia and metaplasia that contributes to the cascade of smooth muscle contraction, leading to lumenal contraction and narrowing. Bronchodilator therapy remains a mainstay of heaves treatment, supporting the recommendation that resolution of severe airway distress requires administration of rapid-acting bronchodilators.[18]

Aerosolized, short-acting β_2-adrenergic agonists (albuterol, pirbuterol, fenoterol) are rapidly effective bronchodilators indicated for "rescue therapy" for horses demonstrating respiratory difficulty at rest. Albuterol sulfate (360-900 μg) improves pulmonary function by 70 percent within 5 minutes of administration.[19,20] When severe airway obstruction is present, drug administration at 15-minute increments for up to 2 hours may be implemented for sequential bronchodilation. Beneficial effects from short-acting β_2-adrenergic agonists last approximately 1 hour in severely affected horses, resulting in the need for longer acting preparations. Combination therapy with corticosteroids will reduce the tolerance that develops to these agents in addition to enhancing β_2-adrenergic receptor protein expression.[17] The recently released Torpex (Boehringer Ingelheim Vetmedica) (Fig. 16-2) provides the clinician with a valuable therapeutic tool to manage severely affected dyspneic horses. With practice, horse owners easily learn to effectively administer this drug using the novel nasally placed device. This drug serves as an important rescue therapy during an episode of severe distress or before exercise commencement.

Long-acting bronchodilator preparations are ineffective for use as rescue treatment in patients suffering from severe airway obstruction because of their delayed onset of activity and slightly reduced peak activity compared with albuterol sulfate.[19,20] Indications for longer acting preparations are for prolonged bronchodilation after rescue therapy and for maintenance therapy for horses with mild to moderate disease. These agents can maintain

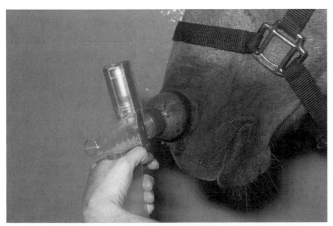

Figure 16-2 Aerosolized albuterol (Torpex, Boehringer Ingelheim Vetmedica) can be administered as a rescue therapy using the recently released intranasal device.

stability of the patient with administration two to three times per day. In addition, pre-exercise administration with long-acting bronchodilators will prevent exercise-induced bronchoconstriction. The most commonly administered agents in this class are salmeterol xinafoate and ipratropium bromide.

Salmeterol xinafoate is a chemical analogue of albuterol with profound lipid solubility and an elongated side chain. Activity of this side chain allows the salmeterol molecule to bind to an exosite proximal to the region of the β_2 adrenoceptor, thereby allowing salmeterol to repeatedly contact the β_2 receptor while being anchored to a site adjacent to the receptor. Additional benefits of salmeterol include enhanced lipophilicity that contribute to enhanced pulmonary residence time, β_2 affinity, β_2 selectivity (safety), and potency when compared to albuterol. Salmeterol xinafoate (210 μg) improves pulmonary function by 55% within 60 minutes of administration, with efficacy lasting for up to 8 hours, even in severely affected horses.[21]

Iprotropium bromide is a surface-acting antimuscarinic agent that exhibits little to no systemic absorption (quaternary ammonium structure) from the respiratory or gastrointestinal system. Ipratropium (180–360 μg) improves pulmonary function by 50 percent within 1 hour and the duration of effect is approximately 4 to 6 hours in severely affected patients. Since minimal systemic absorption occurs, few adverse effects are recognized after administration of ipratropium. In contrast to atropine, ipratropium does not reduce mucociliary clearance mechanisms.

Atropine (5 mg/450 kg horse IV) is a rapid and powerful bronchodilator in horses suffering from heaves. Since several adverse effects (ileus, central nervous system toxicity, tachycardia, increased viscosity of mucous secretions, impaired mucociliary clearance) can develop following the administration of atropine, this agent is reserved for use as rescue therapy for severe and life-threatening airway obstruction.

Orally administered bronchodilator therapy is available in a variety of forms. At the time of this writing, the most appropriately administered therapy is clenbuterol (0.8–0.13 $\mu g/kg$ PO bid). An incremental dose schedule, as recommended on the label, should be followed, since rapidly transitioned high doses are more likely to induce side effects such as tachycardia, sweating, and muscle fasciculations. Terbutaline and oral albuterol have poor bioavailability; thus, these products cannot be recommended for routine administration.

Complicating Factors

Horses with severe airway obstruction may develop secondary bacterial infection, contributing to compromise of pulmonary function. Subsequently, horses demonstrating marked nasal exudate, fever, and/or abnormal hematologic findings should be treated with antimicrobial therapy in addition to corticosteroids and bronchodilators.[3] Commonly administered antimicrobial agents are potentiated sulfas because of excellent spectrum of activity against common airway pathogens, ease of administration, and distribution in pulmonary tissue.

Pharmaceutical Management of Recurrent Airway Obstruction (Box 16-4)

Because heaves-affected horses can present in a variety of clinical conditions, it is important to address each case individually. For instance, individuals suffering respiratory distress at rest will require administration of systemic corticosteroid therapy due to poor drug distribution of aerosolized corticosteroids. Short-acting aerosolized bronchodilators provide immediate relief of airway obstruction (rescue therapy). Long-acting bronchodilators provide prolonged relief of airway obstruction. Precedent albuterol therapy will enhance pulmonary drug distribution of corticosteroids. In contrast to corticosteroids, aerosolized bronchodilators remain effective independent of severity of disease. Aerosolized bronchodilator therapy can be used for relief of airway obstruction until systemic corticosteroids become effective for control of disease. Individuals suffering from severe obstructive disease that is difficult to control respond favorably to aggressive bronchodilator therapy, which has more favorable clinical impact than increasing corticosteroid dosage. Increasing the corticosteroid dose does not provide dose-dependent enhanced efficacy; however, complications associated with corticosteroid administration are dose-related. Therefore, the lowest effective dose of corticosteroid is recommended for treatment of obstructive airway disease.

Prognosis and Expectations

Currently, there is no cure for recurrent airway obstruction in horses. Based on the severity of disease observed at initial evaluation, the prognosis and athletic ability will vary. For instance, horses with severe dyspnea observed at rest that have not been treated during the course of disease are more likely to have developed pulmonary remodeling and permanent compromise of pulmonary function. The spectrum of cases depends on the individual severity of disease in addition to therapeutic implementation. The primary goal of disease management is reduced allergen exposure. With strategic drug administration, these horses have a favorable prognosis for maintaining a good quality of life with continued, albeit limited in some cases, level of athletic activity. Horses with heaves should be observed to have improved breathing within 2 to 5 days of initiation of treatment and environmental modification. Failure to

---

Box 16-4

Management of Recurrent Airway Obstruction

Severe Respiratory Distress at Rest

Remove horse from allergen environment. Maintain at pasture and remove hay (especially round bales) and straw. Use pelleted feed and shavings.

Systemic corticosteroid therapy with dexamethasone (0.02-0.05 mg/kg IV q 24 hours).

If severe (life-threatening) respiratory distress is present, atropine (5 mg/450 kg horse IV).

Rapid-acting, aerosolized, bronchodilator therapy with albuterol sulfate (360 μg) administered every 15 minutes for up to 2 hours. Then continue as needed every 4 to 6 hours.

When breathing becomes comfortable, continue with aerosolized long-acting salmeterol xinafoate (210 μg tid-bid) or ipratropium (180–360 μg tid-bid) in combination with aerosolized corticosteroid therapy beclomethasone (3750 μg bid) or fluticasone (2000 μg bid). Treatment with aerosolized corticosteroids should be continued for approximately 14 days, until pulmonary inflammation has resolved. Bronchodilator therapy should be discontinued when bronchoconstriction has resolved, determined by pulmonary auscultation and/or exercise tolerance.

Moderate to Severe Disease

Remove or modify allergen-inducing environment.

Administer rapid-acting aerosolized bronchodilator therapy, albuterol sulfate (360 μg) followed (5 min) by an aerosolized corticosteroid (beclomethasone or fluticasone) twice daily.

Maintain on long-acting bronchodilator therapy salmeterol (210 μg tid-bid) or ipratropium (180–360 μg tid-bid) in combination with aerosolized corticosteroid therapy. Corticosteroid therapy should be continued for approximately 14 days. Bronchodilator therapy may be discontinued when bronchoconstriction has resolved, determined by normal pulmonary auscultation.

Pretreatment with aerosolized bronchodilator therapy (albuterol) will avoid exercise-induced bronchoconstriction.

---

improve within 7 days of treatment suggests that the therapeutic plan should be reassessed. Minimal improvement within 14 days of treatment suggests reassessment of diagnosis, including alternative differentials for pulmonary disease in the geriatric horse such as infectious pneumonia or pulmonary neoplasia.

Infectious Pulmonary Disease

When the clinician is presented with a geriatric equine patient exhibiting respiratory distress, recurrent obstructive airway disease may not always be the culprit. Bacterial pneumonia should be strongly considered, either as a primary etiologic agent or as a secondary invader due to overwhelming pathogen challenge or systemic immunosuppression. Geriatric horses may suffer from subclinical or undiagnosed pituitary pars intermedia dysfunction and elevated serum cortisol will contribute to immunosuppression and secondary bacterial pneumonia. Although upper respiratory disease associated with chronic sinusitis is more commonly associated with PPID, lower airway disease may also develop.

Bacterial pneumonia in adult horses is considered similarly, independent of host age, with the predominant invading organism being *Streptococcus equi* var. *zooepidemicus*. This pathogen is classified as a β-hemolytic streptococcal pathogen comprising a portion of the normal flora of the upper respiratory tract of healthy horses. Bacterial challenge with *S. zooepidemicus* typically occurs secondary to epithelial disruption after viral invasion.[22] Specifically, viral respiratory disease predisposes the host to bacterial invasion as a result of ciliary destruction, resulting in severe impairment of mucociliary clearance mechanisms. *Streptococcus equi* var. *equi* is less often an invader of the lower respiratory tract and therefore not usually a component of infectious pneumonia in horses. Rarely, *Streptococcus pneumoniae* results in bacterial pneumonia in horses despite the fact that this is a primary invader in many cases of human pneumonia. Further complications associated with equine bronchopneumonia arise when secondary invaders include gram-negative pathogens. A recent retrospective investigation demonstrated that greater than 50 percent of the cases of infectious pulmonary disease suffered from mixed populations of bacteria, based on transtracheal aspirate culture results.[22] These results indicate that multiple isolates are a common finding for equine bronchopneumonia. In an examination of gram-negative isolates, *Escherichia coli*, *Enterobacter* spp., *Klebsiella* spp., and *Pseudomonas* spp. were classified, in order of frequency.

Similar to younger horses, geriatric patients suffering from bacterial pneumonia should be investigated for the presence of secondary anaerobic pathogens. Retrospective investigations have revealed that an apparent rise in the prevalence of anaerobic pathogens such as *Bacteroides* spp. and *Clostridium* spp. has occurred with time.[22] When anaerobic pathogens are identified on culture results, they are generally considered secondary invaders. Since anaerobic proliferation will contribute to disease progression, every effort should be made to implement effective antibiotic protocols. Pulmonary contamination with this class of pathogens is attributed to oropharyngeal aspiration. Polymicrobial infection with anaerobic pathogen involvement is not uncommon and should be considered in geriatric horses suffering from bronchopneumonia.

Clinical Signs

Independent of age, horses presenting with infectious pulmonary disease will provide the clinician with a similar composition of clinical signs that include fever, respiratory distress, and coughing. An inducible cough is commonly present and can be demonstrated by compression of the proximal trachea. Irregular respiratory patterns are common and variable. Elevated respiratory rate is a frequent and sensitive abnormality observed in horses with infectious pulmonary disease.

Differentiation of infectious from noninfectious disease in geriatric horses with clinical signs of lower respiratory disease is the primary goal of physical examination. As discussed, the predominant noninfectious disease affecting geriatric horses is recurrent airway obstruction. Bacterial pulmonary disease occurs secondary to upper airway viral pathogens. Horses suffering from serious gastrointestinal disease and neutropenia may develop pulmonary fungal disease with the predominant pathogen being *Aspergillosis* spp. Parasitic pneumonitis is an uncommon manifestation of disease in older horses, it is more likely observed in yearlings or horses stabled with donkeys. However, after systemic immunosuppression or significant parasitic challenge, this disease may exist in geriatric patients. Parasitic pneumonitis can be complicated by secondary bacterial organisms.

Diagnosis (Box 16-5)

Initial diagnostic testing in horses with lower respiratory disease should involve a complete physical examination with pulmonary auscultation. Horses not demonstrating respiratory distress will require examination with a rebreathing bag to enhance auscultable respiratory sounds. Altered pulmonary sounds may include an increase audibility of inspiratory and expiratory sounds; these findings are in contrast to normal horses, which demonstrate minimally detectable expiratory sounds. When fluid and bronchoconstriction predominate, crackles and wheezes will be present, respectively. Percussion of the entire thorax is performed to identify fluid or pulmonary consolidation. Pleural fluid accumulation is detected by identification of a fluid line during thoracic percussion, below which a reduced pulmonary inflation and fluid accumulation result in pronounced dullness. In horses with pleural inflammation, friction rubs may be localized or generalized, depending on disease distribution.

Demonstrable changes on hematology associated with infectious pulmonary disease will include an inflammatory leukogram characterized by mature neutrophilia, increased fibrinogen concentration, and hyperglobulinemia. Elevated fibrinogen concentration may

> **Box 16-5**
>
> **Diagnosis of Infectious Pulmonary Disease**
>
> Physical examination: Pyrexia in combination with nasal discharge or respiratory distress indicates pulmonary involvement.
>
> Hematology to include complete blood cell count, serum chemistry analysis, and urinalysis to rule out other multisystemic disease.
>
> Thoracic radiographic and ultrasonographic examination will confirm pulmonary involvement and classify disease severity.
>
> Transtracheal aspiration: cytology and aerobic and anaerobic culture and sensitivity.

be profound for individuals with severe disease, especially when disease is long standing. Normal fibrinogen concentrations are accepted by most laboratories to be less than 400 mg/dL.

Thoracic radiographs provide diagnostic and prognostic information for patients with infectious pulmonary disease. Not only will pulmonary radiographs demonstrate specific abnormalities, they can also be used to document temporal changes that occur during disease progression and resolution. Individuals with infectious pulmonary disease generally have abnormal pulmonary radiopacities demonstrated by a diffuse bronchointerstitial to alveolar pattern. The most common radiographic pattern observed in horses with bacterial pneumonia is cranioventral distribution of increased radiodensity. When anaerobic, gas-producing organisms are present, consolidated regions of lung may contain focal, fluid-filled, round structures consistent with gas–producing organisms confined within a pulmonary abscess.

When percussion and auscultation are consistent with the presence of pleural effusion, ultrasonography is indicated to determine volume and characterize accumulation and to identify the optimal site for thoracocentesis. Fluid samples obtained from thoracocentesis are submitted for cytologic examination and bacterial culture (aerobic and anaerobic) and sensitivity. In cases of thoracic neoplasia, cytologic evaluation may identify exfoliating neoplastic cells. Pathogenic organisms responsible for the development of pleuropneumonia are best isolated from samples obtained via transtracheal aspiration, since infectious pleural disease results from extension of primary bacterial bronchopneumonia. The clinician working to establish a diagnosis of pulmonary disease in a geriatric equine should recognize that a complete evaluation is essential, as complicating circumstances may obscure the primary disease process (i.e., necrotic foci centrally located within a tumor).

Identification of specific pathogens is determined by aerobic and anaerobic culture of transtracheal aspirate samples. Cytologic evaluation of transtracheal aspirate samples will reveal degenerate neutrophils with intracellular and extracellular organisms. Gram staining is performed to assist therapeutic considerations pending bacterial culture and sensitivity results. In contrast, cytologic patterns consistent with recurrent airway obstruction will contain mature, nondegenerate neutrophils without intracellular microorganisms. Occasionally, neoplastic cells may be identified by transtracheal aspiration or bronchoalveolar lavage.

Pathogenesis

The most common coarse of infectious pulmonary disease is immunosuppression or disruption of the mucosal barrier resulting in secondary pathogenic invasion and disease. As previously mentioned, geriatric horses are more likely to suffer from primary immunosuppression due to PPID. Accompanying signs observed with PPID may include poor wound healing, chronic parasitic infestation, laminitis, hirsutism, and hyperhidrosis. Unlike younger athletic horses, long-distance transport is not a common event for geriatric horses; therefore, pleuropneumonia is uncommon in this age group of horses. However, a systematic and complete evaluation of the individual with pulmonary disease is imperative to establish the correct primary etiologic diagnosis.

Therapy and Prognosis

Antimicrobial selection for bacterial pneumonia is ideally based on sensitivity results obtained from aerobic and anaerobic cultures. Although the predominant pathogen in most cases of equine bronchopneumonia is *Streptococcus zooepidemicus*, additional pathogens may be present, especially with chronic disease. Since most cases of pneumonia are polymicrobial, the clinician is justified in selecting broad-spectrum antimicrobial coverage. Intravenous penicillin (potassium or sodium salt) is administered four times daily (22,000 IU/kg IV) or intramuscular procaine penicillin G (22,000 IU/kg) twice daily will provide adequate gram-positive coverage. In those individuals suspected to have polymicrobial infection ampicillin (20 mg/kg IV three to four times daily) provides a broader antimicrobial spectrum than penicillin. Beta-lactam treatment in combination with gentamicin (6.6 mg/kg IV or IM once daily) will significantly augment gram-negative pathogen coverage.[23] Aminoglycosides are nephrotoxic; therefore, serum creatinine, urinalysis, and potentially the urinary ratio of GGT (γ-glutamyltransferase) to creatinine should be monitored throughout the course of drug administration. The normal GGT-to-creatinine ratio is less than 25.

Further evaluation may include monitoring for serum peak and trough aminoglycoside drug levels. An alternative treatment with broad-spectrum coverage is trimethoprim-sulfadiazine (or methoxazole) 15 to 30 mg/kg twice daily. Intravenous preparations are available for hospitalized patients, whereas orally administered treatments are appropriate for horses treated on the farm. When anaerobic isolates are suspected, based on gas echos or putrid odor, metronidazole (15 mg/kg three times daily by mouth) is added to the antimicrobial regimen. Rifampin (10 mg/kg) administered by mouth twice daily is an alternative consideration,[22] particularly when abscess formation is a concern. Favorable anaerobic coverage, combined with excellent lipid solubility, allows for deep penetration into abscesses, thereby supporting selection of this drug as a component of therapy targeted for resolution of pulmonary abscess formation. Fluoroquinolones have become a popular choice for treatment of equine respiratory disease. Evidence to support this drug choice includes good gram-negative spectrum of activity and lack of nephrotoxicity, unlike the aminoglycosides. Fluoroquinolones have poor coverage for anaerobic pathogens and should be combined with a beta-lactam for adequate gram-positive antimicrobial coverage. Advantages of fluoroquinolone administration are good tissue penetration and patient tolerance, even when administered for extended periods of time.

In any patient, inadequate duration of antimicrobial therapy will contribute to treatment failure associated with infectious pulmonary disease. Patient monitoring should include frequent evaluation of the pulmonary system and vital parameters (respiratory rate and character and rectal temperature). Rectal temperature should be monitored as antibiotic therapy is withdrawn. If nonsteroidal anti-inflammatory therapy is administered, pyrexia may be masked; therefore, clinical evaluation of other pulmonary factors is necessary. When the appropriate antibiotics are administered for an adequate length of time, prognosis for complete recovery of infectious pulmonary disease is good.

Some individuals benefit from administration of immunomodulatory therapy, such as inactivated *Propionibacterium acnes* (EqStim, Neogen; 1 mL/250 lbs IV every other day for three treatments), for enhanced efficiency of pathogen clearance. Case selection is important to therapeutic success with immunomodulatory therapy and includes individuals with chronic infection or lymphopenia.

Complications associated with infectious pulmonary disease may include incomplete disease resolution due to poor drug penetration into necrotic or abscessed pulmonary tissue. Incomplete disease resolution may be a sequel to PPID, which again underscores the need for hormonal function analysis, in addition to effective antimicrobial therapy in geriatric patients with pneumonia.

An additional infectious pulmonary disease to consider is parasitic pneumonitis. Individuals demonstrating eosinophilic pulmonary infiltrates with an appropriate history of being housed with a donkey will benefit from larvicidal therapy with ivermectin 200 μg/kg orally. Diagnosis is based on history and pulmonary cytologic findings. Horses rarely develop a patent infection, thereby limiting the value of fecal analysis using the Baermann technique. All individuals, including donkeys, should be maintained on an effective rotating deworming program.

Box 16-6 lists treatments for infectious pulmonary disease.

Prophylaxis against Infectious Pulmonary Disease

Management is considered by most authors to be the primary factor associated with normal pulmonary immune defense mechanisms.[22] Ventilation is a specific example of a factor that, when inadequate, will prove detrimental to the pulmonary system of intensively housed horses during winter months. Low humidity and a dust-free environment contribute to health and well-being of the pulmonary system. Stress minimization should be employed whenever possible, particularly

---

Box 16-6

Treatment of Infectious Pulmonary Disease

1. **Appropriate Broad-Spectrum Antibiotic Therapy**

Beta-lactam procaine penicillin G (22,000 IU IM bid)/gentamicin (6.6 mg/kg IV or IM daily)

Trimethoprim sulfamethoxazole (15-30 mg/kg IV or PO bid)

Beta-lactam/enrofloxacin 5-7.5 mg/kg IV daily

2. **Nonsteroidal Anti-inflammatory Therapy**

Phenylbutazone 2.2 mg/kg PO bid PRN for pain and pyrexia

Flunixin meglumine 1.1 mg/kg IV or PO sid-bid for pain and pyrexia

Ketoprofen 2.2 mg/kg IV daily

3. **Immune Modulatory Therapy**

Propionibacterium acnes (EqStim) 1 mL/250 lbs IV every other day for three treatments

4. **Anthelminthic Therapy for Parasitic Pneumonitis**

Ivermectin 200 μg/kg PO

with the introduction of new horses onto the property. Immunization programs focusing on enhanced mucosal immunity, such as intranasal influenza vaccination, will reduce the likelihood of primary viral disease.

Pulmonary Neoplasia

Thoracic neoplasia is an uncommon disease affecting equine patients with an overall incidence of approximately 0.62 percent, based on a major retrospective study conducted in the United States spanning a 19-year period.[24,25] Several studies have demonstrated similar results, concluding that the importance of thoracic neoplasia in equine patients is considered by most investigators to be low. Primary pulmonary neoplasia is an uncommon disease, whereas metastatic disease most commonly results from lymphoma; the University of Pennsylvania identified 54.2 percent of the thoracic neoplasia cases to be metastatic lymphoma.[25] Metastatic spread of tumor cells results from hematogenous filtering, which occurs at the level of pulmonary capillaries. Diagnosis of primary versus metastatic disease may be difficult; therefore, it is important to establish a lack of neoplasia elsewhere in the body to support the diagnosis of primary pulmonary neoplasia[24] (Box 16-7).

Although primary pulmonary neoplasia remains an uncommon finding, the equine pulmonary neoplasias have been classified and include granular cell tumor, bronchial myxoma, adenoma, adenocarcinoma, aplastic bronchogenic carcinoma, pulmonary carcinoma, and potentially undifferentiated sarcoma. The granular cell tumor may not always be pathologic to the host, illustrated by the fact that granular cell tumors are sometimes reported as incidental findings at necropsy.[24] Characteristics of this tumor include a whitish rounded appearance that is well defined and located within major bronchi or with the distal bronchial tree. Pulmonary tumors that have been reported in horses as primary or metastatic disease include pulmonary chondrosarcoma,

pleural mesothelioma, thymoma, and malignant lymphoma. The majority of these tumors develop in older equine patients, although lymphoma may occur in younger individuals, similar to descriptions for this tumor type in other species.[25,26]

When the clinician is presented with a geriatric horse demonstrating primary pulmonary disease, neoplasia should be included in the list of differential diagnoses. If metastatic disease is present, diagnosis may be based on the primary tumor, with pulmonary involvement being identified secondarily. However, if overt pulmonary disease is demonstrated, appropriate diagnostic testing such as bronchoscopy, thoracic radiographs, ultrasonography and potentially thoracocentesis will aid in determining a definitive diagnosis. Ventral edema may indicate the presence a neoplastic mass or malignant effusion. Eighty percent of horses suffering from thoracic lymphoma exhibited some degree of ventral edema (Fig. 16-3).[25]

Primary pleural tumors are rare; however, pleural mesothelioma may develop occasionally, as a primary disease. Clinical manifestation includes remarkable pleural effusion; in some cases, more than 40 L of malignant effusion can be seen. Although effusive pleural disease strongly suggests the diagnosis of mesothelioma, specific diagnosis is based on cytologic findings. Other neoplastic diseases, such as lymphoma, melanoma, and carcinoma may yield voluminous pleural exudate. Pleomorphic mesothelial cells may be identified in cytologic analysis of pleural effusion in horses with pleural mesothelioma.[25]

A relatively common tumor type that often involves the equine thorax is lymphoma. Four tumor types have been described: mediastinal, multicentric, gastrointestinal, and cutaneous.[27,28] A generalized form may develop as an extension of multicentric disease. Combinations of these tumor types occur and may complicate an accurate

---

Box 16-7

Suspect Thoracic Neoplasia

1. Physical examination: identify abnormalities such as weight loss, epistaxis, and ventral edema.
2. Hematology (complete blood cell count, chemistry profile, urinalysis) to determine systemic involvement.
3. Ancillary diagnostic testing: thoracic radiographs, rectal palpation, abdominocentesis, thoracocentesis.
4. Perform biopsy of tumor or regionally enlarged lymph nodes.

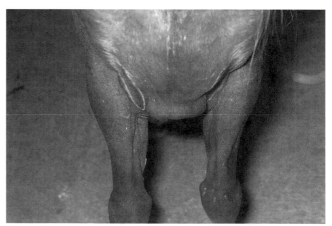

Figure 16-3 Ventral edema is a common finding associated with thoracic neoplasia in horses. Note the presence of pectoral edema in this individual diagnosed with metastatic, multicentric lymphoma.

diagnosis of the primary tumor site. The cutaneous form appears most drug responsive. Multiple reports of steroid-responsive disease exist. In addition, hormonal influences can potentiate disease: removal of a granulosa cell tumor resulted in disease resolution in one mare. Lymphoma may be accompanied paraneoplastic conditions such as hypercalcemia and thrombocytopenia. A recent report described a mare with generalized dermal lesions, alopecia, and pruritus secondary to multi-centric lymphoma. The presence of some of these paraneoplastic conditions should prompt the clinician to investigate the presence of an occult tumor.

In a 1973 review of 54 cases of equine lymphoma, the lung was involved in 16.6 percent of the cases, and thoracic lymph nodes were involved in 35.2 percent of the cases. As previously reported, malignant lymphoma was the most common neoplasm of the thoracic cavity, present in approximately 54 percent of the cases.[24] Although not always exfoliative, cytologic examination was diagnostic of neoplasia in 75 percent of these cases, whereas a definitive diagnosis was based on biopsy of peripheral lymph nodes in some instances. In a report from Bristol, thoracic lymphoma accounted for 74 percent of the cases of thoracic neoplasia.[26] Variation in disease prevalence between these studies was also represented in the frequency of metastatic adenocarcinoma. The University of Pennsylvania study reported a 20% incidence and the Bristol study identified an 11 percent prevalence of equine adenocarcinoma.[24] Primary sites for this tumor type included kidney, uterus, thyroid, and ovary with secondary pulmonary involvement due to metastatic dissemination.[25]

Metastatic gastric squamous cell carcinoma may invade the equine thorax and produce significant pleural effusion. Similar to other thoracic neoplasms, cytologic analysis of pleural fluid is valuable for making an antemortem diagnosis. Metastatic squamous cell carcinoma of the thorax was found in 14 percent and 5 percent of the cases in the University of Pennsylvania and Bristol studies, respectively.[24] In addition to cytologic analysis, monoclonal antibodies directed against cytoskeletal elements of epithelial origin have been successful in making the diagnosis of squamous cell carcinoma.[24,25]

Mature to older horses that demonstrate ill thrift, respiratory distress, epistaxis, and/or bleeding tendencies should have thoracic hemangiosarcoma on the list of differential diagnoses. Hemangiosarcoma comprises approximately 9 percent of thoracic neoplasia in horses.[25] Although this is not a common pulmonary neoplasm, hemangiosarcoma should be considered in horses with an appropriate history and clinical signs. Hemothorax, anemia, variable degrees of respiratory distress, and dyspnea were observed in cases within the retrospective study. Tentative antemortem diagnosis was determined via transcutaneous thoracoscopic approach

with direct visualization of visceral hemorrhages located on the visceral and parietal pleural surfaces. Histopathologic examination of suspect lesions identifies neoplastic endothelial cells, establishing a definitive diagnosis. Occasionally, diagnosis can be determined on cytologic examination of hemorrhagic pleural effusions. Horses with malignant hemangiosarcoma typically have many sites of metastatic invasion, including liver, spleen, muscle, brain, and eyes.

Neoplastic disease involving the equine thorax, particularly in gray horses and occasionally horses with other color patterns, may be associated with metastatic melanoma. A recent report described the overall incidence of melanoma in the equine population to remain unknown, since many clinicians make this diagnosis based on phenotypic characteristics alone. However, in the hospital population of the University of Pennsylvania, the prevalence of metastatic disease in those horses suffering from melanoma was approximated to be 14 percent.[27] The diagnosis of metastatic disease is consistent with the diagnosis of dermal melanomatosis, which is more commonly present in older gray horses with multiple dermal melanomas. Amelanotic melanoma warrants a poor prognosis and is extremely uncommon in horses, requiring microscopic identification of melanin granules to determine a definitive diagnosis. In addition, melanocytes may express S-100 protein, which is thought to demonstrate sequence homology with other domestic species.[24] Sequence comparisons may help make the diagnosis in equine cases, therefore representing an additional diagnostic tool for use in the horse.

Other pulmonary metastatic tumors expressed in horses include mammary carcinoma, seminoma, and malignant pheochromocytoma. Diagnostic evaluation in horses has been restricted to a morphologic diagnosis since many molecular techniques demonstrating unique malignant-associated proteins are not yet available for use with equine samples.

Conclusion

Disease associated with thoracic neoplasia in equine patients is often subclinical initially. Early manifestations are nonspecific, with clinical signs including depression, weight loss, inappetence, and fever. Disease progression will suggest pulmonary disease including cough, epistaxis, and potentially dyspnea. Cytologic evaluation of tracheobronchial aspirate, bronchoalveolar sample, or biopsy of pulmonary tissue or mass will aid in the antemortem diagnosis of neoplasia. In cases of primary pulmonary disease involving geriatric patients, the differential list should include neoplastic disease. Unfortunately, therapeutic protocols are not available for resolution of neoplastic disease in geriatric equines. By characterizing various tumor types and making every effort to diagnose neoplasia early in the course of disease, we will be better equipped to make therapeutic recommendations that will and prolong the life of the patient and enhance the quality of the patient's life.

REFERENCES

1. Bracher V, von Fellenberg R, Winder NC, et al: An investigation of the incidence of chronic obstructive pulmonary disease in random populations of Swiss horses. Equine Vet J 23:136, 1991.
2. Martin J, Sasse H, Slocombe R, et al: International Workshop on Equine Chronic Airway Disease, Michigan State University. Equine Vet J 33:5, 2001.
3. Dixon PM, Railton DI, McGorum BC: Equine pulmonary disease: a case control study of 300 referred cases: part 1. Examination techniques, diagnostic criteria, and diagnoses. Equine Vet J 27:422, 1995.
4. Marti E, Gerber H, Essich G, et al: The genetic basis of equine allergic diseases 1. Chronic hypersensitivity bronchitis. Equine Vet J 23:457, 1991.
5. Horohov DW: Equine T-cell cytokines: protection and pathology. Vet Clin North Am Equine Pract 16:1, 2000.
6. Giguere S, Viel L, Lee E, et al: Cytokine induction in pulmonary airways of horses with heaves and effect of therapy with inhaled fluticasone propionate. Vet Immunol Immunopath 85:147, 2002.
7. Mair TS: Obstructive pulmonary disease in 18 horses at summer pasture. Vet Rec 138:89, 1996
8. Seahorn TL, Groves MG, Harrington KS, et al: Chronic obstructive pulmonary disease in horses in Louisiana. J Am Vet Med Assoc 208:284, 1996.
9. Sandersen C, Bureau F, Turlej R, et al: Homodimer activity in distal airway cells determines lung dysfunction in equine heaves. Vet Immunol Immunopath 80:315, 2001.
10. Franchini M, Gill U, von Fellenberg R, et al: Interleukin-8 concentration and neutrophil chemotactic activity in bronchoalveolar lavage fluid of horses with chronic obstructive pulmonary disease following exposure to hay. Am J Vet Res 61:1369, 2000.
11. Dixon PM, Railton DI, McGorum BC: Equine pulmonary disease: a case control study of 300 referred cases: Part 2. Details of animals and of historical and clinical findings. Equine Vet J 27:422, 1995.
12. Savage CJ: Evaluation of the equine respiratory system using physical examination and endoscopy. Vet Clin North Am Equine Pract 13:443, 1997.
13. Thomson JR, McPherson EA: Chronic obstructive pulmonary disease in the horse. Equine Vet J 15:207, 1983.
14. Dixon PM, Railton DI, McGorum BC: Equine pulmonary disease: a case control study of 300 referred cases: Part 3. Ancillary diagnostic findings. Equine Vet J 27:422, 1995.
15. Veil L: Small airway disease as a vanguard for chronic obstructive pulmonary disease. Vet Clin North Am Equine Pract 13:549, 1997.
16. Lugo J, Stick JA, Peroni J, et al: Safety and efficacy of a technique for thorascopically guided pulmonary wedge resection in horses. Am J Vet Res 63:1232, 2002.
17. Rush BR, Raub ES, Rhoads WS, et al: Pulmonary function in horses with recurrent airway obstruction after aerosol and parenteral administration of beclomethasone and dexamethasone, respectively. Am J Vet Res 59:1039, 1998.
18. Lavoie JP: Update on equine therapeutics: inhalation therapy for equine heaves. Comp Cont Educ Pract Vet:475, 2001.
19. Derksen FJ, Olszewski MA, Robinson NE, et al: Aerosolized albuterol sulfate used as a bronchodilator in horses with recurrent airway obstruction. Am J Vet Res 60:689, 1999.
20. Rush BR, Hoskinson JJ, Davis EG, et al: Pulmonary distribution of aerosolized technetium Tc 99m penetrate after administration of a single dose of aerosolized albuterol sulfate in horses with recurrent airway obstruction. Am J Vet Res 60:764, 1999.
21. Henrikson SL, Rush BR: Efficacy of salmeterol xinofoate in horses with recurrent airway obstruction. J Am Vet Med Assoc 218:1961, 2001.
22. Warner AE: Bacterial pneumonia in adult horses. In Smith BP, editor: Large Animal Internal Medicine, 3rd ed. St. Louis, Mosby, 2002, pp 491–496.
23. Bertone JB: Antimicrobial therapy for respiratory disease. Vet Clin North Am Equine Pract 13:501, 1997.
24. Del Piedro F, Wilkins PA: Equine thoracic neoplasia. In Smith BP, editor: Large Animal Internal Medicine, 3rd ed. St. Louis, Mosby, 2002, pp 507–509.
25. Sweeny CR, Gillette DM: Thoracic neoplasia in equids: 35 cases (1967–1987). J Am Vet Med Assoc 195:374, 1989.
26. Mair TS, Brown PJ: Clinical and pathologic features of thoracic neoplasia in the horse. Equine Vet J 25:220, 1993.
27. MacGillivray KC, Sweeney RW, Del Piero F: Metastatic melanoma in horses. J Vet Intern Med 16:452, 2002.
28. Savage CJ: Lymphoproliferative and myeloproliferative disorders. Vet Clin North Am Equine Pract 14:563, 1998.

CHAPTER 17

Reproductive Disorders

Elaine M. Carnevale

Advances in veterinary care and management have allowed increasing numbers of mares and stallions to be maintained until old age (>20 years). However, with increasing age, reproductive potential declines. Although changes in other body systems can affect reproduction in the old horse, age appears to be directly associated with altered reproductive function and reduced fertility.

The Mare

Reduced fertility has been documented with advanced age in the mare, with a decrease in pregnancy rates and an increase in pregnancy loss rates.[1] The reported decline in fertility could be lower in a natural population. Potentially, old mares with low fertility are not bred during subsequent years, although more fertile counterparts remain within the reproductive pool. In recent years, research has provided insight into reproductive aging. Understanding how reproductive function differs in old and young mares will assist in developing optimal management procedures.

Anatomic Changes

Previous injuries, infections, and foaling can predispose the old mare to further reproductive problems. The presence and extent of any conformational changes associated with aging vary with an individual mare. In pluriparous mares, stretching of the vulval lips and vestibular-vaginal sphincter can impair competence of the posterior reproductive tract; and with reduced body fat and musculature, the old mare is more susceptible to pneumovagina and ascending infections. Loss of fat in the perineal area, especially in mares with a flat or short croup, will result in a "sinking" of the anus and tilting of the vulva, again increasing ascending infections. Repeated pregnancies stretch the broad ligament that suspends the uterus from the abdominal wall and increase uterine weight, resulting in a more pendulous uterus. Reduced tone of the abdominal musculature and reduced body fat can further result in tilting of the uterus into the abdominal cavity. Subsequently, expulsion of fluid and debris from the uterus is impaired. The ventral tilt of the vagina can predispose to pooling of urine in the anterior vagina. When the cervix relaxes during estrus, urine can enter the uterus and cause inflammation and subfertility. With repeated foaling, the potential for cervical tears, adhesions, and scarring is increased. In old maiden mares, the cervix is often fibrotic and fails to open adequately during estrus. Subsequently, drainage of fluid from the uterus is impaired, and endometritis can result.

Because old mares have a higher incidence of conformational or anatomical abnormalities than young mares, old broodmares should be evaluated for problems before breeding. Maintenance of good body condition, potentially including exercise to strengthen abdominal muscles, is important to help prevent some pathologic conditions, such as pneumovagina and urine pooling. Evaluation for surgical correction of anatomical problems should be done before breeding the old mare. The extent of abnormalities in some mares may prevent them from carrying a pregnancy to term. These mares should be retired from breeding or evaluated as embryo or oocyte donors.

Uterus

Uterine pathology has been historically implicated as a major cause of age-associated subfertility. Aging of the equine uterus is associated with structural and functional changes. Contractile activity is important to remove debris from the uterus and to maintain uterine health. Contractile activity of the uterus is less effective in old mares, as demonstrated in a number of experiments. After pretreatment with estradiol, the physical clearance of inoculated bacteria, charcoal, and microspheres from the uterus was reduced in old versus young mares.[2] In another study,[3] uterine contractility, as measured with ultrasound, was reduced; and uterine tone tended to be lower in mares 15 years of age or older than in mares 5 to 7 years. Consequently, intrauterine fluid accumulations were more extensive in the old than in the young mares. These studies demonstrated age-associated changes in uterine function. Reduced contractile activity can affect clearance of debris from the uterus after breeding and increase the potential for uterine infections.

The uterus must provide an adequate environment for sperm and embryo survival during estrus and early pregnancy and for placental and fetal development during late pregnancy. Endometrial biopsies were used to classify changes that occurred in aging uteri. When researchers[3] compared biopsy scores for old mares (≥15 years) and young mares (5-7 years), the uteri of old mares had more inflammatory cell infiltrations, more fibrosis, and less glandular density.

Fibrotic changes were frequently observed in the endometrium of old mares.[4] Cells of the stroma of the lamina propria deposit collagen around the endometrial glands or in association with the basement membrane of the luminal epithelium. In the mare, periglandular fibrosis could compromise gland function, because of a mechanical separation from the underlying capillary network.[4] Changes in uterine histology were correlated with increased age in maiden and nonmaiden mares, suggesting that uterine pathologic conditions occurred independent of previous pregnancies and were associated with aging.[5] Ricketts and Alonso[6] correlated chronic infiltrative endometritis (mononuclear cell infiltrations) and chronic degenerative endometrial disease (glandular degenerative changes) with mare age. Correlations between age and endometritis were minimal, but correlations between increasing age and degenerative changes were high. Old maiden mares had chronic degenerative endometrial disease that was determined to be more closely associated with age than

with parity. Results of the studies confirm that degenerative changes occur in the uteri of old mares; these changes could affect the potential of old mares to carry pregnancies to term.

Uterine pathologic conditions can be diagnosed in mares using various procedures, such as ultrasonography, biopsy, cytology, culture, and endoscopy. Consequently, uterine pathology is frequently diagnosed in old mares; however, less obvious causes of fertility failure can be overlooked. Results of experiments suggest that, although uteri in old mares are compromised, other causes of reduced fertility are present. Waelchli[7] classified the uteri of mares into four grades based on endometrial histologic findings. Significant associations were detected between fertility and histologic categories. Mares older than the median age (11 years) had significantly higher category scores and lower fertility than younger mares. However, within a histologic category, there was a tendency for lower fertility in older mares, suggesting that factors other than the uterus influenced fertility. In an experiment by Ball et al,[8] embryos were collected on day 7 or 8 after ovulation and transferred into the uteri of normal, young recipients (3-8 years) or subfertile, old recipients (10-23 years). Pregnancy rates between groups were not different at day 28 (10/20 and 8/10, respectively). The study demonstrated that uteri of older, subfertile mares could maintain pregnancy until at least day 28. Therefore, although changes occur in the uterus, other age-associated factors also affect fertility.

Uterotubal Junction and Oviduct

Clinical and experimental findings suggest that oviductal pathology affects breeding success in the old mare. The oviduct's role in fertility is limited to the first 6 days of pregnancy. During that time, the oviduct functions in the selection and storage of sperm, collection of the oocyte after ovulation, fertilization, and early embryo development. Between 5 and 6 days after ovulation, the embryo will leave the oviduct and enter the uterus.

Age-associated changes in oviductal function could affect fertilization rates of ovulated oocytes. Scott et al.[9] inseminated mares with normal reproductive histories and mares susceptible to chronic uterine infections. Susceptible mares had fewer sperm in the oviduct, and few of these sperm were motile. In addition, pathologic changes were noted in the caudal isthmic epithelium. Although mares were not selected based on age, old mares are frequently susceptible to uterine infections, suggesting that sperm transport could be impaired in many old mares. Fertilization rates of ovulated oocytes have been compared for young and old mares. Results varied, however, with fertilization rates similar[10,11] or lower[12] for old as compared with young mares. It should be noted that, under experimental conditions, mares were inseminated with optimal numbers of sperm from fertile stallions. Differences in fertilization rates could be more pronounced when mares of different ages are inseminated with less fertile stallions or with limited sperm numbers.

During ovulation, the oocyte with surrounding follicular cells must be captured by the infundibulum and transported to the ampulla, where fertilization will occur. The ability of the infundibulum to collect and transport the oocyte could be altered by infundibular adhesions and inflammation, which are more frequent in old than in young mares.[13] Ovulated oocytes or embryos were collected less frequently from the oviducts of old than of young mares,[10,11] suggesting that movement of the oocyte from the follicle and into the oviduct was less effective in old mares.

The ability of the oviducts of old mares to sustain embryo viability has been debated. Proteins synthesized and secreted by oviductal epithelial cell explants were not different for young and old mares during estrus and 4 days after ovulation.[14] However, in another study using cells collected 2 days after ovulation, cells collected from fertile, young mares (2-7 years) and subfertile, old mares (17-24 years) had differences in secretory patterns.[15] More cells tended to be present in embryos that were cultured on the oviductal cells from young than old mares.[12] The authors suggested that oviductal function could affect early embryo development. The relevance of oviductal secretory patterns on fertilization and early embryo development is still to be determined.

Ovarian Function

Ovarian failure, caused by the depletion of oocytes, has been implicated as the primary cause of reproductive failure in women and most domestic animals. Changes in the population of primordial follicles associated with aging have not been determined in mares. Young (2-4 years) pony and horse mares had an average of 36,000 primordial follicles and 100 growing follicles,[16] but variability among mares was high for the number of primordial follicles (5600-75,000) and growing follicles (20-300). Ginther[1] deduced that a mare would deplete her reserve of follicles in 25 years if she had an original number of approximately 40,000 primordial follicles, cycled continuously, and used 100 follicles per cycle.

Although the depletion of primordial follicles has not been documented in the old mare, this scenario is suggested by changes in ovarian activity. In a slaughterhouse study,[17] mares older than 15 years had significantly less ovarian activity than younger mares as demonstrated by reduced ovarian weight and fewer follicles (2-10 or 10-20 mm). Vanderwall et al.[18] reported ovarian inactivity in 4 of 10 mares 25 to 33 years of age and 2 of 25 mares 20 to 30 years of age during two ovulatory seasons; none of 21 young mares (3-12 years) was anovulatory. During an 80-day interval during the ovulatory season, all (n = 19) pony mares 5 to 7 or 15 to 19 years of age had at least three sequential ovulations; fewer mares 20 years of age or older (8/16) had three ovulations. Three of the old mares ovulated twice, two old mares ovulated once, and three mares did not grow a follicle greater than 5 mm in diameter or ovulate during the 80-day interval.[19] The failure of old mares to grow follicles and ovulate was potentially caused by depleted oocyte reserves.

Reduced numbers of viable follicles in the ovaries of old mares can have clinical significance. A wave of follicles is recruited for each cycle with the eventual selection of the dominant follicle. Fewer follicles in a wave may result in an altered selection process, and a less viable oocyte could be ovulated.

Cyclic Characteristics

In the old mare, alterations occur in cyclic activity during the transitional period and ovulatory season. Time to the first ovulation of the year was delayed in old mares. The spring transition from anestrus until ovulation is characterized by elevated concentrations of follicle stimulating hormone (FSH) but insufficient luteinizing hormone (LH) to induce ovulation. During the spring transitional period, the number of follicles imaged on ovaries was lower for old than for young mares.[20] Mares older than 19 years of age ovulated approximately 2 weeks later than mares younger than 14 years.[21] The age-associated delay in the first ovulation of the year could be partially dependent on factors other than age. Nutrition and body condition have been shown to affect the time to ovulation in the spring. During the spring, when old mares (>19 years) were fed a special, highly digestible diet, they ovulated approximately 2 weeks earlier than old mares on isocaloric control (oats).[22]

During the natural breeding season, follicular and endocrine activity was compared among cyclic ponies of different ages.[23] The interval between ovulations and the length of the follicular phase (luteolysis to ovulation) were longer for old mares (≥20 years) than for younger mares (5-7 or 15-19 years). The longer interval to ovulation in old versus young mares was caused by a smaller mean diameter of the dominant follicle at the time of natural luteolysis (approximately 15 days after ovulation) and a slower growth rate for the preovulatory follicles of old than of young mares. Although mares 15 to 19 years old also had a slower follicular growth rate than young mares, they ovulated smaller follicles than younger mares (35 and 39 mm, respectively). Therefore, although the interval between ovulations was not different between the young and middle-aged groups, differences in cyclic characteristics were observed. After administration of prostaglandin at 8 days after ovulation, mares 20 years of age and older, versus those 5 to 7 years old, required significantly longer to grow a dominant follicle and ovulate (means of 19 and 11 days, respectively). The length of the luteal phase (ovulation to progesterone <1 ng/mL) and mean concentrations of progesterone were not different between young and old mares. Results of this study demonstrate differences in cyclic activity between mares of different ages. These differences can result in difficulties when synchronizing old and young mares for procedures such as embryo transfer. Although there is more variability in cyclic characteristics in old mares, the cycles of an individual mare often will be similar. Therefore, good records and careful observations are valuable.

The nature of reproductive senescence in pony mares was studied at the University of Wisconsin.[19] The researchers concluded that cessation of reproduction occurs in the mare as follows: (1) elongation of the follicular phase with reduced ovarian activity, (2) sporadic ovulations with elevated concentrations of FSH and LH, and (3) persistent ovarian inactivity (follicles <5 mm and no ovulation) with elevated concentrations of FSH and LH. Elevated concentrations of FSH and LH in mares with no ovarian activity were similar to those in ovariectomized mares.

Mares with an elongated follicular phase and reduced follicular activity often have only one or two follicles imaged with ultrasonography during a cycle. The interval from luteolysis to ovulation is increased because of a small follicle at the time of luteolysis and slow follicular growth. Mares with intermittent follicular activity will usually have one or two follicles imaged during estrus. A corpus luteum is present during diestrus, but follicles usually are not imaged. Luteal regression occurs at the anticipated time after ovulation (14-16 days). After regression of the corpus luteum, no follicles are imaged on the ovaries and the uterus is flaccid. Once a follicle 10 mm or greater is imaged, the mare will usually continue to grow the follicle and ovulate. Mares in reproductive senescence have a flaccid uterus and small ovaries with no follicles larger than 5 mm. The mares can show signs of estrus, although a follicle is not present. Methods to stimulate follicular growth and ovulation in these mares are typically unsuccessful. However, other potential causes for ovarian inactivity (e.g., Cushing's syndrome, stress, poor nutrition) should be investigated. The progression of reproductive senescence in the mare is consistent with ovarian failure. In the author's experience, when mares repeatedly have elongated estrous intervals and reduced follicular activity, most will progress to reproductive senescence in 2 to 4 years.

Preovulatory Follicle

Functional differences in preovulatory follicles between young and old mares currently are being researched. Differences in the follicular milieu could alter the developmental potential of oocytes and could affect fertility.

Ovulatory failure has been documented in old mares. Often when abnormal follicles are imaged with ultrasonography, they appear to be in the process of ovulating, with thickened and irregular borders. However, ovulation of the follicle is rapid,[24] and follicles maintaining this structure probably do not ovulate the oocyte. In the author's laboratory, aspiration of the contents of atypical ovulatory sites resulted in recovery of a bloody follicular fluid and degenerating oocytes. McKinnon et al.[25] noted altered ultrasonographic characteristics of the ovulatory site in old mares, and attempts to recover oviductal embryos were unsuccessful. The authors suggested that follicles were luteinizing without ovulating. The appearance of atypical follicles, in which follicular evacuation appeared to be delayed or incomplete, was more frequent for old mares than for young mares during the breeding season.[19] The incidence of anovulatory hemorrhagic follicles was also higher for old than young mares during the fall months.[24] In some old mares, ovulatory failure appears to occur repeatedly during the ovulatory season. No treatment is known to correct ovulatory failure in the old mare.

Embryo Viability

The equine embryo enters the uterus on day 5 or 6 after ovulation. Embryos can be collected from the uterus by nonsurgical uterine lavage for embryo transfers. Age of the donor affects the success of embryo transfer. Recovery of embryos was less successful from old mares (18-28 years, 30%) than young mares (2-8 years, 61%).[26] More embryos collected from uteri of old than normal (younger) mares were abnormal.[27,28] After transfer, more embryos collected from maiden than old mares (87% and 49%, respectively) and from young than old mares (2-8 years, 70% and 18-28 years, 56%)[26] resulted in pregnancies. After the establishment of pregnancies in recipients, embryo death occurred more often for embryos from old than young donors.[26,29] Although embryo transfer is not as successful for old mares as it is for young mares, the procedure has provided a valuable method to obtain foals from mares that cannot carry a pregnancy to term.

Reduced embryo viability in old mares occurs before the embryo enters the uterus. Embryos were collected on day 4 from the oviducts of subfertile mares (mean age, 19 years) and normal mares (mean age, 6 years) and transferred into recipients. Fewer embryos from the subfertile mares resulted in pregnancies on day 14.[11] In a series of experiments at the University of Wisconsin,[10] oviductal embryos were collected from young and old mares. At 1.5 days after ovulation, fertilization rates between age groups were not different, although fewer ova from old than young mares had cleaved. Three days after ovulation, embryos collected from the oviducts of old versus young mares had fewer cells and more morphologic abnormalities. Although fewer oocytes or embryos were collected from old than from young mares, fertilization rates of collected ova (cleaved or uncleaved) were not different. The studies indicated that within 36 hours after ovulation, differences are present between embryos from young and old mares, including a delayed rate of development and more morphologic abnormalities for embryos from old mares.

Oocyte Viability

Intrinsic defects of the oocyte have been suggested as a cause of age-associated subfertility in mares; however, until recently, experimental or clinical techniques have not been available to evaluate the viability of oocytes from mares of different ages.

In an experiment by Carnevale and Ginther,[30] oocytes were collected by transvaginal, ultrasound-guided follicular aspirations from young (6-10 years) and old (≥20 years) pony mares 24 hours after the administration of human chorionic gonadotropin. Oocytes were cultured in vitro for the completion of maturation and transferred into the oviducts of young recipients. All recipients were artificially inseminated with semen from the same stallion. The number of transferred oocytes from young and old donors that developed into embryonic vesicles was compared. Significantly fewer oocytes from old (8/26, 31%) than young (11/12, 92%) donors developed into embryonic vesicles as imaged by ultrasonography on day 12. Therefore, although the oocytes from old mares were transferred into the oviducts of young recipients for fertilization and early embryo development, a significant reduction in fertility was associated with oocytes from old mares as compared with young mares. Results of this study implicate the oocyte as a cause of reduced fertility in the old mare. Although oocyte transfer rates were lower when oocytes from old versus young mares were used, the 30 percent pregnancy rate still represents a viable alternative for obtaining pregnancies from old mares.

Light and electron microscopy were used to compare oocytes, collected 24 hours after the administration of human chorionic gonadotropin, from young and old mares.[31] Although the percentages of most organelles were similar for oocytes from young and old mares, some oocytes from old mares had large vesicles, nuclear abnormalities, and irregular shapes. Structural differences may represent degenerative changes in oocytes that result in

reduced oocyte viability. Although some oocytes from old mares appeared abnormal, other oocytes were similar to those collected from young mares.

Breeding the Old Mare

Breeding management should be optimized for the old mare. Selection of a fertile stallion is important to increase the chance of conception. Dental care and good nutrition are essential to maintain the body condition needed for optimal reproductive success.

The old mare should be carefully evaluated before breeding. Reproductive pathologies, such as urine pooling, cervical lacerations or scarring, uterine cysts, and endometritis, should be diagnosed. In addition, a uterine biopsy will help determine the ability of the mare's uterus to carry a pregnancy to term and will help the owner to determine whether breeding the mare is an acceptable risk.

The uterus can be evaluated with ultrasonography before breeding to ensure that it is free of fluid accumulations within the lumen. Insemination of the old mare is best timed around ovulation. Repeated inseminations are more likely to result in the establishment of uterine inflammation and infection. Two theories for choosing an insemination dose have been proposed for mares that are susceptible to uterine infections. Insemination of susceptible mares can be done using a minimal number of sperm, potentially minimizing the uterine reaction to insemination. However, because the old and/or susceptible mare is probably less able to establish good numbers of sperm within the oviduct after insemination, the author prefers to inseminate with standard or moderately increased numbers of sperm. After insemination, removal of fluid and debris from uteri of many old mares is impaired; therefore, the uterus should be examined for the presence of intraluminal fluid collections. If fluid is imaged, the uterus can be treated through administration of ecbolics, uterine lavage, or antibiotic infusions, as determined to be necessary. Insemination of the old mare with adequate sperm while maintaining a uterine environment capable of sustaining the developing embryo can be difficult.

The developing follicle and the ovulatory site should be closely examined using ultrasound to determine whether ovulation occurred and whether the corpus luteum appears normal. Although some cycles may not be fertile in the old mare, care should be taken during each cycle to optimize fertility and minimize the response to breeding.

Some old mares will be unable to conceive or carry a pregnancy to term. In these mares, procedures such as embryo or oocyte transfer can be attempted. Embryo transfer requires the old mare to conceive and to support the embryo for the first 6 to 8 days of pregnancy. The embryo will then be flushed from the old donor's uterus and transferred into a young, fertile recipient. Embryo transfer is successful for many old mares. However, if reproductive pathologies prevent a successful embryo transfer, oocyte transfer can be attempted. During oocyte transfer, an oocyte is aspirated from the preovulatory follicle of the donor. The oocyte is then transferred into the oviduct of a young recipient that is inseminated. With oocyte transfer, the old mare is required only to grow a follicle with a viable oocyte. Oocyte transfer has been used successfully to obtain pregnancies from many old mares that were previously considered infertile.

The Stallion

Limited research has been done on disorders associated with aging in the stallion. In contrast to the mare's single oocyte, a normal stallion will produce billions of gametes per ejaculate. Therefore, early reproductive changes associated with aging could go unnoticed in many stallions. As stallions age, there is an increase in the incidence of physical ailments that can affect reproduction. Problems can be directly associated with the reproductive tract, such as testicular or penile injuries, or indirectly, such as hind leg lameness.

Stallion fertility has been reported to decline on average at 15 years of age.[32] Pickett et al.[33] reported that sperm output and total scrotal width increased until 5 years of age and remained relatively constant until 12 years; after this time, sperm output declined. Researchers from Australia[34] reported that stallions older than 13 years had low sperm concentrations and high percentages of dead sperm; however, sperm morphology was normal. The oldest stallions in the study were 26 years old.

Testes

Morphologic changes have been demonstrated in the testes of aged stallions. Jackson and Dowsett[35] noted morphological evidence of germ cell loss in stallions older than 15 years. Fibrosis and atrophy of the seminiferous tubules were reported as the most characteristic changes in testes of old stallions.[36] The population of Leydig cells increased in volume and number in the testes of old stallions (13-20 years).[37] Leydig cells of the older horses had more lipid, large accumulations of lipofuscin, and the suggestion of membrane degradation in regions of smooth endoplasmic reticulum and mitochondria. The increase in Leydig cell numbers and lipofuscin granules are probably the cause of the darker, reddish-brown color of testicular parenchyma in adult and aged stallions.

Endocrine Factors

Normal spermatogenesis in stallions depends on a functional hypothalamic-pituitary-testicular axis.[38] Gonadotropin-releasing hormone (GnRH) is synthesized and released from the hypothalamus. The pulsatile discharge of GnRH stimulates the production of LH and FSH from the anterior pituitary. LH and FSH function at the level of the testes to stimulate production of steroid hormones and sperm. Leydig cells under the stimulation of LH produce testosterone and estrogens in the stallion. Steroids and proteins from the testes enter the system circulation and create a feedback loop with the hypothalamus and pituitary. Increasing evidence also suggests the involvement of paracrine and autocrine factors in the regulation of testicular function.[38] Exogenous administration of testosterone can result in the suppression of LH and reduced production of endogenous testosterone. The final result is usually decreased sperm production. The administration of exogenous GnRH induces the discharge of LH from the stallion's anterior pituitary, and LH causes the subsequent secretion of testosterone by Leydig cells. When human chorionic gonadotropin (hCG) is administered to the stallion, hCG mimics the action of LH and causes Leydig cells to produce testosterone.[33] Reproductive endocrinology and diagnostic testing of the stallion recently has been reviewed.[39]

Limited research has been done to study changes in the hypothalamic-pituitary-testicular axis associated with old age in the stallion. Effects of age and fertility were compared for stallions from less than 1 to 25 years of age.[40] Slow increases in immunoreactive inhibin, LH, FSH, and testosterone were observed with aging in the adult stallions. Data suggested that the production of inhibin and other testicular hormones in the stallion are not detrimentally affected by aging. The increasing serum concentrations of testosterone and LH are in agreement with increasing volume and number of Leydig cells within the testes of older stallions.[37]

Age-associated correlations between changes in fertility and endocrine factors have not been clearly defined. However, endocrine changes associated with idiopathic testicular dysfunction have been outlined.[39] Hormonal imbalances are initially recognized as an increase in circulating concentration of FSH and decreases in circulating concentrations of estrogens and inhibin. As the stallion becomes infertile, the testes are markedly decreased in size; FSH and LH levels are high, and steroids and inhibin are low. In a study by Roser,[41] endocrine profiles of fertile (5-18 years), subfertile (5-14 years), and infertile (14-18 years) stallions were compared. Concentrations of FSH and LH were higher, and concentrations of inhibin and estradiol were lower in the infertile group. Circulating concentrations of testosterone were similar among the groups. After the administration of hCG, the increase in testosterone was significantly reduced for infertile versus fertile and subfertile stallions. The authors suggested that the poor testosterone response in the infertile stallions indicated a disorder at the level of the Leydig cells.

Gonadotropin-releasing hormone and hCG were administered to control (7 ± 3 years) and old (22 ± 4 years) stallions.[42] Higher concentrations of LH were observed at 80 minutes after GnRH administration for old versus control stallions; however, resulting concentrations of testosterone were not different. Administration of hCG resulted in lower testosterone concentrations for old than control stallions. The poor response to hCG in old stallions was similar to that observed for infertile stallions.[41] The authors suggested that the lower testosterone production in old stallions could have been caused by some testicular degeneration, although palpable consistencies of the testes were not different.[42] The authors further speculated that the reproductive endocrine system in old stallions was not functioning optimally. Since basal testosterone concentrations were not lower for old than control stallions, the setpoint of LH release could be different in old than young stallions to maintain adequate basal testosterone. It is generally accepted that alterations in spermatogenesis of older stallions is a result of Sertoli cell problems resulting from a paracrine malfunction.

Testicular Degeneration

Testicular degeneration can occur in stallions of any age and can have many causes. Age-related testicular degeneration has been documented in other species and has been postulated to occur in the stallion. Senile changes within testicular parenchyma could be the result of degenerative vascular changes in the testes.[43] Testicular degeneration is associated with a decrease in total scrotal width. Palpable characteristics of degenerating testes have been described as having two patterns. In the first, the testes become progressively softer and smaller until only a small amount of tissue can be palpated within the scrotum. In the second pattern, the testes become lobulated and/or constricted and progressively smaller, until only a firm mass remains.[33] Some cases of testicular degeneration are reversible. However, degenerative changes that are caused by aging are probably progressive. Use of hormone therapy, most notably GnRH, has been examined as a treatment for testicular degeneration[44]; but the efficacy of GnRH treatment has not been established.

Management of the Old Stallion

Special attention should be given to the feeding and dental care of the old stallion. Other conditions, such as lameness, could affect breeding performance and should be monitored.

Many stallions have been successful breeders until old age. Use of the stallion should be limited by his libido

and seminal characteristics. Advancing age could dictate that fewer mares are booked per breeding season. Optimal management and selection of fertile mares will help to increase pregnancy rates. Monitoring testicular size and consistency and conducting annual breeding soundness evaluations will help the stud manager to recognize changes in reproductive ability. The approval of frozen semen by many breed registries has allowed the preservation of valuable male genetics and has resulted in an elongation of a stallion's reproductive lifetime. For best results, semen should be frozen while a stallion is in his reproductive prime. The semen can be used at a later date if age-associated changes occur in fertility.

REFERENCES

1. Ginther OJ: Reproductive Biology of the Mare, 2nd ed. Cross Plains, WI, Equiservices, 1992.
2. Evans MJ, Hamer JM, Gason LM, et al: Factors affecting uterine clearance of inoculated materials in mares. J Reprod Fert Suppl 35:327, 1987.
3. Carnevale EM, Ginther OJ: Relationships of age to uterine function and reproductive efficiency in mares. Theriogenology 37:1101, 1992.
4. Kenny RM: Cyclic and pathologic changes of the mare endometrium as detected by biopsy, with a note on early embryonic death. J Am Vet Med Assoc 172:241, 1978.
5. Held JP, Rohrbach B: Clinical significance of uterine biopsy results in the maiden and non-maiden mare. J Reprod Fert Suppl 44:698, 1991.
6. Ricketts SW, Alonso S: The effect of age and parity on the development of equine chronic endometrial disease. Equine Vet J 23:189, 1991.
7. Waelchli RO: Endometrial biopsy in mares under nonuniform breeding management conditions: prognostic value and relationship with age. Can Vet J 31:379, 1990.
8. Ball BA, Hillman RB, Woods GL: Survival of equine embryos transferred to normal and subfertile mares. Theriogenology 28:167, 1987.
9. Scott MA, Liu IKM, Overstreet JW: Sperm transport to the oviducts: Abnormalities and their clinical applications. AAEP Proc 41:1, 1995.
10. Carnevale EM, Griffin PG, Ginther OJ: Age-associated subfertility before entry of embryos into the uterus in mares. Equine Vet J Suppl 15:31, 1993.
11. Ball BA, Little JA, Weber JA, et al: Survival of day-4 embryos from young, normal and aged, subfertile mares after transfer to normal recipient mares. J Reprod Fert 85:187, 1989.
12. Brinsko SP, Ball BA, Miller PG, et al: In vitro development of day 2 embryos obtained from young, fertile mares and age, subfertile mares. J Reprod Fert 102:371, 1994.
13. Henry M, Vandeplassche M: Pathology of the oviduct in mares. Vlaams Diergeneesk Tijdsch 50:301, 1981.
14. McDowell KJ, Adams MH, Williams NM: Characterization of equine oviductal proteins synthesized and released at estrus and at day 4 after ovulation in bred and nonbred mares. J Exp Zool 267:217, 1993.
15. Brinsko SP, Ignotz GG, Ball BA, et al: Characterization of polypeptides synthesized and secreted by oviductal epithelial cell explants obtained from young, fertile and age, subfertile mares. Am J Vet Res 57:1346, 1996.
16. Driancourt M-A, Paris A, Roux C, et al: Ovarian follicular populations in pony and saddle-type mares. Reprod Nutr Dev 22:1035, 1982.
17. Wesson JA, Ginther OJ: Influence of season and age of reproductive activity in pony mares on the basis of a slaughterhouse survey. J Anim Sci 52:119, 1981.
18. Vanderwall DK, Woods GL, Freeman DA, et al: Ovarian follicles, ovulations and progesterone concentrations in aged versus young mares. Theriogenology 40:21, 1993.
19. Carnevale EM, Bergfelt DR, Ginther OJ: Follicular activity and concentrations of FSH and LH associated with senescence in mares. Anim Reprod Sci 35:231, 1994.

20. Carnevale EM, Hermenet MJ, Ginther OJ: Age and pasture effects on vernal transition in mares. Theriogenology 47:1009, 1997.

21. Vanderwall DK, Woods GL: Age-related subfertility in the mare. Proc AAEP 36:85, 1990.

22. Carnevale EM, Thompson KN, King SS, et al: Effects of age and diet on the spring transition in mares. AAEP Proc 42:146, 1996.

23. Carnevale EM, Bergfelt DR, Ginther OJ: Aging effects on follicular activity and concentrations of FSH, LH, and progesterone in mares. Anim Reprod Sci 31:287, 1993.

24. Carnevale EM: Folliculogenesis and ovulation. In Rantanen NW, McKinnon AO, editors: Equine Diagnostic Ultrasonography. Baltimore, Williams & Wilkins, 1998.

25. McKinnon AO, Squires EL, Pickett BW: Reproductive Ultrasonography. Fort Collins, CO, Colorado State University, 1988.

26. Vogelsang SG, Vogelsang MM: Influence of donor parity and age on the success of commercial equine embryo transfer. Equine Vet J Suppl 3:71, 1989.

27. Woods GL, Baker CB, Hillman RB, et al: Recent studies relating to early embryonic death in the mare. Equine Vet J Suppl 3:194, 1985.

28. Schlafer DJ, Dougherty EP, Woods GL: Light and ultrastructural studies of morphological alterations in embryos collected from maiden and barren mares. J Reprod Fert Suppl 35:695, 1987.

29. Squires EL, Imel KJ, Iuliano MF, et al: Factors affecting reproductive efficiency in an equine embryo transfer programme. J Reprod Fert Suppl 32:108, 1982.

30. Carnevale EM, Ginther OJ: Defective oocytes as a cause of subfertility in old mares. Biol Reprod Monogr 1:209, 1995.

31. Carnevale EM, Uson M, Bozzola JJ: Comparison of oocytes from young and old mares with light and electron microscopy. Theriogenology 51:299, 1999.

32. Hurtgen JP: Semen collection in stallions. In Samper JC, editor: Equine Breeding Management and Artificial Insemination. Philadelphia, W.B. Saunders, 2000.

33. Pickett BW, Amann RP, McKinnon AO, et al: Management of the stallion for maximum reproductive efficiency, II. Animal Reproduction Laboratory Bulletin No. 05, Fort Collins, CO, Colorado State University, 1989.

34. Dowsett KF, Pattie WA: Variation in characteristics of stallion semen caused by breed, age, season of year and service frequency. J Reprod Fert Suppl 35:645, 1987.

35. Jackson A, Dowsett K: Proliferative cell nuclear antigen in the equine testis: Effects of age and experimental treatment. Biol Reprod Monogr 1:631, 1995.

36. Fukuda T, Kikuchi M, Kurotaki T, et al: Age-related changes in the testes of horses. Equine Vet J 33:20, 2001.

37. Johnson L, Neaves WB: Age-related changes in the Leydig cell population, seminiferous tubules, and sperm production in stallions. Biol Reprod 24:703, 1981.

38. Roser JF: Endocrine and paracrine control of sperm production in stallions. Anim Reprod Sci 68:139, 2001.

39. Roser JF: Reproductive endocrinology of the stallion. In Samper JC, editor: Equine Breeding Management and Artificial Insemination. Philadelphia, W.B. Saunders, 2000.

40. Stewart BL, Roser JF: Effects of age, season, and fertility status on plasma and intratesticular immunoreactive (Ir) inhibin concentrations in stallions. Dom Anim Endocrinol 15:129, 1998.

41. Roser JF: Endocrine profiles in fertile, subfertile, and infertile stallions: testicular response to human chorionic gonadotropin in infertile stallions. Biol Reprod Monogr 1:661, 1995.

42. Parlevliet JM, Bevers MM, van de Broek J, et al: Effect of GnRH and hCG administration on plasma LH and testosterone concentrations in normal stallions, aged stallions and stallions with lack of libido. Vet Q 23:84, 2001.

43. Varner DD, Schumacher J, Blanchard TL, et al: Diseases and Management of Breeding Stallions. Goleta, CA, American Veterinary Publications, 1991.

44. Brinsko SP: GnRH therapy for subfertile stallions. Vet Clin North Am Equine Pract 12:149, 1996.

CHAPTER 18

Urinary Tract Disorders in Geriatric Horses

Thomas J. Divers,

Gillian A. Perkins

Urinary tract disorders are not particularly common in geriatric horses, especially in comparison with the frequency of disorders of the respiratory, musculoskeletal, dental, and endocrine system. Urinary tract disorders of the geriatric horse can generally be divided into those affecting the kidneys,[1] lower urinary tract disorders,[2] and those causing polyuria.[3]

Diseases of the Kidneys

Renal Failure

The most common renal disorders that result in clinical signs in geriatric horses are those that cause renal failure or renal neoplasia. Chronic renal failure is not as common in geriatric horses as it is in geriatric small companion animals, but it may occur from either chronic tubulointerstitial disease or glomerulonephritis, with the latter being the most common. Chronic tubulointerstitial disease causing renal failure may be the result of pyelonephritis or noninfectious interstitial fibrosis. Pyelonephritis is most common in older broodmares, especially those with poor pelvic conformation. In order to cause renal failure, both kidneys must be involved. In some cases, there may be only unilateral or mild bilateral involvement, in which case weight loss is a result of chronic infection and not uremia. Renal calculi may be found in association with the pyelonephritis in some cases. Noninfectious interstitial fibrosis causing renal failure may be a result of nephrotoxic drugs, intermittent obstruction, and/or persistent systemic hypertension. Geriatric horses with chronic muscu-

loskeletal pain, such as laminitis, are particularly susceptible, since they are frequently on prolonged doses of nonsteroidal anti-inflammatory drugs and may be chronically hypertensive. The cause of the renal pathology in many cases cannot be determined.

Glomerulonephritis resulting in renal failure may occur in geriatric horses but is more common in middle-aged (8-15 years) horses. The particular antigen involved in the immunologic disease is generally not identified, although streptococcal antigens are generally blamed.[1,2] In some cases, it is not clear whether the primary and initiating pathologic condition was a glomerular disease or a tubulointerstitial disease.

The clinical signs associated with chronic renal failure (CRF) are most commonly weight loss, decreased appetite and vigor, polyuria/polydipsia, and nonpainful edema (with glomerulonephritis). Fever is often, but not uniformly, present with pyelonephritis, and affected horses may exhibit signs of mild abdominal pain.

The diagnosis of CRF is based on abnormal elevations in serum creatinine and urea nitrogen, along with isosthenuric urine (1.008-1.014). Hypochloremia is the most consistent abnormal serum electrolyte finding. Hyponatremia, hyperkalemia, and hypercalcemia are present in many cases.[3] Large numbers of white blood cells, casts, and bacteruria may be noted with pyelonephritis. When pyelonephritis is suspected, a midstream voided urine sample or catheterized urine sample should be collected in a sterile container and submitted to the laboratory for culture, colony count, and sensitivity. It is imperative that a colony count be performed to determine the significance of a positive culture; more than 10^4 organisms/mL is generally considered significant. The most common offending organisms are *Streptococcus zooepidemicus*, *Escherichia coli*, *Enterobacter* spp., and *Proteus* spp. Urine protein and creatinine should be quantitated if glomerulonephritis is suspected; a protein-to-creatinine ratio of greater than 3 is supportive of glomerulonephritis. A biopsy of the right kidney can be performed to confirm the diagnosis. Ultrasonographic examination of both kidneys should be performed to determine size of the kidneys (glomerulonephritis and fibrosis may be smaller than normal [approximately 9×15 cm], while pyelonephritis may be larger than normal), echogenicity, nephroliths, pelvic dilatation, and ureteral dilatation. Rectal examination is not as helpful as ultrasonographic examination but may identify ureteral dilatation and ureteral stones.

Treatment of CRF is generally supportive.[1] All nephrotoxic drugs should be removed if possible. Fluid therapy should be provided if the patient is dehydrated or if an acute component of the CRF is believed to be involved. Intravenous fluids should be routinely administered if pyelonephritis is suspected. Affected horses should always have access to fresh water and, except in the case of horses with glomerulonephritis, should also have electrolytes in water available (6-10 g/L of both NaCl and glucose).

Ideally, affected horses should be on a moderate-protein, high-calorie, low-calcium, low-phosphorus, and low-potassium diet, but this varies depending on the disease process and serum electrolyte findings. It is most important that horses be fed adequate calories regardless of the other nutritional considerations. Nutritional supplements include vitamin E, vitamin C, B vitamins, and 2 ounces of dietary linseed or canola oil. Systemic blood pressure should be monitored and if the horse is hypertensive, treatment to lower the blood pressure should be given. Calcium channel blockers and angiotensin-converting enzyme inhibitors are expensive, have limited pharmacokinetic studies in the horses and are, therefore, often impractical. Administration of acepromazine granules has been used in horses with CRF and hypertension.[1]

Horses with pyelonephritis should be treated with an appropriate (safe, effective, and relatively inexpensive) antibiotic for at least 4 weeks. Urine should be cultured during and after the course of antimicrobial therapy. Therapy is generally not curative if there is a nephrolith or persistent lower urinary tract disorder, such as neuromuscular dysfunction.

Renal Tumors

Renal cell carcinomas are the most common renal tumors of geriatric horses.[4] The tumor has been reported in horses as young as 9 years of age. Hematuria and weight loss are the most common signs. Ultrasonographic examination may demonstrate the tumorous mass and permit successful biopsy. In most cases, the neoplasia has spread locally and intraperitoneally, preventing successful surgical removal. If the carcinoma is thought to be localized to a single kidney, surgical removal of that kidney is recommended.

Diseases of the Lower Urinary Tract

Incontinence, Infections

Geriatric horses are predisposed to urinary incontinence by both age and use. Older broodmares may develop urinary incontinence secondary to poor conformation and cystitis, or from urethral injury associated with foaling or breeding. Affected mares develop perineal scalding and dysuria. Rectal examination may reveal a normal size bladder or, more likely, an enlarged bladder with detrusor muscle dysfunction. The bladder is usually easy to express. Ultrasonographic examination should be performed of the entire urinary tract, although a distended bladder with "sludge" is generally all that is found. A catheterized urine sample for culture, sensitivity, and colony count should be collected.

Treatments consist of long-term administration of appropriate antimicrobials and correction of any predisposing neurologic or anatomic defect. A Caslick's maneuver should be performed for poor pelvic conformation. If the bladder is of normal size and the urethral tone is diminished (this can be determined by urethral pressure measurements),[5] phenylpropanolamine can be administered once the cystitis is resolved. When the bladder is chronically distended, long-term cure is rare. If the mare is pregnant, she may be able to carry that foal to term, although there is added risk to the foal due to the chronic infection and antibiotic administration. There should be an attempt to acidify the urine, but this is often unsuccessful. Fifteen to 20 g of NH_4Cl and $CaCl$ given orally every 8 hours to decrease "sludge" formation, or a formulated pelleted ration with an abnormally high strong anion-to-cation ratio are the most successful methods of acidifying the urine. Vitamin C is not consistently effective in acidifying the urine of horses, even when given in large amounts.

Older geldings and stallions are predisposed to bladder dysfunction associated with sterile sludge accumulation.[6] The exact cause of this is unknown, but it is in most cases secondary to thoracolumbar spondylitis, pain, and unwillingness to "stretch out" and completely empty the bladder. We hypothesize that over a prolonged period of time, large amounts of calcium carbonate crystals builds in the floor of the bladder, chronically and usually permanently, damaging the detrusor muscle. Affected horses are initially examined many months later because of urinary incontinence. On rectal examination, the bladder is distended and ultrasonographic examination reveals a large amount of echogenic material in the bladder. The first catheterized urine sample is usually found to be sterile, but all following samples will have significant bacteruria. Treatments consist of analgesics for the spondylitis, flushing out the sludge with sterile saline, long-term antibiotics, bethanechol (12-20 mg SQ q8h) and $NH_4Cl/CaCl$ in an attempt to lower the urine pH. There is frequently a good initial response, but within weeks, the clinical signs and findings recur.

Calculi, Neoplasia, Hematuria

Cystic calculi, causing exercise-induced hematuria and occasionally dysuria or obstruction, may occur in geriatric horses but may occur with equal frequency in younger adult horses. Likewise, hematuria occurring at the end of urination associated with ureteral vascular "leaks" may be seen in geriatric geldings or stallions but no more frequently than in middle-aged adult males.

Bladder tumors are rare in horses and when diagnosed are usually in older horses.[7] Hematuria and weight loss are the most common clinical signs. The neoplasia is usually easily identified on cystoscopic examination and a biopsy sample can be obtained. Squamous cell carcinomas are most common with an occasional and rare transitional cell carcinoma. Early diagnosis should offer the opportunity for surgical removal and/or local chemotherapy. Piroxicam, a systemically administered nonsteroidal anti-inflammatory drug, has been used successfully in the horse (80 mg PO SID).

Polyuria

Polyuria is a common abnormal clinical sign in geriatric horses. It is most commonly caused by Cushing's disease but may be caused by chronic renal failure, psychogenic polydipsia, or, rarely, diabetes insipidus. Observation of other clinical signs, urinalysis, serum chemistries, and measurement of adrenocorticotropic hormone and antidiuretic hormone will generally reveal the cause of the polyuria.

REFERENCES

1. VanBiervliet J, Divers TJ, Porter B, et al: Glomerulonephritis in horses. Compendium 24:892, 2002.
2. Divers TJ, Timoney JF, Lewis RM, et al: Equine glomerulonephritis and renal failure associated with complexes of group-C streptococcal antigen and IgG antibody. Vet Immunol Immunopathol 32:93, 1992.
3. Tennant B, Bettleheim P, Kaneko JJ: Paradoxic hypercalcemia and hypophosphatemia associated with chronic renal failure in horses. J Am Vet Med Assoc 180:630, 1982.
4. Brown PJ, Holt PE: Primary renal cell carcinoma in four horses. Equine Vet J 17:473, 1985.
5. Kay AD, Lavoie JP: Urethral pressure profilometry in mares. J Am Vet Med Assoc 191:212, 1987.
6. Holt PE, Mair TS: Ten cases of bladder paralysis associated with sabulous urolithiasis in horses. Vet Rec 127:108, 1990.
7. Fischer AT Jr, Spier S, Carlson GP, et al: Neoplasia of the equine urinary bladder as a cause of hematuria. J Am Vet Med Assoc 186:1294, 1985.

CHAPTER 19

West Nile Virus and the Geriatric Horse

Maureen T. Long

West Nile virus, a mosquito-borne flavivirus, was an old-world virus of Europe, Asia, Africa, and the South Pacific until 1999, when it was discovered as the cause of encephalitis and death in birds, humans, and horses of the New York City area. The first evidence of progression of West Nile virus into the Southeastern United States occurred in horses from Southern Georgia and Northern Florida in late June 2001, and clinical disease in horses was preceded by heavy bird losses. The 2002 arbovirus season was unprecedented. West Nile virus spread rapidly across the central part of the United States, causing the largest epidemic and epizootic in history. For 2002, 2741 cases of West Nile virus meningoencephalitis and 1267 cases of West Nile virus fever were reported in humans. More than 124,854 dead birds were reported in the United States, with 31,514 birds testing positive for the virus. An unprecedented 14,717 horses were identified as having West Nile encephalomyelitis, covering 40 states. At least one third of those horses died during the acute phase of the disease.

Biology

West Nile virus is antigenically related to viruses of the Japanese encephalitis complex and includes two lineages, designated lineage 1 and lineage 2. The original NY99 isolate is most closely related genetically to that which was isolated from a goose in Israel in 1996, and this is a lineage 1 virus. Lineage viruses are mainly found in Africa and appear to cause mild disease in humans and quite possibly limited disease in horses. Also contained within this complex are St. Louis encephalitis, Murray Valley encephalitis, and the extremely closely related subtype of West Nile virus, Kunjin. Several of these viruses are pathogenic for horses. According to the Centers for Disease Control and Prevention, several problematic trends are noted with this group of flaviviruses, including encroachment into new geographic areas, development of new viral variants or subtypes of these flaviviruses in these new areas, increase in the frequency of human and horse outbreaks, increase in severity of human infection, and significantly high avian losses associated with these outbreaks. In addition, new modes of transmission and new clinical syndromes are features of the North American outbreak.

Common among many flaviviruses is a predilection for neural tissue. These viruses cause a polioencephalomyelitis (infection of gray matter) with lesions increasing in number in the diencephalon, progressing through the hind brain. There is spinal infection and pathologic lesions, with the most severe lesions frequently progressing caudally into the lumbar spinal cord. This regional distribution also is found in cases of Japanese encephalitis in humans and horses. Specific areas of the gray matter at risk of viral localization include nerve cell bodies of the mid- and hind-brain and ventral horns of spinal cord. Thus, Parkinson-like symptoms, polio-like syndromes, and weakness are hallmarks of short- and long-term clinical signs. Two reports exist in which horses developed a transient low-level viremia during acute infection. Based on further experimental testing performed by the Centers for Disease Control and

Prevention and National Veterinary Services Laboratory, this viremia is not thought to be high enough for transmission.

Clinical Disease

Several West Nile virus outbreaks have occurred in horses in both old and new world locales. Of note are outbreaks in Egypt (1963), Israel (1996-2000), France (1962-1965), Spain (1996), Italy (1998), the state of New York (1999-present), and the Southeastern United States (2001). The first equine cases in North America were diagnosed in 1999 in New York, and through the next four seasons more than 15,500 cases were identified. In these outbreaks, horses primarily presented with sudden or progressive ataxia. Fever, periods of hyperexcitability, apprehension, somnolence, listlessness, and depression are the primary signs reported. Fever was reported in the French outbreak but not in the Italian outbreak. These two outbreaks were characterized mainly by spinal cord signs of ataxia and muscle rigidity, usually more severe in the hind limbs. Complete, flaccid paralysis when present could involve one or all four limbs. Infrequently, head tilt was observed. Mortality in the 2000 equine outbreak was approximately 30%, and few residual problems are reported in surviving horses.

In these earlier descriptions of equine disease, no breed, age, or sex predilection was described. During the first year of the U.S. encroachment, no bias in signalment was detected in horses affected in the New York outbreak. In 2001, however, 734 horses were confirmed with West Nile encephalomyelitis, and analysis of these data reveals a statistically higher number of older horses confirmed with West Nile encephalomyelitis. In addition, a statistically higher mortality rate occurred in these horses. The higher mortality rate may have reflected bias against long-term or expensive therapy in the older horse. This age predilection has also been demonstrated in humans. The average age for meningoencephalomyelitis is 78 and the mortality rate is higher among older than among younger patients. By comparison, the average age for West Nile fever, a mild, nonfatal form of the disease, is 55 years. Interestingly, older men (59%) are more likely to develop meningoencephalomyelitis, as compared with women, and rates are 64 percent versus 12 percent overall. Although this bias in humans may be related to life-style, significantly more equine males than females were reported to be affected in hospital populations and overall during the 2001 outbreak.

Age-associated enhanced susceptibility to viral diseases has been described in humans and many rodent models. Influenza has been one of the most commonly documented viral diseases in which increasing age leads to increased susceptibility. Although this same susceptibility is not documented in horses, this derangement in immunity has been associated with changes in both innate and adaptive immune responses. In nonspecific immune responses, there is a down-regulation of interferon-α responses and the interferon-α receptor itself. Natural killer activity also is less in elderly humans and in rodent models. Regarding specific immunity, there is senescence of long-term memory cells leading to a smaller repertoire of T-cell responses. In addition, CD8 responses are of shorter and less intense duration. All of these components are responsible for maintenance of innate and long-term immunity to viral diseases.

Differential Diagnoses

Infectious central nervous system diseases that share clinical signs of West Nile virus include alphaviruses, rabies, equine protozoal myeloencephalitis, equine herpes virus-1, less likely botulism, and verminous meningoencephalomyelitis (*Halicephalobus gingivalis*, *Setaria*, *Strongylus vulgaris*). Noninfectious causes to consider include hypocalcemia, tremorogenic toxicities, hepatoencephalopathy, and leukoencephalomalacia. In cases of alphaviral encephalitis and rabies, signs of cerebral involvement are commonly characterized by a change in consciousness as characterized by behavioral alterations, depression, seizure, and coma. Cortical blindness can also be present. Cranial nerve signs are also common, including head tilt, pharyngeal/laryngeal dysfunction, and paresis of the tongue. Signs in common with West Nile virus are the muscle fasciculations, hyperesthesia, excitability, blindness, somnolence, weakness of the tongue, and progression to recumbency. Differentiation from rabies can be quite problematic if signs include ataxia, weakness, or gait abnormalities. Alphaviruses, rabies, *H. gingivalis* infection, hepatoencephalopathy, and leukoencephalomalacia are usually progressive, with cortical signs. Although there are periods of somnolence, blindness, and some cranial nerve deficits, West Nile virus horses either become rapidly recumbent or stabilize in 72 to 96 hours. Spinal disease due to equine protozoal myeloencephalitis is a more difficult differential if horses with West Nile virus are not febrile and do not exhibit excessive muscle fasciculations. Although West Nile virus infection throughout the spinal cord is fairly symmetrical, horses can present with asymmetrical or multifocal cranial nerve and gait deficits. Equine herpesvirus myeloencephalopathy is a white matter infection in which clinical signs vary from subtle gait deficits to profound hind limb weakness, ataxia, and paraplegia. Urinary incontinence, tail elevation, and anal and tail hypotonia are common.

Treatment

Treatment of West Nile virus encephalomyelitis is supportive and largely anecdotal. The survival rate of this infection is high for acute encephalitis, and in many cases horses appear to begin recovery between 3 and 5 days after the onset of signs. Thus, it is difficult to accurately assess the affect of any pharmacological intervention in the face of resolving clinical signs. Flunixin meglumine (1.1 mg/kg IV bid) early in the course of the disease does appear to decrease the severity of muscle tremors and fasciculations within a few hours of administration. The recumbent horse poses special medical problems. To date, much of the mortality in West Nile virus horses results from euthanasia of recumbent horses for humane reasons. Recumbent horses are mentally alert and frequently thrash, sustaining many self-inflicted wounds and posing a risk to personnel. Therapy of recumbent horses is generally more aggressive and includes dexamethasone (0.05-0.1 IV sid) and, sporadically, mannitol (0.25-2.0 g/kg IV). Detomidine (0.02-0.04 mg/kg IV or IM) is effective for prolonged tranquilization. Low doses of acepromazine (0.02 mg/kg IV or 0.05 mg/kg IM) provides excellent relief from anxiety in both recumbent and standing horses. Until equine protozoal myeloencephalitis is ruled out, prophylactic institution of antiprotozoal medications is also recommended. Other supportive measures include oral and intravenous fluids and antibiotics for treatment of infections that frequently occur in recumbent horses (e.g., wounds, cellulitis, pneumonia).

Prevention

Prevention of West Nile virus in the geriatric horses is problematic. Mosquito abatement is just as important if not more so than prophylaxis. Data from the 2002 outbreak suggest that vaccine breaks in individual animals may be more likely to occur in the older horses. Likely the same factors that regulate response to the virus also regulate vaccine responses in the geriatric patient. Concerns regarding efficacy and safety also will extend to future modified live vaccines. Mosquito abatement should focus on environmental management and individual animal protection. Environmental mosquito abatement should consist on elimination of standing water, control of organic debris, and institution of air movement. Breaking the mosquito cycle in standing water requires cleaning of standing water vesicles once per week. Placement of aerators or larvicidal fish in ponds and large stock tanks are excellent means of larval control. Mosquitoes breed and develop in stagnant water that contains organic debris. Stables and farms contain high amounts of organic debris. Finally, installing fans in stables to increase air movement is another effective method of mosquito control.

CHAPTER 20

Liver Disease in the Geriatric Horse

Nicola J. Menzies-Gow

Effect of Aging on the Liver

Aging is associated with marked changes in the physiology of many organs and tissues. These alterations in structure and function are considered nonpathologic but can affect normal physiologic processes in the elderly.[1] However, aging affects the various organs of a given organism in different ways, resulting in varying rates of functional decline, all combining to diminish the overall ability to meet increased demand, for example in a stress situation.[2] Several aspects of aging of the liver have been studied. Aging does not appear to affect the different functions of the liver within a species, or the same function between species, similarly.

Most lipophilic chemicals, including drugs, carcinogens, and naturally occurring compounds undergo enzyme-mediated oxidative, hydrolytic, or conjugative biotransformations in the liver. It is generally accepted that the sensitivity to the effects of drugs and other foreign chemicals is often greater in young and elderly individuals than in adults as the result of several factors, including differences in the rates of biotransformation and excretion[3] and age-related reduction of hepatic blood flow, mainly consecutive to fibrosis, without intrahepatic shunting.[4] Data generated from humans[5] and several veterinary species including dogs,[6] and cattle[7] indicate that many enzyme-mediated metabolic pathways show marked age-related changes. Little is known about the effects of aging on the hepatic drug metabolizing capacity of horses despite their relatively long lifespan.[8] However, one study demonstrated that the rate of hepatic oxidative, hydrolytic, and conjugative biotransformations did not decline as a function of age.[8]

Aging in rats is associated with increased hepatocellular uptake function, decreased hepatocyte metabolic function, and unchanged excretion function.[1] Several human studies have shown that liver volume is reduced with advancing age,[9] whereas in rats, it appears to increase with age.[1] The equine liver also shrinks with age, increasing the size of the space between the caudal lobe of the liver and the vena cava known as the epiploic foramen. The decrease in hepatic volume is thought to be due to a reduction in hepatic cell volume as opposed to a reduction in their number.[10] Biliary transport declined with age, but hepatic storage capacity did not decrease in rats.[11] Glucose-6-phosphatase catalyses the final reactions in both gluconeogenesis and glycolysis. It is found mainly in glycogenic tissues such as the liver, where it plays an important role in the synthesis of glucose. With age, enzyme activity[12] and hepatic glucose production[13] decline in rats. Although hepatic mixed function mono-oxygenase activity does not decline with age in mice[14] or horses,[15] the phagocytic function of rat hepatic Kupffer cells decreases with age.[16] Aging also sensitizes the liver to the effect of various hepatocarcinogens through suppression of apoptosis that diminishes the ability of the liver to purge itself of already transformed cells, which then may progress to malignancy.[17] Finally, there is a significant age-related increase in the non-heme iron concentration in the equine liver.[18]

Effect of Aging on Equine Clinical Pathology Data

The aging process may cause metabolic alterations, regardless of the presence or absence of disease, that potentially affect interpretation of clinical data in the aged subject. However, there appear to be no age-related differences in equine serum biochemical analysis, and the only hematologic alteration associated with advanced age was that aged horses had a greater mean corpuscular volume than young animals.[19]

Liver Diseases in the Horse

Disease versus Dysfunction

Hepatic insufficiency or dysfunction refers to the inability of the liver to perform its normal functions properly. Because of the large reserve capacity of the liver, most hepatic functions are not impaired until greater then 80 percent of the hepatic mass is lost.[20] This, combined with the significant regenerative capacity of the liver, means that mild to moderate hepatic disease may be present without accompanying hepatic dysfunction and that clinical signs associated with liver disease without failure are unusual in all cases except for neoplasia or infection.[21] In one study, subclinical hepatic disease was detected in 3 percent to 8 percent of horses 15 years or older presented to a referral hospital for postmortem examination for unrelated reasons.[22] Thus, hepatic disease in the horse can be divided into those conditions that frequently result in hepatic failure, including pyrrolizidine alkaloid toxicity, acute hepatitis, cholangiohepatitis, and chronic active hepatitis, and those that rarely result in hepatic failure, including corticosteroid administration, hypoxia, hepatic neoplasia, abscessation, and parasite damage.[21]

When there is significant loss of hepatic function, some functions fail before others.[23] Compartmentalization of hepatic cytosolic enzymes, conversion of ammonia to urea, and conjugation of bilirubin tend to be lost earlier, whereas synthesis of clotting factors and albumin production are not lost until later.[24]

Specific Hepatic Diseases Affecting the Aged Horse

Pyrrolizidine Alkaloid Toxicity: Megalocytic hepatopathy is caused by ingestion of pyrrolizidine alkaloid containing plants, most commonly *Senecio jacobaea* (ragwort). The development of clinical signs of hepatic dysfunction may be delayed for weeks to years after consumption of the toxin. In addition, there is individual susceptibility, as not all horses consuming the plants develop clinical signs.[25] The plants are not palatable, and consumption usu-

ally only occurs if pastures are heavily contaminated, if there is not an alternative feed source available, or if there is significant hay contamination. Consumption of the plants at a dose of 2 percent to 5 percent of body weight over a short period of time can result in acute toxicity.[26] More commonly, however, there is a cumulative toxic effect after chronic low-level exposure. Ingested pyrrolizidine alkaloids are metabolized by the liver to toxic pyrrole derivatives that cross-link with DNA, inhibiting protein synthesis and cellular replication and resulting in periportal megalocyte formation and fibrosis.[27]

Acute Hepatitis: Acute hepatitis, Theiler's disease, or serum hepatitis has been associated with administration of biological products, including tetanus antitoxin,[28] vaccines, and antiserum[29,30] 4 to 10 weeks before the onset of hepatic dysfunction. Lactating mares that receive tetanus antitoxin at parturition seem to be more susceptible.[28] However, there are cases with no history of biological product administration, and the exact cause of the disease remains unknown. The onset of clinical signs is acute to subacute and often progresses over 2 to 7 days. Horses may be found dead or present with signs of depression, lethargy, and anorexia that progress to hepatic encephalopathy.[28] The disease typically occurs sporadically, but outbreaks involving multiple horses on a single farm have been reported. Occurrence may be seasonal, with more cases presenting in summer and autumn.[28,30] It is characterized histologically by acute hepatic centrilobular necrosis and mild periportal inflammatory infiltration.[31]

Cholangiohepatitis: Cholangiohepatitis is severe neutrophilic inflammation of the bile passages and adjacent hepatocytes caused by ascending bacterial infection from the gastrointestinal tract. Gram-negative organisms are most commonly isolated.

Cholelithiasis: Cholelithiasis occasionally results in hepatocellular disease in the horse. The calculus may develop within the intrahepatic ducts or the common bile duct. There is precipitation of the normally soluble constituents of bile secondary to unconjugation by the enzyme β-glucuronidase. The unconjugated bilirubin then combines with calcium to form calcium bilirubinate that precipitates. β-glucuronidase is synthesised by the bile duct epithelium, hepatocytes, and certain bacteria. Many horses with cholelithiasis have concurrent cholangitis; cholelith formation in horses most likely occurs after bacterial infection. Bacterial culture of choleliths almost always reveals enteric gram-negative infection; thus, the infection probably ascends from the gastrointestinal tract.

Chronic Active Hepatitis: Chronic active hepatitis is an idiopathic, progressive hepatopathy characterized by biliary hyperplasia and periportal inflammation. There appear to be two forms of the disease. In the first form, neutrophils predominate in the periportal inflammation and in some cases coliform organisms have been isolated, suggesting that chronic active hepatitis may be a manifestation of chronic cholangitis secondary to ascending infection from the gastrointestinal tract.[32] In the second form, a mononuclear inflammatory infiltrate predominates, and the possibility of an autoimmune or hypersensitivity reaction has been postulated.[27]

Hepatic Neoplasia: Primary hepatic neoplasia is rare in horses; cholangiocellular carcinoma,[33] hepatocellular carcinoma, hepatoblastoma, and mixed hamartoma have been reported. Hepatic neoplasia is more likely to be metastatic, most commonly lymphosarcoma.[34]

Clinical Signs

Clinical signs of hepatic dysfunction occur when a significant percentage of the liver is no longer functional, either as an acute disorder or when chronic insults to the liver have surpassed the abilities of cellular regeneration.[35] They vary greatly, are nonspecific, and depend on the extent and duration of the hepatic disease.[27] The clinicopathologic features of 50 cases of equine hepatic disease were reviewed.[36] There was a wide range of clinical signs and at least half of the animals exhibited depression, anorexia, icterus, abdominal pain, cerebral dysfunction, or weight loss. Life-threatening complications included gastric impaction, bilateral laryngeal paralysis, and coagulopathy. Less commonly reported clinical signs include hepatogenic photosensitization and diarrhea, and rarely reported clinical signs include ventral edema, steatorrhea, tenesmus, generalized seborrhea, pruritus, endotoxic shock, polydipsia, and pigmenturia.[27]

Weight Loss: Weight loss is the most common clinical sign associated with hepatic dysfunction and is caused by anorexia and the loss of the normal hepatocellular metabolic activities.[27]

Icterus: Icterus is caused by hyperbilirubinemia with subsequent deposition of the pigment in the tissues, causing yellow discoloration seen most easily in the mucous membranes, nonpigmented skin, and the sclera.[27] Hepatic disease results in impaired uptake and conjugation of bilirubin resulting in increased serum concentrations of unconjugated (indirect) bilirubin and, less commonly, impaired excretion of conjugated bilirubin into the biliary tract resulting in overflow into the circulation.

Hepatogenic Photosensitization: The photodynamic agent phylloerythrin is formed in the gastrointestinal tract as a result of bacterial degradation of chlorophyll, absorbed into the circulation, and normally conjugated and excreted by the liver.[37] Hepatic dysfunction results in accumulation of phylloerythrin, particularly in the skin. Subsequent exposure of phylloerythrin to ultraviolet light causes free radical formation and cellular damage. This is seen clinically as initial erythema, followed by vesiculation, ulceration, necrosis, and sloughing of nonpigmented areas of skin.[27]

Hepatic Encephalopathy: Hepatic encephalopathy is a complex clinical syndrome with clinical signs that vary according to the degree of hepatic dysfunction. The earliest signs (stage 1) are probably overlooked in most horses, as there is only subtle mental impairment.[38] Clinical signs including depression, head-pressing, circling, mild ataxia, aimless walking, persistent yawning, and other manifestations of inappropriate behaviour[27] are seen as the disease progresses (stage 2). These signs can wax and wane and may be precipitated by feeding.[39] Somnolence develops subsequently, during which the horse is rousable but responds minimally or excessively to the usual stimuli. Often there is aggressive or violent behaviour interspersed with periods of stupor (stage 3). Finally, the horse becomes recumbent and comatose (stage 4). Seizures are atypical but occasionally occur during the late stages.[38]

Bilateral laryngeal paralysis and gastric impaction are thought to be due to neuromuscular dysfunction and a peripheral manifestation of hepatic encephalopathy, but the underlying pathogenesis is unclear. No gross or histopathologic abnormalities have been reported in the laryngeal musculature or its innervation.[36] Disturbing the function of gastrointestinal neurotransmitters and reducing gastric emptying[40] has been postulated to induce gastric impaction.

Four hypotheses have evolved to explain the development of these neurologic signs. It is possible that all of these combine to create hepatic encephalopathy.

Gastrointestinal-Derived Neurotoxins. The oldest hypothesis for hepatic encephalopathy involves the synergistic effects of accumulating toxins, as well as metabolic abnormalities such as hypoglycemia.[41] The toxins are derived from metabolism of nitrogenous substrates in the gastrointestinal tract and are normally removed from the circulation by the liver. Ammonia is thought to play a central role in the pathogenesis.[42] It has a toxic effect on neurons by inhibiting the Na-K dependent adenosine triphosphatase, via competition with potassium, causing depletion of adenosine triphosphate.[42] Ammonia is also associated with a disturbance in central nervous system energy production, caused by alterations in the tricarboxylic acid cycle that result in decreased in α-ketoglutarate formation and increased glutamine.[43] Astrocytes in the brain also detoxify ammonia by converting it to glutamate and glutamine. Glutamine accumulation in astrocytes causes cell swelling and cerebral edema. Prolonged exposure of neuronal tissue to ammonia results in down-regulation of the receptors for the excitatory neurotransmitter glutamate and so decreased excitatory neurotransmission.[44]

Ammonia can induce encephalopathy experimentally, and congenital enzyme deficiencies resulting in hyperammonemia in humans show signs of encephalopathy.[45] Therapies aimed at decreasing ammonia absorption from the gastrointestinal tract ameliorate the signs of encephalopathy, but they also decrease production and absorption of other putative toxins.[46] However, plasma ammonia concentration correlates poorly with the severity of the encephalopathy, and intravenous administration of ammonia does not induce the electroencephalographic changes typical of hepatic encephalopathy.[47] In addition, changes in brain neurotransmitters during experimental hyperammonemic encephalopathy are different from those occurring during hepatic encephalopathy, and seizures are a common feature of congenital and experimental hyperammonemia but are rare in hepatic encephalopathy.[48]

Other toxins implicated are mercaptans, fatty acids, and phenols. They are increased in hepatic failure but not in concentrations that alone would induce encephalopathy.[27] In combination, they may act synergistically. Experimentally, however, these compounds induce seizures, and blood and brain concentrations correlate poorly with the severity of the hepatic encephalopathy.[49]

False Neurotransmitter Accumulation. Serum glucagon is increased in liver failure, leading to muscle catabolism and release of amino acids. However, hepatic metabolism of aromatic amino acids (phenylalanine, tyrosine and tryptophan) is reduced, and since branched-chain amino acids (valine, leucine, and isoleucine) continue to be metabolized by muscle and adipose tissue, there is a relative increase in aromatic and a decrease in branched-chain amino acids.[27] This altered ratio of amino acids and increased brain glutamine concentration (presumably a consequence of ammonia retention) promotes an influx of aromatic amino acids into the brain and an efflux of glutamine by exchange transport processes at the blood-brain barrier.[47] Phenylalanine can compete with tyrosine for tyrosine hydroxylase, resulting in decreased production of dopamine.[50] The displaced tyrosine may be decarboxylated to tyramine, which is then converted to the false neurotransmitter octopamine. Accumulated tyrosine also competes for dopamine β-oxidase and reduces the formation of noradrenaline. Phenylalanine and tryptophan are ultimately converted to phenylethanolamine

and serotonin, a false neurotransmitter and a neuroinhibitor, respectively.[27] False neurotransmitters, although structurally similar to catecholamines, are less potent in eliciting postsynaptic membrane potential. The excess of inhibitory neurotransmitters (serotonin) and their receptors and the deficiency of excitatory neurotransmitters (dopamine and noradrenaline) may cause encephalopathy.

The concentration of branched-chain amino acids (leucine, isoleucine and valine) and the concentration of aromatic amino acids (phenylalanine and tyrosine) can been expressed as a ratio. This ratio has been correlated with the degree of hepatic encephalopathy in horses. The ratio in normal horses was 4.0, whereas animals showing signs of hepatic encephalopathy had a mean ratio of 1.3.[51] Administration of branch-chain amino acids to horses with clinical signs of hepatic encephalopathy will sometimes alleviate signs of the disease, at least temporarily.[52] In rats, however, intraventricular administration of octopamine failed to reduce consciousness,[53] and in human beings dopaminergic drugs have not proved useful.

Augmented Activity of True Neurotransmitters. This theory suggests that hepatic encephalopathy involves augmented activity of inhibitors neurotransmitter including γ-aminobutyric acid (GABA), and depressed function of the excitatory glutaminergic system.[27] When the liver fails, GABA, produced by enteric bacteria, is not catabolized by the liver, crosses the blood-brain barrier, and binds to GABA receptors contributing to the neural inhibition of hepatic encephalopathy.[54] Increased plasma GABA has been documented in humans with hepatic encephalopathy and an increased density of GABA receptors has been reported in rabbits with hepatic failure.[55]

Endogenous Benzodiazepines. The most recently proposed hypothesis is that the neurologic inhibition in hepatic encephalopathy is the result of increased cerebral concentration of an endogenous benzodiazepine.[56] The GABA receptor is divided into a GABA receptor unit, a benzodiazepine unit, and a chloride ionophore that contains receptors for barbiturates. Increased endogenous benzodiazepines may bind to GABA receptors, resulting in increased neuronal inhibition. Clinical studies in human beings show improved consciousness and reduced electroencephalographic abnormalities in patients treated with benzodiazepine receptor antagonist flumazenil.[57]

Coagulopathy

The liver synthesizes numerous factors involved in coagulation and fibrinolysis. Synthesis of fibrinogen and the vitamin K-dependent clotting factors (II, VII, IX, X, and protein C), which have short half-lives and need vitamin K that is fat-soluble and is dependent on bile acids for proper absorption, are particularly sensitive to hepatic disease.[27] In addition, hepatic Kupffer cells are responsible for removing activated coagulation factors and fibrin degradation products from the circulation.[58] Failure of these functions promotes coagulation and interferes with platelet function and fibrin clot formation, respectively. Thus, hepatic disease may result in abnormal hemostasis, seen clinically varying from petechial and ecchymotic hemorrhages to hemorrhage after trauma to spontaneous hemorrhage.[20]

Diagnosis of Hepatic Disease

Diagnosis of hepatic disease is based on history, clinical signs, and finding of clinical pathology, hepatic ultrasonography, and histologic examination of a liver biopsy specimen.

Clinical Pathology

Hematology. Anemia may accompany chronic disease and bacterial infection, as in cholangiohepatitis or abscessation, or may show leukocytosis with a left shift. However, most commonly, no hematologic abnormalities are detected in horses with liver disease.

Liver Enzymes. Acute hepatocellular necrosis or changes in hepatocyte membrane permeability result in the release of soluble cytosolic enzymes into the circulation.[27] Thus, increased serum activities of these enzymes may be indicative of hepatic disease. However, it must be remembered that increases in serum enzyme activities are not correlated with the severity of hepatic dysfunction. The enzymes most commonly used to diagnose equine hepatic disease are gamma glutyl transferase (GGT), sorbitol dehydrogenase, aspartate transferase, alkaline phosphatase (ALP), and lactate dehydrogenase.

One of the most useful enzymes is GGT.[21,59] It is present in most duct tissue and so is found in the equine liver, kidney, pancreas, and udder. Pancreatitis is rare in the horse and in renal disease the enzyme is lost into the urine.[24] Thus, increased serum GGT activity is specific for liver disease, and occurs in chronic intra- and extra-hepatic cholestasis.[21] A rising or a persistently increased activity carries a poor prognosis.[60] Liver disease without an increase in GGT would be rare but may occur with chronic (nonactive) hepatic fibrosis and selective hepatic masses.

The enzyme sorbitol dehydrogenase is very sensitive and liver specific,[61] but it has a relatively short half-life outside the animal, necessitating analysis within hours of sampling. Aspartate transferase is not liver specific and is found mainly in skeletal muscle. It is a sensitive indicator of hepatocellular disease and remains elevated for more than 6 days after an acute hepatic insult but has poor predictive value because of its lack of specificity.[21] ALP is present in bone, intestine, placenta, and macrophages as well as the liver. The enzyme is not released during acute hepatocellular death, as it is mitochondrial membrane-bound, but chronic cholestasis results in increased production and release of ALP. Thus, serum activities of ALP may be increased in chronic liver disease, but lack of hepatic specificity reduces its usefulness.[38] Lactate dehydrogenase is present in many tissues, including liver, muscle, erythrocytes, intestinal cells, and renal tissue, and has five isoenzymes. Lactate dehydrogenase-5 levels may be elevated with hepatic or muscle disease and so is useful as a screening test for hepatocellular disease only if creatine kinase is simultaneously measured.

Bile Acids. Bile acids are normally produced by the liver, excreted in the bile, and reabsorbed in the ileum before being excreted again. Thus, they recirculate through the enterohepatic circulation. If the liver fails to remove the majority (90%) of the bile acids on first passage, serum concentrations will increase. Sample collection at the time of feeding has no significant effect of serum bile acid concentration,[62] but fasting for more than 3 days causes an increase in concentration of three times the baseline value. Elevation of total serum bile acid concentration has both sensitivity and specificity for detecting hepatic dysfunction, rather than just disease, in the horse.[21] Changes in bile acid concentration occur early in liver disease and continue through the terminal stages.[24] Serum bile acid concentration is also a good prognostic indicator; concentrations greater than 50 μmol/L are associated with a grave prognosis.[63]

Bilirubin. Hyperbilirubinemia may result from liver disease, hemolytic disease, or anorexia.[24] Horses with hepatic dysfunction most often have significant increases in both indirect and direct bilirubin due to reduced hepatic uptake and conjugation and reduced biliary excretion, respectively. The increase in indirect bilirubin is most pronounced in the majority of cases of hepatic disease except those in which there is significant biliary obstruction, in which case the percentage of direct bilirubin is often greater than 30 percent of the total.[21] Cholestatic hepatic disease will also result in bilirubinuria due to renal excretion of excess soluble conjugated bilirubin.

Protein. The liver produces all of the serum albumin, but the half-life of equine albumin is about 19 days. Thus, hypoalbuminemia is not common in horses with severe liver disease[23] and if present is a poor prognostic indicator.[24] Total protein is almost never low in equine hepatic disease, as there is an increase in serum globulin concurrent with any decrease in albumin.[24]

Ammonia. The liver is primarily responsible for removing ammonia from the circulation and converting it to urea for renal excretion. Thus, blood ammonia concentration may be increased with chronic hepatocellular disease. No correlation exists between blood ammonia concentration and the severity of liver disease, but hyper-ammonemia is correlated with the presence of liver disease and with hepatic encephalopathy.[60,64]

Glucose. Changes in blood glucose concentration rarely occur in equine liver disease.[36] However, hypoglycemia due to reduced hepatic gluconeogenesis[60] or hyperglycemia due to insulin insensitivity or increased release of cortisol in response to the stress associated with the underlying hepatic disease[36] may occasionally be detected.

In conclusion, the single positive test results of greatest diagnostic value are the presence of increased serum GGT activity, increased serum sorbitol dehydrogenase activity, increased serum bile acids concentration, increased total bilirubin concentration, and hypoalbuminemia.[65] However, negative results are invariably poor predictors of the absence of liver disease, and no single, combination, or sequential noninvasive test can fully discriminate between horses with and those without liver disease.[65]

Hepatic Ultrasonography: The equine liver can be imaged ultrasonographically in the 7th to 16th intercostal spaces on the right and in the 6th to 9th intercostals space on the left ventral to the lung margins. Atrophy of the right liver lobe with age may result in the ultrasonographic window over the right hemithorax decreasing in size or being absent.

Hepatic ultrasonography can be used to determine the general size of the liver; to evaluate the parenchyma; to detect focal abnormalities such as abscesses, neoplasia, choleliths[38]; and to guide biopsy. Focal or diffuse lesions can alter the normal parenchymal pattern and result in an increased or decreased echogenicity of the diseased area.[66] Cholelithiasis can be imaged ultrasonographically in 75 percent of cases as hyperechoic foci within thick distended bile ducts and increased hepatic echogenecity.[67,68] It must be acknowledged, however, that it is a specific but not very sensitive technique for identifying hepatic disease. In one study, only 33 percent of cases of equine liver disease diagnosed on biopsy had ultrasonographic evidence of hepatic abnormalities.[69] Nevertheless, horses in which abnormalities are found are significantly less likely to survive compared with those judged to be ultrasonographically normal.[69]

Under ultrasound guidance, the biopsy instrument can be directed into these areas to ensure that the sample is representative of the disease process within that organ. Hepatic biopsies are not innocuous procedures, but ultrasound guidance has helped to reduce the risks involved with the biopsy technique.[66]

Liver Biopsy: Hepatic biopsy is extremely useful in establishing the presence of liver disease, determining a definitive diagnosis and thus guiding treatment and prognosis.[70,71] In most cases, liver biopsy will detect evidence of hepatic disease if the condition is diffuse. If the disease is focal, however, for example metastatic neoplasia, then normal liver may be sampled.[60] Hepatic biopsy material can also be submitted for bacterial culture[68] to determine the underlying bacterial pathogen and its antibiotic sensitivity. However, organisms are cultured in only approximately 50 percent of cases with an underlying bacterial etiology.

The biopsy site can either be determined with the help of ultrasonography or located on the right side at either the 11th or the 12th intercostal space. The height of the biopsy site is determined by drawing a line from the tuber coxae to a point halfway between the elbow and the point of the shoulder. The site is surgically prepared and local anaesthetic instilled. A stab incision is made and the biopsy needle is directed slightly cranially and ventrally. The needle will enter the thoracic cavity and then pass through the diaphragm, resulting in movement of the needle with respiration, before entering the liver. Clotting times should be evaluated prior to hepatic biopsy to minimize the risk of hemorrhage.

Treatment

Hepatic Encephalopathy: Treatment of hepatic encephalopathy is largely supportive and aimed at reducing the production or absorption of toxic metabolites from the gastrointestinal tract.[38] Continuous intravenous administration of dextrose and polyionic fluids with correction of acid-base imbalance is recommended to reduce hepatic workload and to allow time for hepatic regeneration.[72] Mineral oil, neomycin, and lactulose have been used to decrease absorption and production of hepatic toxins, by reducing the numbers of enteric anaerobes and gram-negative urea-splitting organisms.[38] In a study on healthy ponies, however, oral lactulose did not affect plasma ammonia levels.[73] Horses that are agitated, restless, or uncontrollable can be sedated with xylazine or acepromazine, but the benzodiazepine diazepam should be avoided because it enhances the effect of GABA on central inhibitory neurones and may exacerbate the signs of hepatic encephalopathy.[44]

Dietary Therapy: The primary goal in the management of chronic hepatic disease is to rest the liver to allow regeneration. A diet designed to relieve the liver's role in energy production and decrease its exposure to metabolic wastes should be fed.[64] The diet should include a readily digestible carbohydrate source, preferably high in branched chain amino acids (e.g., beet pulp), as an energy source, but avoid excessive protein to help decrease gastrointestinal ammonia production and aromatic amine accumulation.[38,64] Multiple small feeds are optimal because of impaired hepatic gluconeogenic capacity. Administration of B vitamins, because they are usually produced by the liver, and supplementary fat-soluble vitamins, because reduced bile salt production may result in defective gastrointestinal absorption, have also been advocated.[64]

Therapy Specific to Individual Diseases: Successful medical treatment of cholangiohepatitis and cholelithiasis requires long-term antibiotic therapy based on culture and sensitivity results. Penicillin-gentamicin, ceftiofur, enrofloxacin, metronidazole, and trimethoprim-sulpha have been used successfully. In one study, median treatment duration was 51 days (range, 17-124 days) and treatment failure was associated with severe periportal and bridging fibrosis.[68] Surgical intervention may be necessary if there is cholelith occlusion of the common bile duct. Chronic active hepatitis characterized by a neutrophilic infiltrate also requires long-term antibiotic therapy, whereas the form characterized by a mononuclear infiltrate should be treated with oral corticosteroid therapy. Colchicine and cyclosporine have been used to suppress cirrhosis of the liver in humans and dogs, but have proved ineffective in cases of pyrrolizidine alkaloid toxicity.[24]

Prognosis

Horses showing clinical signs of hepatic dysfunction have a significantly increased risk of nonsurvival compared to those with hepatic disease, but no dysfunction.[69] Several studies have shown that hepatic encephalopathy may signify a poor prognosis,[36,69] but the fact that 40 percent of horses with hepatic encephalopathy survive for at least 6 months justifies attempts at treatment. If adequate and appropriate supportive treatment is given, the recovery period from hepatic encephalopathy has been reported to be between 4 and 21 days. Ultimately, however, the prognosis for complete and sustained recovery depends on the underlying hepatic disease; acute hepatic disease having a guarded to fair prognosis and chronic hepatic disease a guarded to poor prognosis. The prognosis for pyrrolizidine alkaloid toxicity is ultimately hopeless, but many horses survive for years after a diagnosis is made. The mortality rate is high in acute hepatitis and ranges from 50 percent to 88 percent.[28] In addition, the prognosis is poor if there is severe hepatic fibrosis, as the chance of hepatic regeneration is low,[38] and recorded mortality rates range from 53 percent to 88 percent.

REFERENCES

1. Jourdan M, Vaubourdolle M, Cynober L, Aussel C: Effect of aging on liver functions: an experimental study in a perfused rat liver model. Exp Gerontol 39:1341, 2004.
2. Gagliano N, Arosio B, Grizzi F, et al: Reduced collagenolytic activity of matrix metalloproteinases and development of liver fibrosis in the aging rat. Mech Aging Dev 123:413, 2002.
3. Baggot JD: The Physiological Basis of Veterinary Clinical Pharmacology. London, Blackwell Science, 2001.
4. Zoli M, Magalotti D, Bianchi G, et al: Total and functional hepatic blood flow decrease in parallel with aging. Age Aging 28:29, 1999.
5. Tanaka E: In vivo age-related changes in hepatic drug-oxidizing capacity in humans. J Clin Pharm Ther 23:247, 1998.
6. Kawalek JC, el Said KR: Maturational development of drug-metabolizing enzymes in dogs. Am J Vet Res 51:1742, 1990.
7. Kawalek JC, el Said KR: Comparison of maturation of drug-metabolizing enzymes in calves with functioning or nonfunctioning rumen. Am J Vet Res 55:1579, 1994.
8. Nebbia C, Dacasto M, Carletti M: Postnatal development of hepatic oxidative, hydrolytic and conjugative drug-metabolizing enzymes in female horses. Life Sci 74:1605, 2004.
9. Zeeh J, Platt D: The aging liver: structural and functional changes and their consequences for drug treatment in old age. Gerontology 48:121, 2002.
10. Kelly WR: The liver and biliary system. In Jubb KVF, Kennedy PC, Palmer N, eds. Pathology of Domestic Animals. San Diego, Academic Press, 1993.
11. Kitani K, Zurcher C, Van Bezooijen K: The effect of aging on the hepatic metabolism of sulfo-bromophthalein in BN/Bi female and WAG/Rij male and female rats. Mech Aging Dev 17:381, 1981.
12. Plewka A, Kaminski M, Plewka D, Nowaczyk G: Glucose-6-phosphatase and age: biochemical and histochemical studies. Mech Aging Dev 113:49, 2000.
13. Sumida KD, Arimoto SM, Catanzaro MJ, Frisch F: Effect of age and endurance training on the capacity for epinephrine-stimulated gluconeogenesis in rat hepatocytes. J Appl Physiol 95:712, 2003.
14. Williams D, Woodhouse K: Age related changes in NADPH cytochrome c reductase activity in mouse skin and liver microsomes. Arch Gerontol Geriatr 21:191, 1995.
15. Lakritz J, Winder BS, Noorouz-Zadeh J, et al: Hepatic and pulmonary enzyme activities in horses. Am J Vet Res 61:152, 2000.
16. Sun WB, Han BL, Peng ZM, et al: Effect of aging on cytoskeleton system of Kupffer cell and its phagocytic capacity. World J Gastroenterol 4:77, 1998.
17. Youssef JA, Bouziane M, Badr MZ: Age-dependent effects of nongenotoxic hepatocarcinogens on liver apoptosis in vivo. Mech Aging Dev 124:333, 2003.
18. Ramsay WN: Age-related storage of iron in the liver of horses. Vet Res Commun 18:261, 1994.
19. Ralston SL, Nockels CF, Squires EL: Differences in diagnostic test results and hematologic data between aged and young horses. Am J Vet Res 49:1387, 1988.
20. Coles EH: Liver function. In Veterinary Clinical Pathology. Philadelphia, W.B. Saunders, 1988.
21. Divers TJ: Biochemical diagnosis of hepatic disease and dysfunction in the horse. Equine Pract 15:15, 1993.
22. Williams N: Disease conditions in geriatric horses. Equine Pract 22:32, 2000.
23. Parraga ME, Carlson GP, Thurmond M: Serum protein concentrations in horses with severe liver disease: a retrospective study and review of the literature. J Vet Intern Med 9:154, 1995.
24. Pearson EG: Liver disease in the mature horse. Equine Vet Educ 11:87, 1999.
25. Giles CJ: Outbreak of ragwort (*S. jacobaea*) poisoning in horses. Equine Vet J 15:248, 1983.
26. Pearson EG: Liver failure attributable to pyrrolizidine alkaloid toxicosis and associated with inspiratory dyspnea in ponies: three cases (1982–1988). J Am Vet Med Assoc 198:1651, 1991.
27. Barton MH: Disorders of the liver. In Reed SM, Bayly WM, Sellon DC, eds. Equine Internal Medicine. Philadelphia, W.B. Saunders, 2004.
28. Guglick MA, MacAllister CG, Ely RW, et al: Hepatic disease associated with administration of tetanus antitoxin in eight horses. J Am Vet Med Assoc 206:1737, 1995.
29. Marsden DE: Equine encephalomyelitis. Utah Acad Sci Arts Lett 11:95, 1934.

30. Tennant B: Acute Hepatitis in Horses: Problems of Differentiating Toxic and Infectious Causes in the Adult. St. Louis, American Association of Equine Practitioners, 1978.

31. Aleman M, Nieto JE, Carr EA, Carlson GP: Serum hepatitis associated with commercial plasma transfusion in horses. J Vet Intern Med 19:120, 2005.

32. Carlson GP: Chronic active hepatitis in horses. Presented at the 7th Annual Forum of the American College of Veterinary Internal Medicine, San Diego, 1989.

33. Mueller PO, Morris DD, Carmichael KP, et al: Antemortem diagnosis of cholangiocellular carcinoma in a horse. J Am Vet Med Assoc 201:899, 1992.

34. Chaffin MK, Schmitz DG, Brumbaugh GW, Hall DG: Ultrasonographic characteristics of splenic and hepatic lymphosarcoma in three horses. J Am Vet Med Assoc 201:743, 1992.

35. Byars TD: Liver disease: Contributions to diagnostic and prognostic aids. Equine Vet J 35:522, 2003.

36. McGorum BC, Murphy D, Love S, Milne EM: Clinicopathological features of equine primary hepatic disease: a review of 50 cases. Vet Rec 145:134, 1999.

37. Scott DW: Environmental diseases. In Large Animal Dermatology. Philadelphia, W.B. Saunders, 1988.

38. Morris DD, Henry MM: Hepatic encephalopathy. Compend Contin Educ Pract Vet 13:1153, 1991.

39. Mair TS: Ammonia and encephalopathy in the horse. Equine Vet J 29:1, 1997.

40. Milne EM, Pogson DM, Doxey DL: Secondary gastric impaction associated with ragwort poisoning in three ponies. Vet Rec 126:502, 1990.

41. Zieve L: The mechanism of hepatic coma. Hepatology 1:360, 1981.

42. Bode JC, Schafer K: Pathophysiology of chronic hepatic encephalopathy. Hepatogastroenterology 32:259, 1985.

43. Bessman SP, Bessman AN: The cerebral and peripheral uptake of ammonia in liver disease with a hypothesis for the mechanism for hepatic coma. J Clin Invest 34:622, 1975.

44. Albrecht J, Jones E: Hepatic encephalopathy: Molecular mechanisms underlying the clinical syndrome. J Neurol Sci 170:138, 1999.

45. Flannery DB, Hsia YE, Wolf B: Current status of hyperammonemic syndromes. Hepatology 2:495, 1982.

46. Zieve L: Diseases of the Liver. Philadelphia, J.B. Lippincott, 1987.

47. Gammal SH, Jones EA: Hepatic encephalopathy. Med Clin North Am 73:793, 1989.

48. Scharschmidt BF: Textbook of Medicine. Philadelphia, W.B. Saunders, 1998.

49. Record CO, Mardini H, Bartlett K: Blood and brain mercaptan concentrations in hepatic encephalopathy. Hepatology 2:144, 1982.

50. Alexander WF, Spindel E, Harty RF, et al: The usefulness of branched chain amino acids in patients with acute or chronic hepatic encephalopathy. Am J Gastroenterol 84:91, 1989.

51. Guglick MA, Knight HD, Rogers GR: Use of amino acid patterns in liver disease of the horse. Cal Vet 33:21, 1979.

52. Guglick MA, Knight HD, Rogers GR: Plasma Amino Acid Patterns in Horses with Hepatic Disease. St. Louis, American Association of Equine Practitioners, 1978.

53. Zieve L, Olsen RL: Colonic bacteria: a source of GABA in blood. Proc Soc Exp Biol Med 107:301, 1977.

54. Jones EA, Schafer DF, Ferenci P, et al: The neurobiology of hepatic encephalopathy. Hepatology 4:1235, 1984.

55. Schafer DF, Fowler JM, Jones EA: Colonic bacteria: a source of gamma-aminobutyric acid in blood. Proc Soc Exp Biol Med 167:301, 1981.

56. Maddison JE: Hepatic encephalopathy: current concepts of the pathogenesis. J Vet Intern Med 6:341, 1992.

57. Ferenci P, Jones EA, Hanbauer I: Lack of evidence for impaired dopamine receptor function in experimental hepatic coma in the rabbit. Neurosci Lett 65:60, 1986.

58. Ratnoff OD: Disordered haemostasis in hepatic disease. In Schiff L, Schiff ER, eds. Diseases of the Liver. Philadelphia, J.B. Lippincott, 1987.

59. West HJ: Observations on γ-glutamyl transferase, 5′-nucleotidase and leucine aminopeptidase activities in the plasma of the horse. Res Vet Sci 46:301, 1989.

60. West HJ: Evaluation of total plasma bile acid concentrations for the diagnosis of hepatobiliary disease in horses. Res Vet Sci 46:264, 1989.

61. Bernard WV, Divers TJ: Variations in serum sorbitol dehydrogenase, aspartate transaminase and isoenzyme 5 of lactate dehydrogenase activities in horses given carbon tetrachloride. Am J Vet Res 50:622, 1989.

62. Hoffmann WE, Baker G, Rieser S, et al: Alterations in selected serum biochemical constituents in equids after induced hepatic disease. Am J Vet Res 48:1343, 1987.

63. Mendle VE: Pyrrolizidine alkaloid-induced liver disease in horses: An early diagnosis. Am J Vet Res 49:572, 1988.

64. Byars TD: Chronic liver failure in horses. Compend Contin Educ Pract Vet 5:S423, 1983.

65. Durham AE, Smith KC, Newton JR: An evaluation of diagnostic data in comparison to the results of liver biopsies in mature horses. Equine Vet J 35:554, 2003.

66. Modransky PD. Ultrasound-guided renal and hepatic biopsy techniques. Vet Clin North Am Equine Pract 1986;2:115–126.

67. Reef VB, Johnston JK, Divers TJ, Acland H. Ultrasonographic findings in horses with cholelithiasis: eight cases (1985–1987). J Am Vet Med Assoc 1990;196:1836–1840.

68. Peek SF, Divers TJ: Medical treatment of cholangiohepatitis and cholelithiasis in mature horses: 9 cases (1991–1998). Equine Vet J 32:301, 2000.

69. Durham AE, Newton JR, Smith KC, et al: Retrospective analysis of historical, clinical, ultrasonographic, serum biochemical and haematological data in prognostic evaluation of equine liver disease. Equine Vet J 35:542, 2003.

70. Divers TJ, Bernard WV, Reef VB: Equine liver disease and liver failure: causes, diagnosis and treatment. Presented as the 10th Bain-Fallon Memorial Lecture, Artarmon, Australia, 1988.

71. Durham AE, Smith KC, Newton JR, et al: Development and application of a scoring system for prognostic evaluation of equine liver biopsies. Equine Vet J 35:534, 2003.

72. Divers TJ: Liver Disease and Liver Failure in Horses. St. Louis, American Association of Equine Practitioners, 1983.

73. Scarratt WK, Warnick LD: Effects of oral administration of lactulose in healthy horses. J Equine Vet Sci 18:405, 1989.

CHAPTER 21

The Equine Geriatric Foot

Donna L. Shettko

The aging horse presents a unique set of veterinary problems. Horses older than 20 years of age now account for 7.5 percent of the entire horse stock. Health maintenance, acute care, and rehabilitation of older horses generate a significant case load for the equine practitioner.[1] Horses older than 20 years are classified as geriatric horses. Yet similar to their human counterparts, geriatric patients may be healthy, energetic, and active. Owners of these horses have high expectations for the welfare of their horse. They expect their animals to age with grace, comfort, and health. Veterinarians must ensure that a realistic balance is maintained between the expectations of the owner and the capabilities of their aging horse.

The normal aging process encompasses physiologic, anatomic, metabolic, and behavioral changes in the geriatric horse. Diminished physiologic reserve, impaired healing, poor dentition, degenerative bone and joint disease, laminitis, hoof disease, and nutritional deficiencies are examples of age-specific problems having an impact on the overall health and productivity of the geriatric horse. Behavioral issues within a herd may relegate the geriatric horse to a lesser stature resulting in difficulty with access to feeding or becoming prey to aggressive younger animals. These problems may present acutely or be insidious in their onset. Some of these processes cannot be reversed but may be augmented by therapeutic maneuvers to slow down the progression of disease. Timely management of these issues may lead to a better outcome than if the problems are allowed to progress to a point where reparative care is not possible. In some instances, delay in treatment may result in a less than desirable outcome. While the focus of this chapter is on geriatric equine foot care, a discussion of interrelated physiologic systems is necessary to place this health care issue in the proper context.

Condition of the Equine Foot

The condition of the equine foot is one of the most important factors affecting the longevity of the horse. Equine foot care is part of the daily routine to prevent hoof deterioration, founder, and lameness. The musculoskeletal system is the second most common body system affected when looking at the distribution of the body systems affected in the older horse.[2] Lameness affects the forelimb more frequently than the hindlimb, with 95 percent of cases of lameness located in the forelimb. This is to be expected, as the weight distribution of the horse is 60 percent on the forelimb and 40 percent distributed to the hindlimb.[3] Anatomically, they are located at the level of the carpus or just distal to the carpus.[3] In a study by Borsnahan and Paradis (North Grafton, MA, unpublished data, March 2002), the most common problem leading to lameness was due to an isolated hoof problem. Laminitis was the leading pathologic hoof problem resulting in lameness. These problems may be due to the normal wear and tear of the hoof over time, injury, poor foot care, or normal physiologic changes occurring with aging. These changes may be due to systemic or local orthopedic events. As the equine population ages, the veterinarian must be cognizant of the age-specific problems.

Dental Health

The maintenance of healthy feet in a geriatric horse is closely related to the ability of the horse to ingest and process adequate nutrients essential for a healthy hoof. Dental health is essential to this process. Changes in dentition are natural and expected. They include missing teeth, wave mouth, hooks, and points, all of which affect the horse's ability to properly masticate.[4] When a horse presents with a history that suggests a dental problem, the age, sex, use, diet, and eating habits should be considered. Tooth loss and improper occlusion secondary to the wear and growth patterns of the hysodontal teeth affect the nutritional plane of the horse. The dental changes affect the ability to properly masticate the feed to the proper fiber length needed for optimum absorption. Poor teeth can interfere with the ingestion of any feed, particularly hay. Mastication is the first step in the digestion of nutrients present in feedstuff. Mastication increases the surface area of ingested feeds and breaking down the protective coatings present in some of the feed, allowing greater access by enzymes and other digestive secretions.[4] The age-related changes in dentition lead to a reduction in the digestion and assimilation of the important nutrients needed for hoof growth and maintenance. In comparison to younger horses, fiber digestion in geriatric horses is less.[5]

Nutrition

Good hoof quality is denoted by a dry, hard, and tough structure that is capable protecting the inner foot anatomy. This serves as a base for ambulation. Poor nutrition, faulty metabolism, and an unhealthy environment can all affect hoof quality. The problem is often due to the inability to synthesize essential nutrients. A horse's ration should provide adequate amounts of the essential amino acid DL methionine, biotin, protein, and minerals.[6] Although research is lacking regarding the nutritional requirements of the older horse, it has been suggested that geriatric horses may not have different nutritional requirements than other mature horses. On the other hand, geriatric horses have a higher incidence of underlying disease, metabolic problems, and poor dentition resulting in specialized requirements for feed and nutritional supplementation.

Good nutrition is essential during the process of epithelialization of the horn. Keratinization of these epithelial cells is necessary to promote horn quality. A better quality horn translates into a reduction of foot problems. The B vitamin biotin is required for hoof growth and quality. Biotin is essential in the metabolism of the keratinizing of the epidermal cells. It is an essential cofactor of enzymes involved in synthesis during keratinization.[7] Keratins are the structural proteins of the highly cornified epidermis of the hoof and skin, which provides for the structural basis for the horn.[8] When there is an insufficient amount of biotin, the hoof horn becomes brittle and the hooves chip. A long-term study was conducted to investigate the effects of biotin deficiency.[9] It was found that by supplementing biotin in the diet, there was an increase in the growth rate of hooves.[9] After supplementation, the tensile strength and hoof horn condition improved as determined by histologic and macroscopic examination.[9] Although the exact requirements for biotin are not known, it has been suggested that supplementation with 15 to 30 mg/day of biotin can improve hoof growth and integrity.[10] Older horses supplemented with lower doses of biotin by a factor of 10 demonstrated significantly lower hoof growth than younger horses.[9]

The "B" vitamins, including thiamine and riboflavin, are synthesized by microbes, and those occurring naturally in forages are generally thought to meet the horse's requirement for "B" vitamins. Again, in the process of keratinization the epidermal cells require a sufficient and balanced supply of nutrients, minerals, vitamins, and trace elements.[8] Zinc is a particularly important trace element required for keratinization of the epithelial cells of the horn.

Proteins are the structural component of all organ systems. A continued supply of protein is necessary to maintain a positive nitrogen balance. Thus, continual breakdown, degradation, and turnover of body protein are balanced with adequate dietary protein intake. There is a limited pool of available body stores of protein before catabolism of muscle begins.[11] This balance is exacerbated in the older horse due to a loss of protein stores from a progressive loss of muscle mass during the aging process. This is compounded by alterations in protein absorption and metabolism. Ralston et al[12] reported that the apparent digestibility or crude protein in geriatric horses, older than 20 years of age was less than that of younger horses 2 to 3 years of age. The quality of protein or the amino acid composition in the feed can influence the total amount of protein that is required to maintain muscle mass.[11] Higher quality sources of dietary protein may be required in smaller amounts due to their superior amino acid profiles.[11] This is important to a geriatric horse who has limited ability to consume feed due to poor dentition or difficulty with mastication.

Laminitis

Laminitis is a devastating disease for an animal of any age. The frequency of chronic laminitis seems to be more prevalent in geriatric horses. Presentation of laminitis can be associated with an acute presentation or multiple mild episodes of acute and subacute laminitis culminating in chronic laminitis. Significant physiologic and pathologic alterations occur in chronic laminitis. Why chronic laminitis is more prevalent in geriatric horses is not known, but poor hoof quality, reduced keratin synthesis, improper nutrition, comorbid disease, environmental factors, or lack of appropriate hoof maintenance are contributing factors. A common systemic disease that is associated with increasing age is dysfunction of the pars intermedia of the pituitary gland. In one study, the median age of horses suspected of having pituitary pars intermedia dysfunction (PPID) was 15.5 years and the median age of horse without PPID was 14.5 years.[13] The increased prevalence of laminitis in the older horse and its association with PPID has put the older horse at a higher risk.[14] Horses with laminitis may have PPID without clinical signs commonly associated with the disease. This atypical presentation may delay the diagnosis and subsequent treatment for the underlying cause for the repeated bouts of laminitis but PPID should be investigated in the older horse.

Familiarity with the anatomy and physiology of the horse's foot is important to understand the biomechanics involved in the development of laminitis and subsequent treatment. The predominant forces imposed on the foot include the laminar bond between the coffin bone and hoof wall, consisting of the dermal and epidermal interface of primary and secondary lamina.[15] These forces are opposed by the pivotal downward vertical load off the bony column supporting the weight of the horse and the proximal palmar or plantar tension provided by the deep digital flexor tendon.[15] The normal load imposed on the damaged and weakened laminae amplifies the dynamic motion of the coffin bone within the hoof capsule, resulting in the pulling and shearing at the laminar surface.[15] Mechanical rotational and vertical displacement of the distal phalanx results in abnormal forces being imposed on the hoof wall, coronary band, and subsolar soft tissues. These forces act to disrupt the damaged blood supply and inhibit the ability of the hoof wall to move downward at a normal rate during the growth process.[15] The eventual outcome is altered keratin synthesis and hoof production, abnormal protection of the underlying structures within the foot, and varying degrees of pathologic changes of the coffin bone.[15]

The basic principles of trimming or shoeing horses with laminitis are geared toward stabilizing the coffin bone within the hoof by decreasing the forces acting to create the third phalanx rotation. How to technically achieve these goals varies. Proper or corrective shoeing will diminish pain while returning the foot to its normal conformation and function. Shoeing techniques that stabilize the movements on the distal phalanx and hoof wall are important in allowing proper healing of the laminae and solar interface. Trimming and shoeing the foot in a way that re-establishes or promotes more normal mechanics reduces the pain. In horses with chronic stable laminitis, protection and support of the sole are important to reduce the bruising. If the pedal bone has rotated then trimming is directed at restoring the pedal bone–ground relationship. The principle is to provide uniform support and enhance stability by counteracting rotation or distal displacement of the distal phalanx. Most shoeing techniques are aimed at reducing the tension on the deep digital flexor tendon, redistributing the load on the foot, or facilitating breakover. These measures reduce the shearing of the laminae at the palmar phase of the stride. The optimal approach to managing these horses is to look at each horse as an individual using different shoeing and trimming techniques. The therapeutic approach does not lie in the shoeing method but rather in the underlying principles and attaining the technical goals.

The primary goals of treatment regimens for acute laminitis are to reduce the pain or hypertension cycle, to reduce or prevent permanent laminar damage, to improve dermal laminae capillary hemodynamics, and to prevent movement of the distal phalanx.

Laminitis often causes a widening between the dermal-epidermal junction due to a redundant dorsal hoof wall known as white line disease or "seedy toe." When this area of separation occurs in the hoof wall, it provides a moist, dark environment ideal for the growth of bacteria. Soil and manure are forced up into the interlaminar space, allowing for the invasion of the inner horn by bacteria, fungus, or yeast, resulting in some degree of damage to the structural integrity of the hoof. Treatment is targeted at débriding the decomposed horn and packing the hole. The redundant wall should be removed to the level of the undermined white line to allow regrowth of the healthy wall. A shoe is applied to protect the packing and to prevent further contamination.

Degenerative Joint Disease

Degenerative joint disease (DJD) is seen in the geriatric horse as well as in competitive horses. One type of DJD affects the high load–low motion joints such as the interphalangeal and intertarsal joints.[6] DJD of the interphalangeal and distal intertarsal and tarsometatarsal joints are characterized by periosteal proliferation. Pathologic lesions noted are usually severe and include wide erosions, subchondral bone sclerosis, eburnation, and marginal osteophytes as well as periosteal exostoses.[6] Another type of DJD is comparable to the degenerative changes observed with age in human joints.[6] This type includes a series of articular cartilage changes found during routine necropsies but are of questionable clinical significance.[6] The changes in the articular cartilage seen with this type of DJD group include blisters, wear lines, ulcerations, and superficial erosions.[6]

Owners of geriatric horses should be prepared to provide preventive maintenance and nutritional additives to their animals. Therapeutic modalities for DJD range from chondroprotective agents, anti-inflammatory agents, and shoeing. It is important to keep in mind that the ultimate goal is to keep the horse comfortable and able to work. Initially, an adequate rest period is recommended, followed by a controlled exercise regimen. The exercise program may need to be stopped for an extended period of time. Anti-inflammatories are administered with care but are used to maintain an adequate level of comfort.

Going without shoes is often a choice that owners make to find an economical solution and a medical solution for the shoeing problems seen in the older horse. It is important to remember that shoes act as shock absorbers, which reduce impact and pain.[16] Pads may provide additional benefit in horses with joint pain. The shoeing plan for DJD should including trimming and balancing the hoof and applying shoes that enhance breakover and provide good lateral and medial support. Easing breakover with short hoof length, squared off toes, or rocker-toed shoes may help horses with osteoarthritis. Horses with hind-end problems do better without calks, stickers, or trailers, which can cause torque. Consideration of the frequency of trimming should be made. With the alterations in hoof growth, the frequency of trimming needs to be determined on an individual basis. Overall, more frequent trimming intervals of approximately 4 to 6 weeks is beneficial to maintain the short foot length.

Phalangeal Exostosis (Ringbone)

Phalangeal exostosis, or more commonly called *ringbone*, describes a condition in which new bone of periosteal origin forms, usually on the dorsal, dorsolateral, and dorsomedial aspects of the first and second phalanx and the extensor process of the third phalanx. This condition occurs in both fore and hind limbs with or without proximal interphalangeal and distal interphalangeal joint arthritis. Treatment targeted for early cases is aimed at reducing the inciting cause. In the geriatric horse, the lesion may be long standing. Measures to keep the horse comfortable are the optimal goal. Therapeutics include anti-inflammatories, shoeing, and neurectomy. Shoeing considerations include maintaining balance and easing breakover.

Tendons and Ligaments

Tendon and ligaments also undergo age-related changes. The suspensory ligament along with the superficial digital flexor tendon acts to stabilize the fetlock joint.

The suspensory ligament is one that often fails, resulting in overextension of the fetlock joint and causing the palmar or plantar surface to touch the ground. This problem is usually treated by shoeing modalities. Changing the hoof angle to prevent or treat tendinous injures should be undertaken with care because reduced strain in one tendinous structure may be associated with an increased strain in another. A high hoof angle reduces the tension of the fetlock joint during the stance phase. This reduces the moment arm of the ground reaction force, resulting in lower overall tension in the palmar soft tissues. A low hoof angle predisposes the horse to injury of the distal check ligament by increasing the tension of the fetlock and the distal interphalangeal joints in the later part of the stance phase. The risk of injury to the superficial digital flexor tendon and the suspensory ligament may be somewhat greater with raised heels. The egg bar shoe is a good alterative for treatment of suspensory failure. The egg bar shoe repositions the center of weight-bearing forward.[7] This puts more of the main load back toward the center of the hoof, so that the forces may be more evenly distributed around the hoof capsule. This holds the toe down and keeps the extensor branches of the suspensory ligament tight.[6] Thus, the egg bar shoe helps to support the fetlock in dorsiflexion.[7] And if those interventions are not successful in correcting the problem, surgical options are available.

Caudal Heel Syndrome

Caudal heel syndrome is responsible for an estimated one third of all chronic forelimb lameness in horses.[6] Given the prevalence of this syndrome in the equine population and the emerging elderly population, this syndrome will have to be managed. The cause of navicular syndrome is multifactorial and is often found in association with degenerative disease of the metacarpophalangeal and interphalangeal joints. A broken hoof pastern axis, upright pasterns, and contracted heels have all been implicated in the development of navicular disease. There are three main categories of treatment: reduction or abolition of pain, drugs that affect the blood supply to the navicular bone, and hoof trimming and corrective shoeing. The aim of trimming and shoeing is to restore normal hoof balance, correct hoof problems, and reduce biomechanical forces on the navicular region.[6] Corrective trimming should be aimed at achieving an unbroken hoof pastern axis with neither heels nor toes being too long. The hoof should be trimmed to achieve a normal hoof pastern axis. If the hoof cannot be trimmed to this alignment, special shoes or pads should be applied. Rolling, forcing, or squaring the toe of the shoe and setting it slightly back on the foot enhances breakover, reducing the stress on the deep digital flexor tendon.

As more aging horses remain active, problems specific to this age group of animals becomes evident. Geriatric horses have a higher burden of foot problems. Comorbid disease, degenerative changes, and nutritional factors all contribute to this problem. Recognition of this problem and acquisition of knowledge and clinical skills to address these problems should be in every equine practitioner's armamentarium. Knowledge and insight into the potential problems and the appropriate therapeutic intervention may help to prevent many of these serious and debilitating conditions. Periodic lower extremity evaluations and appropriate therapeutic intervention may help to prevent many of the debilitating conditions and injuries. An important aspect to the treatment plan for the older horse may include this periodic examination.

REFERENCES

1. Williams N: Disease conditions in geriatric horses. Equine Pract 22:320, 2000.
2. USDA/APHIS: Part I: Baseline Reference of 1998 Equine Health And Management. Fort Collins, CO, National Animal Health Monitoring System, 1998.
3. Ross MW, Dyson SJ: Lameness in Horses: Basic Facts before Starting in Diagnosis and Management of Lameness in the Horse. Philadelphia, W.B. Saunders, 2003.
4. Graham BP: Dental care in the older horse. Vet Clin Equine 18:509, 2002.
5. Ralston SL, Nockels CF, Squires EL: Field evaluation of feed formulated for geriatric horses. J Equine Vet Sci 16:334, 1996.
6. Stashak TS: Trimming and shoeing for balance and soundness. In Adams' Lameness in Horses. Philadelphia, Lippincott Williams & Wilkins, 2002.
7. Mulling CK, Bragulla HH, Reese S, et al: How structures in bovine hoof epidermis are influenced y nutritional factors. Anat Histol Embryol 28:103, 1999.
8. Tomlinson DJ, Mulling CH, Fakler TM: Invited review; formation of keratins in the bovine claw: Roles to hormone, minerals and vitamins in functional claw integrity. J Dairy Sci 87:797, 2004.
9. Geyer H, Schulze J: The long term influence of biotin supplementation on hoof horn quality in horses. Schweiz Arch Tierheilkd 136:137, 1994.
10. Reilly JD, Cottrel DF, Main FJ, et al: Effect of supplementary dietary biotin on hoof growth and hoof growth rate in ponies: A controlled trial. Equine Vet J Suppl 26:51, 1998.
11. Frape D: Nonprotein nitrogen. In Equine Nutrition and Feeding, 2nd ed. Malden, MA, Blackwell Science, 1998, pp 38–39.
12. Ralston SL, Squires EL, Nockels CF: Digestion in the aged horse. Equine Vet Sci 9:203, 1989.
13. Donaldson MT, Jorgensen AJ, Beech J: Evaluation of suspected pituitary pars intermedia dysfunction I horses with laminitis. J Vet Med Assoc 224:1123, 2004.
14. Alford P: A multicenter, matched case control study of risk factors for equine laminitis. Prevent Vet Med 49:209, 2001.
15. Hunt RJ: Laminitis in the geriatric horse. Vet Clin North Am Equine Pract 18:439, 2002.
16. Felson DT, Lawrence RC, Hechberg MC, et al. Osteoarthritis: New insights. Part 2: Treatment approach. Ann Intern Med 133:726, 2000.

CHAPTER 22

Neurologic Disease in Geriatric Horses

Joseph J. Bertone

Neurologic disease in geriatric horses occurs for many of the reasons it occurs in younger animals. Some notable exceptions are discussed below. As occurs with almost all diseases, the longer an animal is alive, the more likely it is to have a pathologic condition. The exceptions are often developmental disorders, but even those disorders (e.g., cervical facet osteochondrosis) may not manifest until horses are much older. The predicament in old horse neurology is the interpretation of the findings in the "standard" neurologic examination. The boundaries of normal for many of the neurologic examination tests on younger horses need to be broadened for older horses. In some cases, "normal" for an older horse may be considered "abnormal" for younger animals. In older horses, there are neurologic signs of aging that are at least clinically apparent in horses and well documented in human patients. These include changes in mental status, reflexes, equilibrium, and strength.[1] Most veterinarians would probably agree that these functions are affected in older horses as well.

Severe neurologic signs are as evident in older horses as they are in younger horses. However, it is the author's opinion that subtle, and not so subtle, neurologic signs that are common in older horses and likely associated with aging have been ascribed as disease abnormalities. The findings have driven diagnostics (e.g., the cerebral spinal fluid centesis), and the tests have produced false-positive results (e.g., Western blot for equine protozoal myeloencephalitis). The horses then were managed with medication (e.g., anti-protozal drugs) or euthanized. Unfortunately, it can be assumed that some fraction of these horses had age-associated reduced neuromuscular function or had osteoarthritis, but were ascribed neurologic deficits and were simply old. As a general rule, a lackadaisical response to any pushing, pulling, prodding, or other stimuli is the norm for geriatric horses. Below are some specific issues that the author has found particularly problematic.

Mental Status

Most horses seem quieter with age. There are exceptions. However, in general they seem quieter and less excitable and have reduced attention capacity and environmental acuity. This is seen in most human patients as well.[1]

Reflexes in General

Most reflexes in geriatric horses are slowed, as occurs in human patients, and these may not all slow simultaneously. So a sluggish papillary light reflex, a subdued menace or cutaneous reflex, as long as the finding is bilateral, should not be considered an issue but should be noted (Fig. 22-1). Most of these changes occur in geriatric patients in association with neuraxonal degeneration, accumulation of degenerative axonal bodies, and reduced axonal nutrient flow.[1]

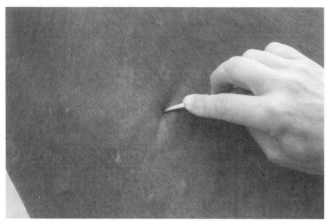

Figure 22-1 Testing the cutaneous reflex on the neck of a horse.

Musculoskeletal System Function, Aging, and the Neurologic Examination

There is a clear decline in motor function with age. This function can be maintained[2] with exercise in human patients, and it is safe to assume in horses as well. In many cases, however, aged horses are relegated to a sedentary pasture life and little is done concerning physical condition. In many cases, not only is function impaired, but there is a loss of total muscle mass even in the face of proper nutrition. In addition, there is an increase in joint pathology seen with age. This will affect strength and possibly create an appearance of weakness in geriatric horses.

Rhythmic Versus Arrhythmic Gaits

An important rule of thumb to keep in mind when performing a gait analysis during the neurologic examination is that when neurologic deficits exist alone, the gait is likely to be *arrhythmic*. If there is musculoskeletal disease alone, then the gait is likely to be *rhythmic*. When both conditions exist, then the degree of rhythmicity is determined by the two deficits' relative severity to each other. Hence, a moderate lameness will add rhythmicity to a gait abnormality when the neurologic deficit is milder and vice versa. Also realize that pain can increase sensory input to cortical centers and improve compensatory abilities in neurologic deficits. This seems to be the theory behind why, in animals with mixed disease after a course of nonsteroidal anti-inflammatory drugs (NSAIDs), many times the neurologic deficit is more pronounced.[3,4] In general, mixed system gait abnormalities tend to be rhythmic but unusual, and the gait arrhythmia is enhanced by a course of NSAID therapy, as long as the lameness is mild. So when in doubt, apply NSAIDs for a few days, and then take the horse for a walk on pavement and listen to and observe the gait. In the author's experience, this rule holds true for aged horses as well.

Age Effects on Tests of Neurologic Integrity

When performing a neurologic examination, one must identify changes that are considered abnormal for the animal at hand. For a test result to be abnormal, the findings have to be outside of what one can assume are within normal limits. However, it is clear that the "normal limits" of a neurologic examination are affected by age[1] and conditioning[5] (hence, use) and, in the authors experience, breed and use of the horse. Pain may improve the findings in a neurologic examination, but with chronic pain, deficits in muscular function can occur as well and appear as weakness.[6]

Circling

Circling is a favorite manipulation for neurologic examination (Fig. 22-2). Unfortunately, in some cases, the examination stops here. Unfortunately, "abnormal findings" associated with this test seem to often bias the further evaluation of the patient. This author recommends that this test be performed after the entire examination is complete, because of its impact on the subjectivity of the neurologic examination. The manipulation involves tight circling of the horse with observation for planting of the medial limb and circumduction of the outer limb.[7] Circumduction is an extended time and lateral excursion of the outer limb arc with hypermetric abduction. This leads to a wide outward and upward arc and delayed landing of the limb. This abnormality is often identified as a general proprioceptive dysfunction.[4] However, the spastic phase of this gait abnormality is reminiscent of an upper motor neuron hyper-reflexia. Also, since this is most often an indicator of a spinal cord

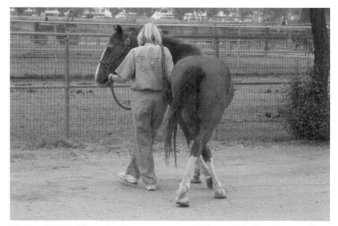

Figure 22-2 The circling maneuver showing the normal medial neck arch.

deficit, and since general proprioceptive and upper motor neuron tracts course so tightly together,[4] it is likely that circumduction associated with spinal cord disease is influenced by upper motor neuron deficits as well. Clearly, this may not be the case with cerebral, cerebellar, or other higher center disease. Many horses have been identified as neurologically dysfunctional based on this response alone. Horses with subtle pelvic limb pain (especially the tarsal and femorotibial joints) do circumduct the affected limb and pivot on the normal limb, albeit in a less exaggerated and more rhythmic and consistent fashion than horses with moderate to severe neurologic deficits. This response apparently protects the abnormal outer limb from flexion (the arc is needed to move an unflexed limb) and from weight bearing (remaining on the nonpainful limb as long as possible). One thing to keep in mind when evaluating this test is whether the horse tilts its trunk to the center of the circle to move the limb (as can be seen with lameness) or whether the horse drops the hip with this procedure (as can be seen with neurologic disease). Again, observation will identify that this response, when associated with the musculoskeletal system, is consistent and rhythmic in the lame horse and inconsistent and arrhythmic in the neurologically impaired horse.

Neck Pain Effects on Circling: "In older horses, musculoskeletal (non-neurologic) circumduction is easily explainable. Old horses are likely to have arthritic pelvic limb changes. However, one must consider that cervical neck pain can also generate non-neurologic circumduction. When a normal horse is turned in a tight circle, the horse will arc its neck to the inside of the circle (Fig. 22-2). If a horse has cervical or thoracic pain and refuses to arc its neck, the horse will demonstrate non-neurologic circumduction. The theory that may explain this phenomenon is that when a quadruped circles tightly, the head and neck moves medially to facilitate the unweighting of the outer leg. The unweighting occurs because the center of gravity moves medially when the head and neck are bent medially. The author has tested this theory using a force-sensitive array floor mat. If the head and neck do not turn medially, the horse does not unweight the outer limb in rapid fashion and the outer foot stays on the ground for a protracted time. Hence, the forward phase of the outer limb is longer because there is a longer time in its initiation and the outward arc is wider to avoid striking the medial limb. This can be evident with any form of cervical issues that reduce the horse's ability to bend medially. Pain in the neck must be evaluated in old horses (Fig. 22-3).

The Sway Test

The sway reaction assessment is performed by having another person walk the horse while the tail is pulled with some force (Fig. 22-4A). An acceptable response is

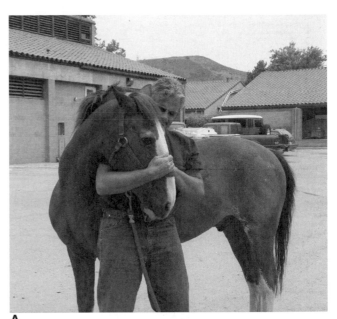

A

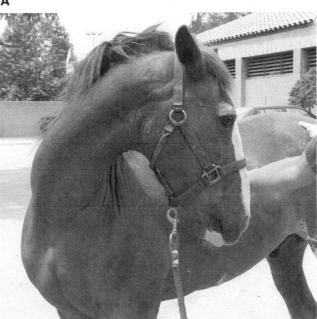

B

Figure 22-3 A, B, Flexion of the neck to assess neck pain.

resistance away from the tail pull. This test can also be performed by pushing at the hip as the horse walks and observing for pressure exerted toward you.[8] However, for safety reasons, this author does not recommend this part of the procedure. This author feels that with a tail pull, an acceptable response is a medial rotation of the hock on the side being pulled and subsequent extension of that limb. This test and the subsequent reaction are measures of upper motor neuron, lower motor neuron, and proprioceptive function. Weakness (upper and lower motor neurons), overabduction, and crossing of the limbs are (non–stand-alone) evidence of a general proprioceptive deficits. Many older horses with no apparent neurologic disease will demonstrate all of these signs with no (other

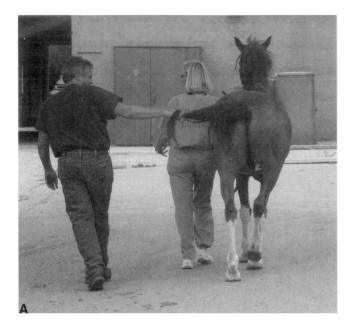

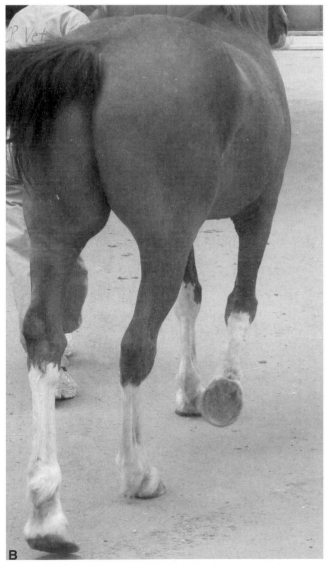

Figure 22-4 A, The sway test. B, Note the outward rotation of the left hind limb.

than age-related) abnormalities (Fig. 22-4,B). Geriatric horses tend to give easier to the force and may completely rotate their hock to nearly the point of collapse. With some excitement, or when the horse is put into a fitness regimen, these signs may disappear in many older horses.

Hopping

Hopping a horse can be done by lifting a front limb and placing force against the shoulder (Fig. 22-5). One does not have to actually make the horse hop to achieve an examination with this test. The younger normal horse will apply resistant force against you almost as soon as you apply pressure to the shoulder. The test is then complete and deemed a normal reaction. Many older horses will allow you to apply pressure until the foot on the ground breaks a plane less than or equal to the sternal midline before resistance is initiated. The normal horse will apply pressure directly and linearly against you. Horses with suspect abnormalities will allow you to push them beyond the sternum. This is evidence of a general proprioceptive deficit. Horses with chronic cervical vertebral malformation stenosis and myelopathy will give to the opposite side. Horses with acute cervical vertebral malformation are more hyper-reflexic and spastic and will push spastically against you. However, the force will be generated in a 45-degree or so angle and backward to your force with collapse of the rear limbs. Given a short period of time, a few weeks at best, this will dissipate and become a more flaccid and weak response in association with upper and motor neuron compensation. It is common to see a more flaccid and weak response in older horses with no other neurologic deficit.

Positional Tests: Positional tests include front and hind limb crossing and extension away from the body (Fig. 22-6). Older horses are more compliant to these

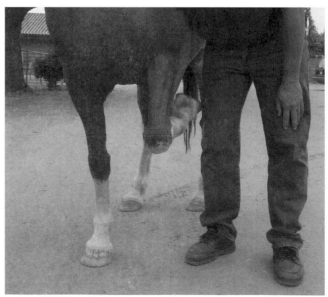

Figure 22-5 The hopping maneuver.

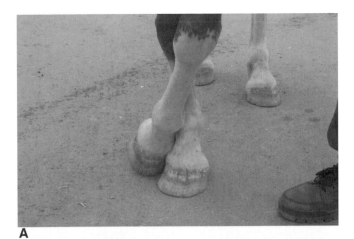

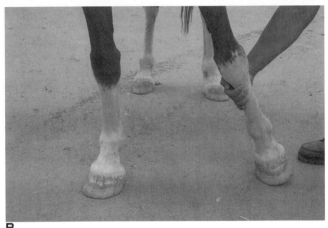

Figure 22-6 A, Front limb positioning, crossing stance. B, Front limb positioning, widening the stance.

tests. The horse in Fig. 22-6 stayed this way for 4 minutes. This horse had no neurological deficits.

Cervical Facet Disease

Cervical facet disease, osteoarthritis, and degenerative changes can affect the neurologic examination, as indicated above. Many of these horses can be managed with NSAID therapy and or intra-articular vertebral facet injection of steroidal medications.

Cervical Pain and Arthritic Disease

As was stated earlier, false circumduction can be evident with any form of cervical disease that reduces a horse's ability to bend medially. Figure 22-7 shows radiographs from a 23-year-old stallion that was unable to rise without help. A cursory (circling) neurologic examination deemed that the horse was significantly neurologically impaired. However, a more careful examination revealed that true neurologic deficits were not evident. In the image, there is severe ventral bridging spondylosis. No histologic findings were evident on spinal cord examination at necropsy. In another case, one can see radiographic (Fig. 22-8, A) and gross

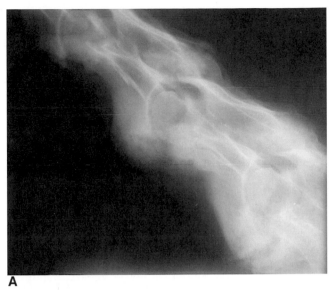

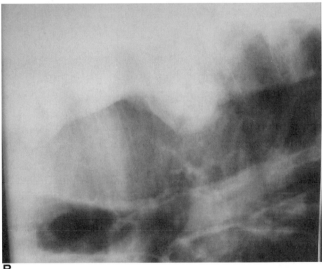

Figure 22-7 *A, B,* Radiographs demonstrating severe cervical vertebral bridging spondylosis in an aged stallion.

pathologic (Fig. 22-8, B) evidence of extensive articular facet disease. This horse was also deemed as having a severe neurologic deficit. On careful examination, no neurologic deficit was evident, and the horse was maintained for pleasure riding with regularly scheduled intra-articular facet injections of steroidal anti-inflammatory drugs over the course of 3 years (Fig. 22-9).[9] One can observe the disappearance of this form of false circumduction when arthritic facet disease is managed using intra-articular cervical facet anti-inflammatory injection. Although these cases represent more severe forms of cervical osteoarthritis, it is almost a given that when old horse cervical vertebrae are evaluated, some form of degenerative disease is evident (Fig. 22-10).

Primary Hypersomnia

Horses need a period of recumbent sleep, which can be avoided for several days, but eventually must be taken.[10]

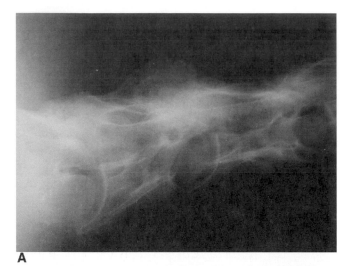

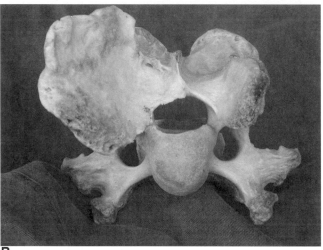

Figure 22-8 A, Radiograph of severe cervical facet disease in an aged gelding. B, Severe cervical facet disease in an aged gelding.

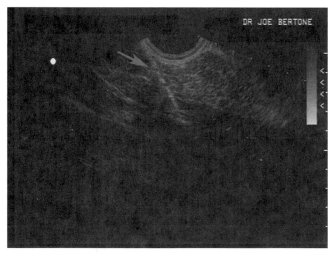

Figure 22-9 An ultrasonographic image demonstrating the needle (arrow) being guided toward the cervical facet.

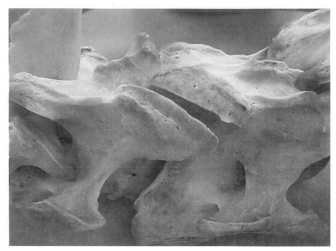

Figure 22-10 A cervical vertebra with capsular calcification evident at the cervical facet.

Horses transition from slow wave sleep (stay apparatus dependent) with marginally opened lids but fixed eyes to paradoxical sleep (loss of muscular function) when they become recumbent.[10] Paradoxical sleep must occur periodically. A period of recumbency is essential for horses to have a normal sleep pattern. Primary hypersomnia is the state whereby sleepiness occurs with no central nervous system defect, either physiologic or psychological, and is likely what is seen in most horses that simply fall asleep and nearly collapse at the wrong time (Fig. 22-11). Often, these horses can be identified by scuff marks and calluses that have formed over the dorsal surface of the fetlock. This behavioral abnormality can be divided into three categories.

Pain-Associated Primary Hypersomnia

In this condition, horses do not lie down because it is painful to do so. Most often, these horses have musculoskeletal issues that create pain on attempting to

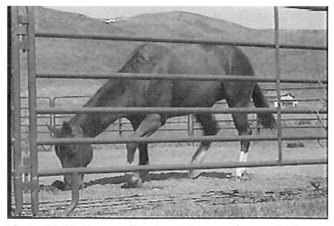

Figure 22-11 Horse collapsing to its nose in association with behavioral primary hypersomnia.

become recumbent or trying to rise. In addition, horses have episodes of primary hypersomnia in association with thoracic or abdominal pain that is elicited with recumbency or on attempting to stand (Fig. 22-12).

Environmental Insecurity–Associated Primary Hypersomnia

Horses do not lie down unless they are comfortable doing so.[10] One can assume that this stems from prey and herd behavior. Horses that are alone or are in an aggressive environment will often not lie down and have been seen to develop hypersomnia. The author has treated several horses with this syndrome by adding a friend to the pasture or stall or by moving the horse to an area where there are more horses. This would probably include horses in an insecure environment that may just require a larger stall or paddock and those horses near loud harassing noise, such as fireworks or speedways.

Monotony-Induced Hypersomnia

This is best represented, theoretically, by the horse in crossties being braided that almost collapses because it nearly goes into paradoxical sleep. This may also be seen more commonly at the odd hours owners tend to braid the horse. The horse is often very comfortable in its environment.

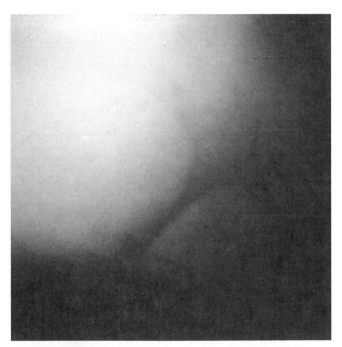

Figure 22-12 Enterolithiasis in a horse with painful primary hypersomnia. An exploratory laparotomy identified extensive adhesions of the large colon to the diaphragm. A few days after recovery from an exploratory laparotomy in which the enteroliths were removed and the adhesions reduced, the horse became recumbent for almost 24 hours. The hypersomnia resolved.

Narcolepsy

One has to clear the air on this issue concerning other sleep disorders. Narcolepsy is associated with excessive sleepiness under conditions of monotonous sedentary activity but also when patients are fully engaged in a task. Cataplexy is an abrupt and reversible decrease in or loss of muscle tone. Both are frequently elicited by emotions such as laughter, excitement, anger, or surprise.[11] The narcolepsy–cataplexy syndrome does occur in horses. However it is rare and breed associated.[12] Horses should not be ascribed as having narcolepsy-cataplexy unless they meet the criteria of the clinical syndrome as listed above. Labeling horses as narcoleptics leads one to look at pathophysiologic mechanisms and therapies that have little to do with the more prevalent condition of *primary hypersomnia* in horses. Others would call the typical clinical syndrome *hypersomnia*. However, in human medicine that name is linked to a specific syndrome associated with excessive sleepiness, associated with some central nervous system disorder.[13] That syndrome also does not explain the vast majority of horses that simply have inappropriate sleepiness.

More appropriately and simply, most horses that fall asleep at the wrong times can be categorized as having *primary hypersomnia*. Hypersomnolence defined as excessive daytime sleepiness seems to be a far more typical syndrome in horses. A review of the authors' cases also indicates that it is more likely to occur in horses older than 15 years of age.

Other Diseases

The risk of equine motor neuron disease increases with age and peaks at 15 years old.[14] In addition, vaccine breaks in West Nile virus and other encephalitides increase in the very young and older horses (information also within this book).

REFERENCES

1. Assal F, Cummings JL: Neurological signs in old age. In Tallis RC, Fillit HM, editors: Brocklehurst's Textbook of Geriatric Medicine and Gerontology, 6th ed. London, Churchill Livingstone, 2003, pp 541–548.
2. Evans W: Exercise for successful aging. In Tallis RC, Fillit HM, eds: Brocklehurst's Textbook of Geriatric Medicine and Gerontology, 6th ed. London, Churchill Livingstone, 2003, pp 855–861.
3. Capra NF, Ro JY: Human and animal experimental models of acute and chronic muscle pain: Intramuscular algesic injection. Pain 110:3, 2004.
4. Svara CJ, Hadler NM: Back pain. Clin Geriatr Med 4:395, 1988.
5. Camicioli R, Nutt JG: Gait and balance. In Goetz C, editor: Textbook of Clinical Neurology, 2nd ed. St Louis, WB Saunders, 2003, pp 317–369.
6. Verbunt JA, Seelen HA, Vlaeyen JW, et al: Pain-related factors contributing to muscle inhibition in patients with chronic low back pain: an experimental investigation based on superimposed electrical stimulation. Clin J Pain 21:232, 2005.
7. Delahunta A: Large animal spinal cord disease. In Veterinary Neuroanatomy and Clinical Neurology. St Louis, WB Saunders, 1983, p 216.

8. Reed SM, Andrews FM: Neurologic examination. In Reed SM, Bayly WM, Sellon DC, eds: Equine Internal Medicine. St. Louis, WB Saunders, 2004, pp 533–541.

9. Nielsen JV, Berg LC, Thoefnert MB, Thomsen PD: Accuracy of ultrasound-guided intra-articular injection of cervical facet joints in horses: a cadaveric study. Equine Vet J 35:657, 2003.

10. Dallaire A: Rest behavior. Vet Clin North Am Equine Pract 2:591, 1986.

11. Guilleminault CG, Anagnos A: Narcolepsy. In Kryger MH, Roth T, Dement WC, eds: Principles and Practice of Sleep Medicine, 3rd ed. St. Louis, WB Saunders, 2000, pp 676–686.

12. Andrews FM, Mathews HK: Seizures, narcolepsy and cataplexy. In Reed SM, Bayly WM, Sellon DC, eds: Equine Internal Medicine. St. Louis, WB Saunders, 2004, pp 560–566.

13. Guilleminault CG, Pelayo R: Idiopathic central nervous system hypersomnia. In Kryger MH, Roth T, Dement WC, eds: Principles and Practice of Sleep Medicine, 3rd ed. St Louis, WB Saunders, 2000, pp 687–692.

14. Nout Y: Equine motor neuron disease. In Reed SM, Bayly WM, Sellon DC, eds: Equine Internal Medicine. St. Louis, WB Saunders, 2004, pp 646–650.

CHAPTER 23

Euthanasia and Grief Support in an Equine Bond-Centered Practice

Carolyn Butler,

Laurel Lagoni

Advances in veterinary medicine make it possible for many horses to live well into old age. As horses age, it is not unusual for owners to invest significant amounts of time, energy, and money in their horses' health care. During this process, owners also invest significant amounts of emotional trust in their veterinarians. When a horse dies, owners do not want their trust betrayed. They want and deserve reassuring words and demonstrations of support in acknowledgement of their horse's death.

Extending veterinary services beyond the medical treatment of animals to also include the emotional support of clients is the hallmark characteristic of a Bond-Centered Practice. The Bond-Centered Practice approach to veterinary care is based on the belief that providing emotional support for people is as much a priority as providing high quality medical treatment for animals. A Bond-Centered Practice is defined as one that supports and responds to the emotions created by the human-animal bond.[1] The Bond-Centered approach is most effectively used in equine medicine when veterinary teams are dealing with the death or euthanasia of a beloved horse.

Many people view their horses as companion animals. This usually means a horse is thought of as a source of emotional and social support and often viewed as a best friend or even a family member (Fig. 23-1). Horses in this category are likely to elicit strong feelings of attachment from their owners, especially geriatric horses who have lived with the same family for many, many years.

Yet, according to researchers at the University of California-Davis, veterinarians characteristically underestimate the importance of their clients' attachments to their animals.[2] If equine veterinarians trivialize the human-animal bond, they can damage relationships between them and their clients. This is especially true when clients experience the deaths of their horses.

Death is an inevitable part of horse ownership. Patient death is also an inevitable part of veterinary medicine. Due, for the most part, to the option of euthanasia, it is estimated that veterinarians experience the deaths of their patients five times more often than their counterparts in human medicine.[3] Therefore, death and euthanasia are issues of central importance to the field of equine medicine.

This chapter does not concern itself so much with the medical aspects of equine euthanasia. Rather, its focus is on how to make the emotional side of the experience more positive, especially when owners want to be present during their horse's euthanasia.

Horse Owners

Horses may be used for ranch work or ridden for competition, therapy, or pleasure. Some owners' livelihoods are dependent on their horses. When people and horses spend time together on a daily basis, there is no doubt that special bonds develop between them.

One survey revealed that most horse-owning households tended to be families with children who were

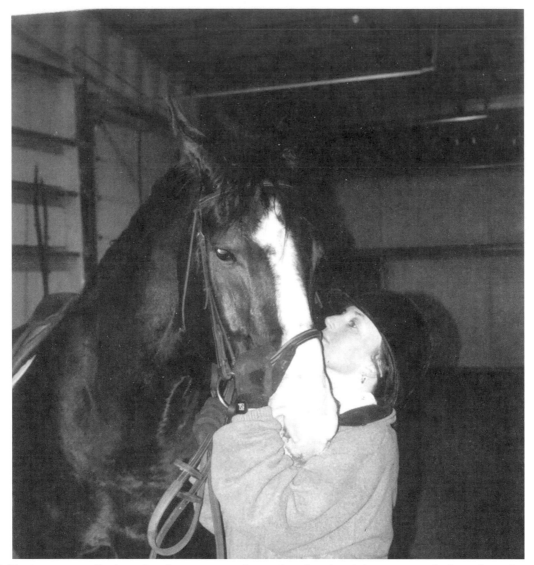

Figure 23-1 Horses are usually thought of as a source of emotional and social support and often viewed as a best friend or even a family member.

more likely to live in rural areas or small towns.[4] In a high percentage of these horse-owning households, a female between the ages of 31 and 50 took care of the horses' daily needs and decided whether or not the animals needed veterinary care. Specifically, 68 percent of women compared to 32 percent of men were the primary caretakers of their horses' needs, and 69 percent of women compared to 31 percent of men decided if their jointly owned animals needed veterinary care.

Many equine veterinarians deal primarily with female clients. In studies, girls and women have reported stronger emotional relationships with their companion animals.[5] Girls and women are socialized to attend to and express emotions more than men. They also expect others to attend to their emotions. It can be expected, then, that female horse owners will

often react differently to the deaths of their animals than male owners. As one long-time equine veterinarian said,

> "Most of my clients are women. I work with show horses a lot. Men are quicker to go with euthanasia. Women are slower to accept [euthanasia] and are quicker to cry."[6]

Another said,

> "Women need to say good-bye. They are generally responsive to a hug or kind words about how special their horse was, an acknowledgement of how well she cared for the horse, or reassurance that she has made the right decision to help the animal die. Most go around the corner of the building while the injection is given and then come back to spend time with the horse once it is down."[6]

Regardless of gender, the majority of horse owners appreciate it when veterinarians extend a caring attitude along with their medical expertise. When veterinarians strive to lend clients their emotional support, they help to relax the societal restrictions about what is acceptable when grieving the deaths of horses and other companion animals (Fig. 23-2).

Euthanasia

Perhaps no other medical procedure has as great an impact on veterinarians, the veterinary team, and the quality of the veterinarian-client relationship as the procedure of euthanasia. When euthanasia is performed well, it can soothe and reassure all involved that the decision to end a horse's life was the right one. However, when euthanasia is done poorly or without sensitivity and skilled technique, it can deepen, complicate, and prolong grief for everyone. Equine veterinarians who wish to perform euthanasia well should keep several techniques regarding grief support in mind. These techniques can be grouped into three categories: pre-euthanasia preparation, client-present facilitation methods, and post-death follow-up care.

Pre-Euthanasia Preparation

In equine medicine, client presence at euthanasia has traditionally been discouraged. However, contemporary equine medicine is beginning to see euthanasia in a new light. Today, many equine veterinarians recognize that, when euthanasia is performed humanely and with the clients' emotional needs in mind, the presence of the client can be a powerful practice-builder and a potent grief intervention tool.

In the old model of equine euthanasia, the standard operating procedure was to talk about the process as little as possible, involve clients as little as possible, and get the deed over with as quickly as possible. Euthanasia was often referred to only indirectly or euphemistically and clients were encouraged to simply "walk away" from their animals so they would not be burdened by the details of their horse's deaths. It was believed that this impersonal, clinical approach to euthanasia helped protect both clients and veterinarians from dealing with emotions, thus making the process as painless as possible for all involved.

This paradigm probably worked for some, but for others it created different kinds of emotional pain. For many clients and veterinarians alike, it created feelings of guilt, shame, depression, and unresolved grief. The old model of euthanasia was particularly hard on veterinarians because it placed the bulk of the emotional burden on their shoulders. Veterinarians were usually the ones to decide when, why, how, and where animals should die. In addition, veterinarians usually refrained from formally acknowledging their patients' deaths and from contacting their clients afterwards. The old model forced everyone to grieve in isolation and, in general, did not

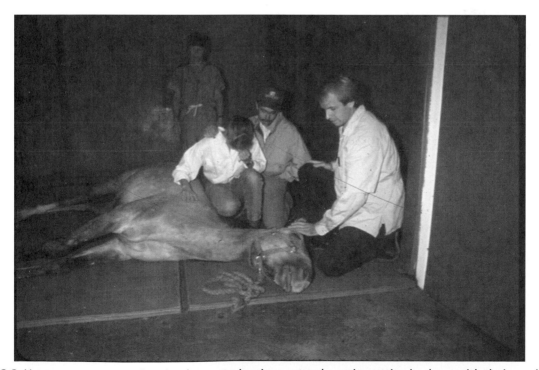

Figure 23-2 Horse owners appreciate it when veterinarians extend a caring attitude along with their medical expertise.

allow either veterinarians or clients to find "closure" for their grief.

In the new model of euthanasia, the standard operating procedure is the opposite of the old. With the new model, it is more common for veterinarians and clients to discuss and talk about euthanasia together, directly, and at length. It is also common to take as long for the procedure as is needed and as is possible, to involve clients in the process as much as possible, and to acknowledge the death and to talk openly about it afterward. The new paradigm is congruent with the research concerning healthy grief resolution and effective practice management.[7,8] The new model is both sensitive and pragmatic.

Not all clients want or require a lot of time or attention when euthanizing their horses. Based on clinical experience, each client makes a different choice. Some choose total involvement and orchestrate fairly complex euthanasia processes, whereas others choose minimal involvement, opting only for a good-bye nuzzle as they leave the euthanasia site.

Client Presence: Once clients decide to be present during euthanasia, they need to be prepared for what lies ahead. Research shows that longer preparation time diminishes the intensity of grief reactions and that anticipatory grief acts as a mitigating influence on postdeath grief.[9,10] Successful client-present euthanasias begin with thorough preparation. Preparation minimizes regrets—the "what ifs," and the "if onlys"—that inevitably follow companion animal death.

Talking to owners about the impending deaths of their animals is challenging. Veterinarians are most helpful to clients when they do not interfere or take sides during the decision-making process and then support them in whatever decision they make. Veterinarians are also helpful when they present accurate information in nonjudgmental ways.

Explaining the Procedure: Clients should be informed about what occurs during euthanasia, regardless of their choice regarding presence or nonpresence. To begin, veterinarians should review the procedure step-by-step. For example, owners should be told what drugs will be given and how they will affect their horses. They should also be told that the drugs will take effect in several seconds and that their horse may fall (perhaps hard) to the ground. Veterinarians should be honest, specific, and thorough in their descriptions of death by euthanasia, as this is the only way owners can make informed decisions about whether or not to be present. They should also focus on the fact that death is quick and painless.

A pre-euthanasia description may be similar to the following. In general, veterinarians should deliver this information in a private setting where clients can sit down and have access to tissues, water, and other comforting items. Veterinarians should use a soft, gentle tone of voice and speak a bit more slowly than usual. The topics usually take about 10 minutes to cover and clients often have questions and comments and may express emotion along the way.

> "Mrs. Brown, I know Sugar is very important to you. I want you to feel you have said good-bye to him in whatever way is right for you. I realize you might want to be there when Sugar is euthanized, so I would like to inform you of what you might expect from this procedure now, if that is okay with you."

With the client's permission, the veterinarian continues.

> "When I euthanize a patient, the first thing I do is place a catheter in the horse's neck. This makes it easier for me to give the drugs. If necessary, I may give Sugar a mild sedative, but when he is actually euthanized, Sugar will die from the injection of a very strong barbiturate. The barbiturate will cause his brain to stop functioning so he will feel no pain. Soon after, the rest of Sugar's body will shut down until his heart stops. I want to assure you that there is no physical pain for Sugar associated with this.
>
> Once the injection is given, Sugar will continue to stand for several seconds, then begin to collapse, and finally fall to the ground. He will not know what is happening and will be dead by the time he hits the ground. He may hit the ground very hard. For a few seconds, he may move his legs a bit or stretch them out stiffly. In addition, Sugar may take several deep gasps, but he will not be aware of this. You may see his eyes moving back and forth for several seconds and his eyes will remain open after death. There is generally no blood from the nose or mouth (unless a particular disease is present that would cause this). Sugar will most likely urinate, defecate, or pass gas within a few minutes. He may also have a heartbeat for a couple of minutes, but generally no breathing. Sugar will be completely unaware of what is happening during this time, but I still want to prepare you that this may be difficult to watch."

The veterinarian continues by saying something like,

> "It will be impossible for me to fully control Sugar's collapse; therefore, I cannot predict which direction he will fall. In some instances, I have had horses rear up or kick. Therefore, it will be important that you stand away from him until he is on the ground. If you wish to pet or talk to him again, you will be able to in a few minutes after I have pronounced him dead. Then, you will need to come in on the safe side of his body, away from his legs. Under no circumstances should you come close to Sugar during the procedure. This is for your safety and for Sugar's benefit. I can't perform euthanasia in the most humane way if I am distracted by your presence. Remember, you should not try to intervene even if it appears I need help. If I need help, my technician will step in."

Veterinarians close the description of what will occur by reassuring owners that they will support them whatever they decide. They say something like,

> "You will need to decide what is best for you based on everything I've told you. I want to ensure your needs are met, so I will respect your decision whether or not you want to be there."

Owners should also decide who else they want to accompany them to the euthanasia. For example, with proper preparation, children often choose to be present when their horses die. It is a good idea to encourage owners to ask someone to attend their animals' euthanasias with them, as even sensitively conducted deaths are difficult to bear alone.

Although client presence has value, encouraging client presence must be done with care. Veterinarians should never talk clients into being present at euthanasia. Some clients very clearly decide to leave their animals in their veterinarian's hands to be euthanized. This option is as acceptable as any other and clients should not be deterred from this decision.

Locations and Logistics: When horses are injured or in distress, veterinarians need to act quickly. Also, on ambulatory services, the luxury of euthanizing sick or injured animals in private usually does not exist. Thus, emergency euthanasias are often performed in pastures, stables, arenas, show rings, or race tracks. The goal in these situations is to help horses die as quickly and painlessly as possible.

The most common place for horses to be euthanized is in clients' pastures and stables. Under most of these conditions, veterinarians do not have the benefit of support staff to help clients make decisions or to comfort them after their horses have died. Therefore, it is helpful to encourage owners to bring friends or family members along with them to the euthanasia site to help them with their decision-making and to provide extra support. This way, veterinarians can focus on medical procedures, while clients receive comfort from others.

Clients may ask veterinarians to euthanize their horses in a stall, especially if they choose to be present. However, it may be hazardous to perform euthanasia in a stall that is not specifically equipped for euthanasia. In addition, it is very difficult to remove a horse's body once euthanasia has been completed. Therefore, stalls should be used only when horses are already down or unable to be moved due to illness or injury.

If euthanasias are conducted in stalls, concrete areas can be padded with hay or other protective padding, but caution should be used, as this material can become slippery. When it is explained, most owners understand why stalls are not the most practical areas for euthanizing horses. They, too, are interested in using areas that will later facilitate the most efficient disposal or rendering of their horses' bodies.

If client-present euthanasias are performed at veterinary hospitals or large animal surgery practices, an ambulatory horse can be moved into a surgery preparation room for euthanasia. There, an intravenous catheter can be placed and a sedative can be given to calm the horse prior to moving him or her into an anesthesia induction stall.

Anesthesia induction stalls are padded (walls and floor) and equipped with a padded wooden gate. This gate is used to keep the animal safely against the wall during the administration of the euthanasia solution. The gate swings up against the horse and pushes him into a space approximately equal to an adult horse's length and width. At this time, a lead rope is loosely looped through a wall tie or iron ring to partially control the animal's movements. The animal may show brief excitability when gently pushed against the wall, but this is momentary, as the euthanasia solution is injected into the catheter immediately (Fig. 23-3).

As the animal goes down, the lead rope is loosened and the gate is slowly moved back. This allows the horse to fall onto the padded floor. A thick strap with loops at each end is placed on the floor before the gate is opened and the horse falls. Later, the strap is attached to a hoist for moving the horse onto a cart and then to the necropsy or body disposal area.

Horses can also be euthanized in an anesthesia recovery stall. Like the induction stall, the recovery room is padded but does not have a swinging gate. Once the animal is in the stall, the lead rope is loosely attached to a wall tie or iron ring to partially control the animal's movements. The veterinarian and technician then ensure that they are safely positioned while working with the animal. If possible, they attempt to guide the animal down slowly. The veterinarian may also try to push the animal toward the wall so the animal can lean against it. This way, the animal slumps down rather than falling with full body weight onto the mat. A horse may still fall hard, but a fall onto a recovery pad is more aesthetically pleasing to witness than one that occurs on concrete. The recovery room also has a hoist that allows an animal to be lifted up onto a cart for transport to necropsy or other body care areas.

With adequate preparation, clients often observe these euthanasias, but they should not be directly involved with the procedures. Clients should stand in the doorway of the anesthesia induction or recovery stall and can enter the stall to spend time with their animals after they are down. They should be offered time to say goodbye to their animals and then escorted out before the hoist is used to move the animal. If possible, a staff member

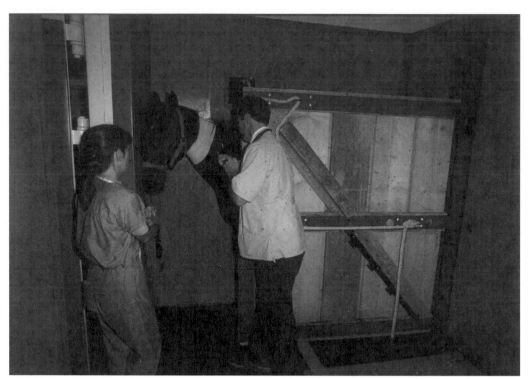

Figure 23-3 Anesthesia induction stalls are padded (walls and floor) and equipped with a padded wooden gate. The gate swings up against the horse and pushes him into a space approximately equal to an adult horse's length and width. A lead rope is loosely looped through a wall tie or iron ring to partially control the animal's movements.

should stay with the horse's body at the euthanasia site. Clinical experience shows that almost every owner takes one last look back at their companion animal before they actually leave. When they see a friendly, familiar face next to their horse, they feel reassured that their companion animal will not be forgotten or treated with disrespect once they leave.

It should be noted that neither of these rooms should be used if animals are suspected to have contagious conditions such as strangles or salmonellosis. If this is the case, the situation should be fully explained to the owner and an appropriate place (based on convenience, safety, and privacy) can be used for the euthanasia, with or without the owner's presence.

On some occasions, the decision is made to euthanize horses during surgery. If the decision is made to euthanize on the surgery table, or if animals die unexpectedly on the table, owners can be offered the opportunity to view their horse's body and to say goodbye. In these cases, owners can be dressed in surgery scrubs and the surgical incisions can be adequately draped so owners are not overwhelmed by the medical aspects of the scene.

Regardless of where and when euthanasia occurs, procedural matters should be dealt with prior to the euthanasia, if possible. Consent forms should be signed and arrangements for payment should be made. If the

owner is a trusted client, a bill can be sent after the event. However, the bill should *never* be included in a condolence card.

Body Care: Whenever possible, decisions about body care should be made prior to euthanasia. Owners should be offered all of the options available to them, and each should be explained with honesty and sensitivity. The cost of each option should also be disclosed. Some horse owners choose to bury or cremate their companion animals, even though it is very expensive to do so.

When offering body care options for large animals, veterinarians can say something like,

> "Mrs. Brown, I can offer you three options for taking care of Sugar's body after he dies. The first option is that you can take him with you and bury him yourself. The most efficient system for this is to prepare the gravesite first and then euthanize Sugar at that location.*
>
> Second, I work with a service that can cremate Sugar's body and either dispose of the cremains for you or return them to you. Some people like to keep their horses' cremains and some like to spread them in an appropriate

---

*Regulatory agencies warn that barbiturates in the rendering food chain and "relay toxicity", where scavenger wildlife ingest barbiturates from an animal carcass and are intoxicated, may be problematic.

location. Just so you know, cremating a horse is a very labor intensive process and can be very expensive.

Your third option is to have us take care of Sugar's body for you. Although I wish I had a more aesthetically pleasing option to offer you, my only option is_____." (Veterinarians should fill in the blank with whatever is accurate, usually disposal by a rendering company.)

Most owners have no choice but to render their animals; however, many of them may feel it would be more meaningful to bury or cremate them. When clients express this dilemma to you, you can help them come up with creative solutions. For example, you may suggest that they make a clay impression of their horse's hoof as a keepsake or take the horseshoes or hair from the tail or mane with them and send the remains to be rendered (Fig. 23-4). There are numerous other creative solutions to this problem. The idea is to give clients permission to take action that is meaningful to them.

Client-Present Facilitation Methods

When the day arrives, a euthanasia appointment should be given first priority over everything except medical emergencies. Whenever possible, it is recommended that all client-present euthanasias be conducted by a team of at least two veterinary professionals. This allows whoever is assisting the veterinarian to also focus on owner needs and allows the veterinarian to concentrate on the medical aspects of the euthanasia procedure. Pagers should be turned off during the actual procedure to avoid unnecessary distractions.

Catheters: If owners have elected to be present, it is highly recommended that a catheter and a sedative be used. Catheters and sedatives are not always necessary to improve the medical procedures involved with euthanasia. However, they often enhance the emotional side of euthanasia, as they make it easier to watch the drugs being administered because the horse does not appear to resist the needle (Fig. 23-5).

If a catheter is used, it should be placed in the jugular vein. This allows easier and safer access to the horse. A catheter not only facilitates rapid administration but also ensures direct injection into the vein without multiple attempts. Horses are given local blocks (1 mL of lidocaine) under their skin, just over the vein, to anesthetize a small area of their necks and to ease placement of a catheter into their jugular veins. Most will feel no discomfort with the insertion of the catheter. If the added cost of using catheters for euthanasias is a concern, nonsterile, previously used ones can be placed. Veterinarians should be sure that used catheters are in working condition before they are used with an owner present.

If a catheter is not used, a 14-gauge needle should be inserted into the jugular vein. The needle should be loosely attached to the first syringe so that it can be removed and the second syringe attached without delay. Veterinarians should be sure to explain to owners that blood will be seen flowing from the needle as the syringes are exchanged. If a technician is available, the solution from both syringes can be injected into both jugular veins simultaneously.

Drugs*: Because client presence during euthanasia has not been the norm in equine medicine, drug combinations that would reliably produce both humane and psychologically acceptable deaths for owners have not been methodically tested. However, successful methods for minimizing the side effects of euthanasia that make the dying process appear difficult to owners, such as vocalizations, reflexive muscle contractions, and agonal gasping, are being developed. With a variety of current methods, unconsciousness is reached rapidly, death occurs quickly, and the process appears to be painless for the animal.

When clients are present, veterinarians should carefully evaluate the usefulness of sedatives or tranquilizers prior to euthanasias, as they may calm animals and smooth out the way animals fall. Several drugs, in various combinations, can be used to sedate or tranquilize horses prior to euthanasia. According to several veterinarians consulted on this topic, a tranquilizer such as acepromazine or sedatives such as detomidine or

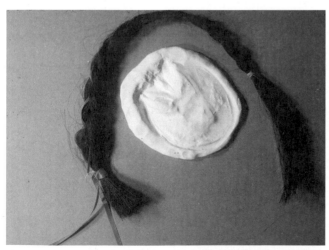

Figure 23-4 A clay impression of the horse's hoof and hair from the tail or mane are examples of meaningful keepsakes that you can suggest to owners.

*Authors' note: We are not veterinarians and wish to make it clear that we are not making recommendations about how veterinarians should use any of the drugs listed in this chapter. Rather, we are reporting what several equine veterinarians and pharmacists we interviewed recommended.

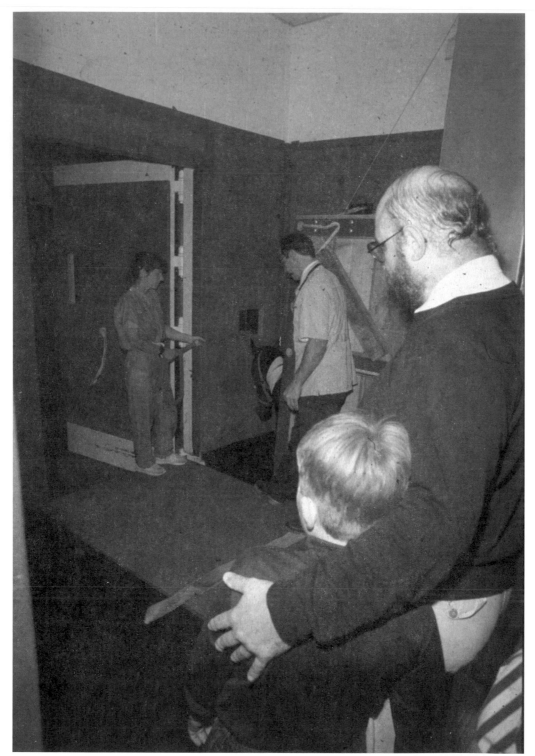

Figure 23-5 If owners are present during euthanasia, it is highly recommended that a catheter and a sedative be used, as they make it easier to watch the drugs being administered.

xylazine (Rompun) can be used. Xylazine, for example, is a short-acting sedative/analgesic that is often used for pain in colicking horses. Ketamine, an anesthetic, can also be used, but must be used in combination with a sedative such as xylazine. Butorphanol, a narcotic

agonist–antagonist analgesic can also be used to calm horses prior to euthanasia. The amount of drug used varies based on the drug, the nature of the situation, and the needs and disposition of the animal. It is important to remember, however, that when using sedatives and tranquilizers prior to euthanasia, it may take longer for the euthanasia solution to take effect. This is particularly true for animals suffering from cardiovascular problems, other serious illnesses, or old age.

Pentobarbital sodium, a Class Two barbiturate, is most commonly used for euthanasia of large animals. The recommended dosage is 40 mg per pound of animal. The drug is administered intravenously as rapidly as possible. It is important to be accurate when preparing the dosage, as clinical experience shows that underdosing animals usually causes them to die more slowly. An inadequate dose, or even slow delivery of the dosage, can result in extreme excitement in the animal. At a client-present euthanasia, this will cause the horse, the owner, and the veterinary team more distress.

In special circumstances, some veterinarians recommend adding an appropriate dose of succinylcholine, a paralytic agent, to the second syringe of pentobarbital. This eliminates gasps, "running in place," and other residual effects associated with euthanasia. This drug should be added only to the euthanasia solution, so that animals are unaware of its paralyzing effect. The 1993 Report of the AVMA Panel on Euthanasia summarizes some of the unacceptable agents and methods for euthanasia. It condemns the sole use of succinylcholine, or any other neuromuscular blocking agent, for the purpose of euthanasia without use of a sedative,[11] because it causes death by suffocation. It is assumed that suffocating an animal that is fully aware of what is taking place would produce great distress and severe anxiety.

Saying Good-Bye: Before a euthanasia procedure begins, owners should be given the opportunity to spend a short time alone with their horses, if they so desire. If owners are left alone to say their last good-byes, veterinarians should state when they will return. For instance, the veterinarian may say, "I will be back in about 10 minutes." If more time can be allowed for clients to say good-bye, it should be provided. Owners often report that they felt rushed through the euthanasia process by their veterinarian and feel this negated the other positive aspects of their experience.

Once the procedure has begun, the drugs should be injected as quickly as possible. During this time, the owner should stand away from the horse and the veterinarian's full attention should be given to bringing the horse down as safely and gently as possible. During this time, it is natural for the veterinarian to talk to the horse, calming it and guiding it down safely.

Once horses have actually died, it is very important to use a stethoscope to listen for a final heartbeat. When it is honest to do so, the animal should be pronounced dead. Veterinarians should do this by walking over to the client and saying something such as,

"Mrs. Brown, Sugar is dead. If you want to, you can go in on the safe side of his body, away from his legs, and spend time with him."

At this time, owners may gasp, cry, sob, or sigh with relief. They may make remarks about how quickly death came and about how meaningful the experience of being present was to them. This is a good time for veterinarians to reassure owners about their decisions to euthanize their animals. It is also a good time for veterinarians to express their own feelings of affection and respect for their patients.

For example, the veterinarian might say "I'm going to miss Sugar, too. He always nuzzled me when I came into his stall." These statements may prompt owners to begin a review of their horse's lives. Many owners appreciate the opportunity to talk a bit about their horses and to reminisce about the life that has just come to an end.

Post-Death Follow-Up Care

After euthanasia, some people want to leave the veterinary facility or euthanasia site quickly, whereas others need more time alone with their horses. Since many owners have invested so much in the physical care of their companion animals, even after death, their animals' bodies remain important to them. If appointments are waiting and owners want to spend time with the body, veterinarians can tell owners they will be back in whatever time frame is reasonable.

Sometimes, family members, especially children, who have not been present at the euthanasia may want to view a horse's body before it is buried, cremated, or sent for rendering. If there is time, horses should be cleaned up or brushed before being presented for owners to see. In addition, all catheters and tape should be removed. When owners are ready to leave, they should be escorted out a side or back door, if possible, so they do not have to exit through busy areas.

Contacting owners after their horses have died is a crucial part of retaining their trust. Sending clients personalized condolence cards or letters should be standard procedure in an equine practice. The content of a condolence should include personal comments about the companion animal who has died. Veterinarians can also confirm that the owner's decision to euthanize their horse was both timely and humane. In addition, mention of any preliminary necropsy results that serve to validate the owner's decision is also helpful to include.

Loss and Grief: When the human-animal bond is broken, owners and veterinarians experience loss. Loss is defined as an ending or as a point of change and transition. Clinical experience shows that most horse owners judge the death of a horse as a significant loss and feel, at the very least, sad and disturbed by the experience

For most horse owners, the actual death of a horse is the main cause of their grief. However, the death of a horse often creates disruptions in other areas of a horse owner's life. These additional disruptions are referred to as secondary losses.[7] Secondary losses have the greatest impact on horse owners who share their leisure activities and daily routines with their companion animals. For example, owners who participate in competitive horse shows lose more than their show partners when their horses die. Along with the primary loss of their horse, they also experience the secondary loss of no longer participating in an enjoyable pastime. Another secondary loss common to horse owners is the end of the supportive relationship the veterinarian has provided them.

Understanding that loss is significant for horse owners in many different ways is important to the delivery of Bond-Centered veterinary care. Understanding, for example, that grief due to a number of secondary losses may last longer or be reactivated more easily enables veterinarians to provide more effective support for clients.

In reviewing his experience with the death of his dog, a 60-year-old client wrote,

> "My veterinarian did a beautiful job explaining what was going to happen to my dog Dusty during the euthanasia. He prepared me in great detail for the procedure and for the handling of his body afterwards. But, he didn't tell me what was going to happen to me.
>
> After Dusty died, I couldn't watch a simple 30-minute television program. I couldn't read the Readers' Digest. There were times when I felt so down, I even thought about killing myself. I couldn't express these feelings to anyone because I thought I was the only person who had grieved this deeply for a dog. I couldn't call my veterinarian, the person who knew the most about my relationship with Dusty, because I figured he would think I was crazy. I know now that, if he would have given me just five minutes of grief education, it would have helped me make sense of many of the feelings and behaviors I experienced after Dusty died."[6] (Box 23-1)

Veterinarians who play a more active role in their clients' experiences with loss, often find that most people know very little about coping with grief. They also find that what clients do know, or think they know, is generally inaccurate.

Research and clinical experience show that what people say and do during bereavement is based on the myths and misinformation about grief that are passed along in families from generation to generation.[12] One of the most prominent of these myths is the belief that the best way to handle loss is to be strong and composed during grief. Another is the belief that staying busy and keeping one's mind off thoughts of the loss is the best way to feel better and to recover more quickly.

These methods of grieving can actually prolong the process of grief and cause grief to become complicated and even pathological. To avoid reinforcing the myths and misinformation, veterinarians need to become knowledgeable about the normal, healthy grieving process.

Veterinarians are more likely to respond to grief in its early, acute phases than in its middle or final stages. Therefore, it is useful for veterinarians to have a basic, working knowledge of the normal manifestations and progression of grief. In a Bond-Centered Practice, grief support begins with a working understanding of normal grief.

Normal Grief: Loss and grief are two of the most common human experiences. As a matter of fact, everyone experiences loss and grief repeatedly during the course of their lives. However, loss and grief are also the two normal life processes about which we probably know the least. This is because, until recently, conversations about loss, death, and grief have been viewed as morbid, morose, and even taboo.

Grief is the natural and spontaneous response to loss. We also know it is the normal way to adjust to endings and to change. Grief is the necessary process for healing the emotional wounds caused by loss. Grief is a process, not an event, and, because grief often starts with just the anticipation of loss, we may not always realize when grieving actually begins.

The end of the grief process is as unclear as the beginning. The progression of normal grief happens over no specific time frame. In fact, normal grief may last for days, weeks, months, or even years, depending on the significance of the loss.

During the process of normal grieving, the level of emotional intensity ranges on a continuum from no reactions at all to thoughts of suicide. The intensity of a person's grief response is based on several factors. These include the nature of the loss, the circumstances surrounding the loss, the griever's "pre-loss" emotional status, and the availability of emotional support before, during, and after the loss. If progressing in a healthy manner, grief lessens in intensity over time.

The grief response is unique to each individual. There is no right or wrong way to grieve. Grief is also unique to different groups, societies, and cultures. In most cases, the variables of age, gender, and developmental status greatly affect peoples' expressions of grief. For instance, research conclusively confirms that women shed more tears and cry more often during grief than men.[13] This is probably due to the fact that men are socialized to maintain their composure during

---

Box 23-1

Five Minutes of Grief Education

Predeath education should focus on preparation, decision-making, and predictions about how grief is likely to manifest. *Education during grief* should take advantage of "teachable moments." For example, if a client says, "I don't know why I'm acting like this. After all, Jeanie is just a horse," you might say, "Yes, Jeanie is a horse, but she is also your true friend. If your best human friend were dying, you'd be very upset. This situation is no different than that. It's very normal to be feeling and behaving this way." *Postdeath education* should normalize and validate grief and give grievers permission to openly express their feelings. Postdeath education is more effective when it is offered a few days after a death, as clients are often in shock immediately after loss has occurred. They also may not have consciously experienced many of the manifestations of grief.[6]

It is appropriate to educate your clients about grief before, during, and after their horses' deaths. The basic content of your educational synopsis should be adapted according to each loss situation. Information about euthanasia procedures or helping children with grief, for example, can be included when appropriate.

Obviously, information about grief is not delivered in the form of long, dry monologues. It is more common for it to be delivered within the context of a conversation, with clients responding, crying, and/or asking questions along the way.

Grief education is most effective when it is supplemented with written materials. The following is an example of 5 minutes of postdeath grief education. Note that the topics covered include typical grief manifestations, a time frame for grief, the individual characteristics of grief, ideas about memorializing, and referral information.

"Mary, we all experience grief when we lose an important relationship, whether our loss is a human family member or a companion animal, like your horse Jeanie. How feelings of grief are expressed varies from one person to the next. Somehow, though, we all find our own personally meaningful ways to get through important losses.

When grieving, it is not uncommon to cry a lot—or to feel like crying a lot. You may feel sadness, depression, anger, guilt, and even some relief in response to your loss. You might find yourself uninterested in your usual activities for a while as you try to adjust to a new life without Jeanie. You may also have a hard time concentrating on even the most basic tasks and your eating and sleeping routines may be disrupted. Some people find that grieving makes them feel extremely tired and they become irritable and even angry about their losses.

Even as time goes by, it may be hard to accept that Jeanie is really dead. You may find that you think about her frequently and miss her deeply. You may even think you see or hear her. These sensations, these emotions, are common during times of loss. All of them are normal.

Grief can be very unpredictable. One minute you may feel fine and the next minute you may feel awful. That's why there is no specific time frame for grieving. It may take days, weeks, or months to come to terms with Jeanie's death. It may take a year or longer to adapt. You'll have your first holiday season without her (her first birthday or competition). Those can be tough times to get through. The important thing is to find your own pace with it.

Expect that others may want you to feel better before you are able, Mary. You will probably find that everyone in your family grieves in their own way. That is to be expected. You all had a different relationship with Jeanie. Your grief will be different, too.

You might find it helpful to think about some ways to memorialize Jeanie. Some people make a scrapbook of pictures or special objects. Others have a funeral, plant a tree or bush in their horse's honor, or make a donation to an equine-oriented organization in remembrance of their animal. Whatever is most meaningful to you will be the best memorial for Jeanie.

When my horse died I talked to others about how much I missed him and that seemed to help me get through the rough times. You might want some additional support along the way, too. There is a support group in town and several grief counselors who understand the special bonds people have with their animals. I'd like to give you some information about them (business cards and brochures). There are also good books available in our library about companion animal death and the grief that often follows (bibliographies).

My staff and I would like to support you, too. We know Jeanie was a true friend and her death has had a significant impact on your life. We want you to know that we will be thinking about you during this difficult time. How should we leave it between us? Would you like to contact us if you'd like to talk further, or would you prefer that one of us call you in the next week or so to see how you are doing?"

---

emotional times, while women are socially conditioned to express their feelings more openly. Research also confirms that children grieve just as deeply as adults. Due to their shorter attention spans, though, they do so more sporadically.

Clinical experience shows that, when the expression of grief is restricted in some way, the healing time for recovery is prolonged. Likewise, when grief is freely expressed, the healing time for recovery from loss is, in general, greatly reduced.

Equine veterinarians can best help horse owners by encouraging them to openly express their grief-related thoughts and feelings. They can also give clients permission to grieve by encouraging them to cry, to ask questions, to view their horse's bodies, and to reminisce about their horse's lives. When permission to grieve comes from an authority figure like a veterinarian, clients are reassured that grief over the death of a horse is not immature, overly sentimental, or crazy. As Dusty's owner said in his essay about his dog's death, a veterinarian's encouragement, along with 5 minutes of grief education, can save clients months and even years of emotional pain, worry, and embarrassment after the death of an animal.

To provide your clients with 5 minutes of education about normal grief, you must understand how normal grievers generally think, feel, and behave. Boxes 23-1 and 23-2 provide an overview of the normal symptoms of grief and suggestions for a brief discussion regarding grief education.

Conclusion

In a geriatric equine practice, it is important for veterinarians to realize that the grief process often begins before death actually occurs. Anticipatory grief occurs prior to an actual death.[7] For horse owners, it begins when they first begin to sense that their relationship with their beloved friend may end sooner than they had hoped. The symptoms of anticipatory grief include any or all of the manifestations of normal grief detailed in Box 23-2.

As a horse continues to age and deteriorate, owners must adjust to many changes in appearance, personality,

---

Box 23-2

Manifestations of Grief

Although grief responses, in general, differ from one person to another, there are many predictable manifestations of grief. These manifestations occur on physical, intellectual, emotional, social, and spiritual levels. Before, during, and after loss, grief may appear in several of these forms:

Physical

Crying, sobbing, wailing, shock and numbness, dry mouth, a lump in the throat, shortness of breath, stomach ache or nausea, tightness in the chest, restlessness, fatigue, exhaustion, sleep disturbance, appetite disturbance, body aches, stiffness of joints or muscles, dizziness, or fainting.

Intellectual

Denial, sense of unreality, confusion, inability to concentrate, feeling preoccupied by the loss, experiencing hallucinations concerning the loss (visual, auditory, and olfactory), a need to reminisce about the loved one and to talk about the circumstances of the loss, a sense that time is passing very slowly, a desire to rationalize or intellectualize feelings about the loss, thoughts or fantasies about suicide (not accompanied by concrete plans or behaviors).

Emotional

Sadness, anger, depression, guilt, anxiety, relief, loneliness, irritability, a desire to blame others for the loss, resentment, embarrassment, self-doubt, lowered self-esteem, feelings of being overwhelmed or out of control, feelings of hopelessness and helplessness, feelings of victimization, giddiness, affect that is inappropriate for the situation (nervous smiles and laughter).

Social

Feelings of withdrawal, isolation and alienation, a greater dependency on others, a rejection of others, rejection by others, a reluctance to ask others for help, change in friends or in living arrangements, a desire to relocate or move, a need to find distractions from the intensity of grief (to stay busy or to overcommit to activities).

Spiritual

Bargaining with God in an attempt to prevent loss, feeling angry at God when loss occurs, renewed or shaken religious beliefs, feelings of being either blessed or punished, searching for a meaningful interpretation of a loved one's death, paranormal visions or dreams concerning a dead loved one, questioning whether or not souls exist and wondering what happens to loved ones after death, the need to "finish business" with a purposeful ending or closure to the relationship (a funeral, memorial service, last rites ceremony, good-bye ritual).

and physical capabilities as well as give up knowing their horses in the ways they used to know them. During this period of anticipatory grief, owners begin the process of saying good-bye and many, either consciously or subconsciously, detach from their horses, investing emotional energy into other companion animals and other aspects of their lives. For the most part, emotional detachment is healthy and represents an owner's attempt to prepare for the death. Still, when death arrives, it is emotionally painful for all involved. This is when Bond-Centered veterinarians shine. The commitment they make to extend their care beyond medical treatment to also soothe their clients' pain helps everyone work together to guide that special horse through the final transition from life to whatever lies beyond.

REFERENCES

1. Lagoni L, Morehead D, Brannan J, et al: Guidelines for Bond-Centered Practice. Fort Collins, CO, Argus Institute for Families and Veterinary Medicine, 2001.
2. Hart LA, Hart BL, Mader B: Humane euthanasia and companion animal death: caring for the animal, the client, and the veterinarian. JAVMA 197:1292, 1990.
3. Hart LA, Hart BL: Grief and stress from so many animal deaths. Comp Anim Pract 1:20, 1987.
4. Troutman M: The Veterinary Services Market Survey for Companion Animals. Overland Park, KS, Charles and Charles Research Group and the American Veterinary Medicine Association, 1988.
5. Staats S, Miller D, et al: The Miller-Rada Commitment to Pet Scale. Antrozoös 9:2/3, 88-94, 1996.
6. Lagoni L, Butler C, Hetts S: The Human-Animal Bond and Grief. Philadelphia, W.B. Saunders, 1994.
7. Rando TA: Grief, Dying, and Death: Clinical Interventions for Caregivers. Champaign, IL, Research Press, 1984.
8. Lagoni L, Hetts S, Withrow S: The veterinarian's role in pet loss: grief education, support, and facilitation. In Withrow SJ, MacEwen EG, editors: Clinical Veterinary Oncology. Philadelphia, J.B. Lippincott, 1989.
9. Ball JF: Widow's grief: The impact of age and mode of death. Omega 7:307, 1977.
10. Parkes CM, Weiss RS: Recovery from Bereavement. York, NY, Basic Books, 1983.
11. 1993 Report of the AVMA Panel on Euthanasia. J Am Vet Med Assoc 202:229, 1993.
12. Loss: An interview with University of Chicago's Froma Walsh. Psych Today 25:64, 1992.
13. Frey WH, Lanseth M: Crying: The Mystery of Tears. Minneapolis, Winston Press, 1985.

CHAPTER 24

Conditions, Diseases, and Injuries of the Older Horses for Horse Owners

Robert E. Holland Jr.

Older horses do not get a lot of attention from researchers or, until recently, from the media, yet they are among the best-loved animals on farms. Just like humans, horses need different care as they age. This chapter gives you an overview of the most common problems in the older horse. This is a good introduction; for more in depth information, see the recommended reading list at the end of this chapter.

Proper care of older horses and ponies (15 years and older) can extend their healthy lifespan and increase their years of use. Owners of older horses and ponies should keep in mind three goals. All start with the letter C. The three C's are *Concern* for their welfare; *Commitment* to their daily care; and *Consistency* in their feeding, use, and treatment.

As an owner, you can look for signs of degenerative problems and work on minimizing their effects. The aging process affects all body tissue, organs, and systems. As horses age, there is a loss of organ reserve capacity and a decrease in the cell volume, bone density, and brain activity. The aging process affects all body tissue, organs, and systems.

As your horse ages, ask your veterinarian to get a baseline complete blood cell count and serum chemistry when your horse is healthy. That way, if your horse has a problem later, it will be easier to see what levels are out of reference range from the normal for your horse. At this time, it is worth having endocrine levels checked, as this can be an indicator of Cushing's disease. Your veterinarian will be able to monitor potential indicators for cancer from these blood levels as well.

Look for any changes in your horse. Is it off feed? Is it acting lethargic? Do you notice a loss or gain of weight? Is it behaving normally? Changes in any of these indicators can mean a problem is developing.

Owners of older horses and ponies can help their aging animals by developing an individual wellness program for each animal in partnership with their veterinarian and doing a few simple things:

1. Proper nutrition is key: Provide a good combination of roughage (from hay or pasture grass) with more concentrated feed. There are several good senior diet formulations currently on the market. Do feeding two or three times a day rather than one large meal, because the older animal's digestive system cannot assimilate food as well as it did when it was younger.
2. Offer clean water at all times. Warm the water in wintertime.
3. Increase the frequency of immunizations against contagious diseases to at least two times a year. I recommend consulting the AAEP Vaccination Guidelines found on the web at www.aaep.org.
4. Set up a schedule for deworming and stick to it religiously.
5. Set up a schedule that includes dental "checkups," shoeing, or trimming.
6. Arrange for a veterinarian to do a blood test and take baseline measurements of the horse now while it is well, so that you can judge the amount of change when it is unwell.

Provide good stabling or pasture board with some shelter from the weather and make sure the equine senior has the company of at least one other calm horse. Because horses are herd animals, no equine should be kept alone without company.

Old horses can, and do, become ill with the very same illnesses that affect younger horses. You will not find a comprehensive list of all of the diseases of horses here, but you will find a description of the most common—and most dangerous—problems that affect older horses.

The following text details some typical problems or conditions of the older horse.

Dental Problems

Older horses tend to have dental problems. Some lose their grinding teeth and can no longer exist on a simple diet of grass and hay. In this case, moistening the feed or a supplement mash will help the horse get the needed calories to maintain proper body condition. Many develop sharp points on their teeth and wave mouth that make chewing very painful. A few have cracked or loose teeth caused by yanking the bits out of their mouths or caused by a poor job of "floating" their teeth. For this reason, it is very important to have your older horse's teeth checked twice per year. This does not mean that you need to have them floated each time, but it is just good dental maintenance to check regularly. This way, problems can be corrected before they become big problems.

Colic in Older Horses

Remember that *colic* is a general term for abdominal pain. There are several types and causes of colic. Two of the most common are changes in feed and parasites.

Changes in Feed

Changing an older horse's diet can cause colic. The frequency, quantity, or types of feed are big factors in colic.

Absentmindedly leaving the door of the feed room ajar can have an equally disastrous effect if any horse gets in and eats everything in the feed bin.

According to University of Kentucky Horse Extension Specialist Craig H. Wood, "Sudden changes in feed (either by type or quantity) or moldy feed can cause colic due to the improper fermentation in the gut or an obstruction. A predominantly concentrated diet can lead to colic if an adequate supply of long stem roughage is not provided. Horses with bad eating habits (such as choke, bolting, or cribbing) are prone to colic. Lack of water can also lead to colic symptoms and may contribute to the formation of an impaction."

Provide adequate roughage in their diet. Make sure fresh, warmed water is always available. Check each hay bale and do not feed moldy or spoiled hay or grain. Check the latches on your feed bins and feed room; also make sure the room and bins are latched at all times. If your pastures and paddocks are overgrazed, it becomes doubly important to remove manure frequently.

Parasitic Worms

The most common cause of colic is the build-up of internal parasites, or the sudden exit of such parasites. Migrating strongyle larvae can damage the blood vessels in the intestines, decreasing the blood supply and leading to necrosis, or death of the cell walls. Large numbers of roundworms can cause an obstruction of the intestines, called an impaction. Even administering a deworming medicine such as ivermectin to a horse overburdened with internal parasites can cause colic.

Proper management is the best way to prevent colic caused by parasites. Avoid situations that predispose your horses to colic. Put all of your horses on a regular deworming program that targets all known parasites. Often a rotation of different dewormers is helpful. Make sure to include tapeworms, as they have recently been found to cause more problems than previously thought. Adding a daily top dressing of Strongid C to the older horses' feed works well.

Trauma/Injuries

Since injuries and wounds account for more than 10 percent of old horse fatalities each year, your horses should be checked over on a daily basis. Even if the horses are simply free to roam across a large pasture, if you establish a set time of day to give them a small treat or bit of sweet feed, then they will come in long enough for you to look them over.

If the wound is severe and bleeding profusely, put a pressure bandage on and call the veterinarian. The sooner the wound is treated and repaired, the better the chance is for the patient's full recovery. Well before the emergency occurs, you should have protected your horse with a routine annual vaccination to protect against tetanus. It is frustrating to know that this preventable disease, also called lockjaw, is the cause of death for many horses every year. After an accident or other trauma occurs, the veterinarian will inject tetanus antitoxin that will give the horse a short period of protection (lasting a week or two).

Any wound between the front legs and in the chest should be considered very serious. If the chest cavity is affected, contamination and infection are likely. A lung may collapse (pneumothorax) and immediate respiratory distress will be evident. If you hear "sucking" noises from the chest, cover the wound with a clean dressing and secure it with an elastic bandage wrapped completely around the horse's trunk. Hopefully, the bandage will apply enough pressure to seal the wound until the veterinarian arrives. If a foreign object is stuck in the horse, leave it in place for the veterinarian to deal with.

Head injuries do not have a good prognosis. Older horses may fracture their skulls after falling, flipping over backwards, or rearing up into a stall door. The presence of blood in an ear canal after trauma is often the first indicator of a fracture. Other signs include severe depression, seizures, and holding the head tilted over. Thankfully, older horses have fewer injuries of this kind than younger horses. It occurs most often when young horses start training.

If you have a wound that looks like it will need stitches, it is very important to call your veterinarian immediately, as a wound cannot be sutured after 3 hours have passed due to risk of infection. This can cause a longer healing time and scarring to occur.

Neurologic Disorders

A number of nervous system disorders can affect horses at any age. If your older horse develops a bit of a problem staggering forward, sideways, or backwards, this can indicate the onset of acute ataxia, or "wobbler" syndrome. Some of the common causes of ataxia are severe head trauma, spinal cord injuries, equine protozoal myeloencephalitis, also called wobblers syndrome, and equine degenerative myelopathy. As a horse gets older, it is often challenged to fight by younger horses trying to change the pecking order. If the old horse takes a bad fall, it may result in ataxia.

Eye Injuries

Consider all eye problems to be medical emergencies best treated by your veterinarian. Do not "borrow" an eye ointment prescribed for another pet or medicine designed for a human. Eye ointments containing corticosteroids can make a minor eye problem very serious in a matter of hours.

Eyelid lacerations and eye puncture wounds are often preventable. Before you bring your older horse into new surroundings, check its stall, trailer, and paddock, for any sharp, protruding objects that might cause wounds of the eye, including eyelid lacerations, scratches, or ulcers caused by a foreign body, such as a splinter or thorn, or tears.

Allergies

Chronic obstructive pulmonary disease, also called COPD or heaves, is primarily an allergy problem. For this reason, its onset may be rapid. The problem is often complicated by secondary respiratory infections (pneumonia) or emphysema. The problem can be very stressful and may be life-threatening to an older horse with an impaired immune system. Fortunately, chronic obstructive pulmonary disease can now be managed medically using new drugs that allow for a comfortable life. Consult your veterinarian for the best course of treatment. Stabling the horse away from the source of the toxins that started its allergy, a dusty hay storage area for example, also helps.

Cancer in Older Horses

Cancer frequency increases with the age of the horse. Gray horses and certain breeds of horses seem prone to developing melanomas and squamous cell carcinoma. Surgical removal of cancerous growths can give older horses many more years of life. Sometimes, noncancerous fatty lipomas can cause problems if they are located on long stalks; they may become wrapped around a piece of intestine and cause colic. Skin cancer or melanomas, especially those around the anus, may spread into the gut and create conditions that predispose the horse to blockages. Watch for any strange bumps or swelling and consult your veterinarian if they do not resolve in a few days. Catching a cancer early increases the chances of recovery.

Tumors

Tumors of the pituitary and thyroid glands are frequently found in older horses. According to a 1989 study by S. L. Ralston et al, blood tests on the aged horses in the study (20, all over the age of 20 years) showed that more than 70 percent of them had tumors. Of the study group, thyroid tumors appeared to be more common in geldings, whereas mares had more pituitary tumors.

A horse with a thyroid tumor often develops a swelling in the throat area. These tumors are slow growing and are not life-threatening.

Cushing's Disease

Cushing's syndrome is often found in older horses. It has several other names, including pituitary pars intermedia dysfunction, hyperadrenocorticism, and equine Cushing's disease. In more than 85 percent of the cases, signs of the disease include a heavy, wavy hair coat that is not shed in the summer. Horses with equine Cushing's disease develop excessive thirst (polydipsia) coupled with excessive urination (polyuria). The water gives them a potbellied appearance. Although their appetites increase, there is generally no corresponding weight gain. Soon chronic laminitis and loss of muscle tone over the topline result.

In horses, Cushing's syndrome comes about when the pituitary gland malfunctions and occasionally develops into a tumor. Because it is inoperable, the problem has the best chance of being successfully treated with drugs. Dopamine (trade names Parlodel or Permax) was the first drug used to treat Cushing's syndrome. More recently, two drugs—cyproheptadine and pergolide—have been used successfully.

Horses with equine Cushing's disease have compromised immune systems; therefore, they are more susceptible to disease and infections. Wounds heal more slowly. Blood tests may reveal high blood sugar level, a high white blood cell count, a reduced lymphocyte count, and an electrolyte imbalance. Allergies may begin to bother the older horse that never bothered it before and create new respiratory problems for it.

Immunosuppressed Horses: Common Issues

There are also four non-life-threatening conditions I often find in older horses that have compromised immune systems, from Cushing's or from other problems: insect hypersensitivity, rain-rot, ringworm, and thrush. Immunosuppressed horses may develop an allergy to insect stings and bites. Ringworm is a fungal infection, whereas rain-rot and thrush are bacterial infections, the latter characterized by a stinking exudate coming from the grooves around the frog on the base of a horse's feet. Painting the affected areas with providone iodine (Betadine) usually takes care of the first two problems, and applying a dressing with copper sulfate crystals (Coppertox) usually clears thrush. However, if the foot has abscessed, opening a drainage tract and treating with penicillin may be called for.

Heart Disease

Compared with humans, horses are rarely troubled by heart disease. Equine heart problems include bacterial endocarditis, when bacterial infection clogs the heart valves. Symptoms include periods of unexplained fever and lethargy with sudden weight loss. A course of antibiotics can occasionally treat the problem.

Atrial fibrillation, or cardiac arrhythmia, occurs when the upper chambers of the heart beat independently or to a different rhythm than the lower cham-

bers. An older horse with this condition will have an irregular heart beat. The condition can be seen in very old horses and ponies (30 years and older). The medication quinidine usually will bring the horse's heartbeats back into a normal rhythm; however, this may not be necessary because some animals can live quite normal lives with this condition. If treatment is undertaken, once a horse's heartbeat is converted to a normal rhythm, the animal will not usually need any further treatment.

Kidney Problems

Symptoms of kidney disease include sudden weight loss and anorexia. Reduced kidney function can cause potentially fatal problems. When the kidneys shut down, stones begin to form. The kidney stones are bits of calcium (in the form of calcium oxalate) that build up the kidneys, the urethra, or the bladder. The stones can be extremely painful and can block the path urine should take. Stones in the kidneys are inoperable, but sometimes those in the bladder or urethra can be surgically removed.

Structural Problems

Cartoonists always draw an older horse with one very noticeable structural problem: a swayback. A real horse often shows the same sign of old age as the ones in cartoons. The ligaments that span the spine stretch and weaken with age. At the same time, if the horse is carrying too much weight or if it loses condition, the large muscles that run down the horse's back weaken, or atrophy, creating the sagging swayback. Surprisingly, some older horses live to a very great age without developing swayback. Those horses have good body condition and are kept in condition with exercise.

Arthritis

Degenerative arthritis is the most common ailment found in old horses. It is not usually a life-threatening disease. It often begins as a subtle stiffness in the joints, but it can get much worse in the form of degenerative joint disease.

Performance horses may develop problems years after their careers have ended. They may suffer from problems such as degenerative joint disease. When an old horse's joints are hot and painful, it is a sign of the inflammation of degenerative joint disease. It marks the degeneration and erosion of the cartilage within the joint coupled with an excess of synovial fluid. If radiographs show that the joint has degenerated, then the prognosis is poor.

Arthritis is directly related to the wear and tear a joint has had during the entire lifespan of the horse. The pain of arthritis comes from the rubbing of osteophytes, bony spurs that have developed within the joint or from erosions (holes) in the soft cartilage lining the joint. I often find arthritis in the knees and hocks of older horses that raced during their early years. It also frequently occurs in poorly conformed horses, sickle hocked or cow hocked horses for example. I would venture to say that all very old ponies and horses have some arthritis by the time they are in their 20s to 40s.

Rest is always recommended when a horse is suffering from an inflamed arthritic joint. However, it is always a balancing act to give an old horse a short period of complete rest followed by a controlled exercise program designed to keep it in condition. You will want to talk to your veterinarian about they way you intend to use the horse in the future. If, for example, it has arthritic hocks, it cannot do sports that require a lot of jumping or sharp turns, especially when it has a flare of the disease.

Hydrotherapy, or running water down the leg, is often helpful. Use cold water on hot, inflamed joints and then later switch to periodic washes of warm water over the legs if chronic pain persists.

Antiarthritis drugs include phenylbutazone (bute) to control the pain and reduce inflammation and nonsteroidal anti-inflammatory drugs such as Banamine, Arquel, and Equiproxen. A relatively new drug, Adequan, is injected into the joint to reduce friction and inflammation. It often has dramatic results with the horse going sound for a long time. Each drug has great benefits but some side effects you should discuss with your veterinarian. Depending on the horse's future uses, the veterinarian may recommend doing arthroscopic surgery.

Arthroscopic surgery involves a tiny incision that allows the vet to examine the interior of the joint for bony spurs, cartilage damage, and inflamed synovial linings. The total operative invasion is smaller, and postoperative recovery times are reduced.

Since arthritis attacks often follow periods of cold, wet weather, offering an older horse a way to get out of the cold will help manage its arthritis. Most of the following chapter is designed to provide common-sense hints and tips for making your older horse as comfortable as possible.

The good conformation of a horse's legs increases the chances that it will remain sound. Simply put, an older horse with good confirmation that has had good care and a full athletic career will usually outlast an older horse with poor confirmation.

If you already have an older horse, you will need to deal with problems of the joints, legs, and feet as they arise. With all live creatures, there is no such thing as a 100 percent perfect, blemish-free individual. By the time a horse reaches old age, it may have some bumps and blemishes such as "windpuffs," which is the common term for a harmless synovial fluid build-up around the digital flexor sheath at the fetlock joint. If there's no heat at the joint (indicating a new problem, inflammation), then the windpuffs are only a cosmetic problem that will not bother the horse.

At some time or other, you may be considering buying an older horse with a foreleg that shows signs of an old splint, but no heat in the area. That is probably not going to be a troublesome problem in the future. It is an old and healed injury.

In approximately 95 percent of cases of front leg lamenesses, the source of the problem is found from the knee down through the foot. Although there are causes of lameness related to the forearm, elbow, and shoulder, they are rare. If the lameness is located in a rear leg, the cause is most apt to be in the hock joint.

Laminitis

Laminitis, or founder, is a common condition that has several causes and is often preventable. Some causes of laminitis are mechanical, such as road founder, or concussion problems from work on hard surfaces. Support laminitis, or bilateral laminitis, is a secondary problem that commonly develops on the "good leg" when the horse tries to avoid its lame leg. Endotoxemia is a high-risk acute condition characterized by sudden lameness, acute swelling, and inflammation of the sensitive lamina inside the foot.

Chronic laminitis involves repeated attacks. With each one, the prognosis for the older horse worsens. The pedal bone in the foot (P3) becomes displaced. I know you have seen a laminitic pony or horse painfully shuffling around on overgrown hooves with long toes and overgrown heels. They desperately try to avoid pain by rocking back and stepping gingerly, landing on their heels. Soon, they develop seedy toe, as the laminae along the white line separate, which opens the foot to infections.

If radiographs show that rotation of the P3 has occurred, after months of treatment and special trimming, only a proportion of horses treated for chronic laminitis will return to some form of athletic activity. Many laminitic horses and ponies are euthanized if they do not respond to treatment.

Navicular Disease

Navicular disease accounts for one third of all forelimb lamenesses. Causes include poor conformation, poor shoeing or trimming resulting in an unbalanced foot, and concussion (for racing and working horses). There is no cure for navicular disease. The goal becomes managing the horse's pain and doing corrective shoeing to shorten the toe. A surgical procedure known as digital neurectomy, also called "denerving" the horse, may eliminate its pain, but it does not cure the disease. The cut nerve results in little or no sensation in the back part of the foot. Afterwards, the horse may step down on something sharp and never even sense that it has a puncture wound. After the surgery, for the rest of the horse's lifetime, it becomes important for the horse's owner or caregiver to check its feet daily. After the surgery, horses usually go sound for at least a few years. Eventually, all such horses are retired due to lameness.

Other Lamenesses

Western working horses may develop a chronic low-grade lameness that looks much like the short, choppy gate of a navicular horse. However, it is usually bilateral, affecting either the front or hind limbs. It leads to osteoarthritis, or low ringbone. This is a progressive disease that may develop into articular arthritis. Dosing the horse with phenylbutazone before each competition or work session may extend its useful career.

Septic arthritis often comes from puncture wounds or wire cuts that go into a joint. Like the other ills and conditions described so far in this chapter, septic arthritis affects horses of all ages. The prognosis for such cases is poor and, as the horse ages, it often results in degenerative joint disease.

Osselet, a form of chronic arthritis of the fetlock that included chronic synovitis, is an occupational hazard of racehorses. Stretching and tearing of the structures inside the fetlock joint results in calcification called osselets. Horses with upright pasterns are predisposed to this condition. It frequently shows up for the first time in young horses being trained for racing.

Problems in the Hind Limbs

Old horses and ponies often have bone spavin of a hock. It is the rear-end lameness problem seen most often. Again, poor conformation such as sickle hocks or cow hocks are predisposing factors in spavins. In Western horses, the quick, sliding stops and tight turns for reining and barrel racing may cause it. It is also a problem found harness-racing standardbreds. The conservative method of treatment is to relieve pain with analgesics (such as bute or aspirin) plus an injection into the joint of Depo-Medrol, a long-acting steroid. Adequan can also be added to the treatment protocol.

A bog spavin looks poor cosmetically, but is not be a serious problem if there is no lameness. It is a swelling of the tarsocrural joint. Similarly, a "capped hock" is swelling at the hock. It is usually a problem seen in young horses that have injured themselves kicking a wall or trailer. By the time you see it in an older horse, there is generally no lameness; it is just a cosmetic problem—a bump that will not go away.

Sometimes, an older horse will lock a stifle. Poorly conformed horses with straight hind limbs are prone to this problem. If your older horse has lost a lot of weight, part of that loss may be in the fat pad that keeps the patella anchored in the stifle. Another name for the problem is an upward flexion of the patella.

The joints that form a horse's pelvic girdle are very strong. An equine hip dislocation is a rare occurrence. According to Dr. Chris Pasquini's *Guide to Equine Clinics—Lameness*, 46 percent of the cases occurred in ponies and miniature horses. In 35 percent of all cases a fall was cited as causing the dislocation, in another 35 percent of the cases, the patient had been kicked. Some of those cases, no doubt, were very old horses or ponies that had fallen in icy, slippery conditions and had gone down hard with their hind ends doing "the splits." Almost half of these horses were euthanized. Even for the survivors, when their hips were put back in place, their long-term prognosis was poor because of the likelihood of a reoccurrence of the problem.

Older Horse Statistics

According to the 1998 USDA National Animal Health Monitoring System Survey, "Overall, the largest percentages of deaths for equines more than 30 years of age [and used in the survey], were attributed to old age (29.5%) followed by colic (17.5%) and injury/wounds/trauma which accounted for 10.5%." Those with leg or hoof problems accounted for 7.1 percent of deaths. Neurologic problems such as equine protozoal myeloencephalitis, wobbler's syndrome, spinal problems, and seizures, accounted for 4 percent of the deaths of horses 20 years or older and 3.4 percent of all of the horses in the survey. More than 11 percent of the old horses (20 years or older) were euthanized during the 1-year survey period.

Given those statistics, your goal should be to slow the rate of degenerative changes to the minimum and do what you can to prevent problems before they become fatal.

If you have healthy old horses and ponies, a carefully thought out wellness program will usually keep them healthy for a long time. Proper care of older horses and ponies can extend their healthy lifespan and increase their years of use. More detailed information can be found in *Understanding the Older Horse* from Bloodhorse Publications.

RECOMMENDED READING

Ball MA: Equine First Aid. Lexington, KY, BloodHorse, 1998.

Easley J: Equine dental development and anatomy. AAEP Proc 42:1-10, 1996. (other papers in same volume also)

Eisenmenger E, Zenter K: Veterinary Dentistry. Philadelphia, Lea and Febiger, 1985.

Harcourt MF, Ambrosiano NW: Building Horse Barns Big and Small. Millwood, NY, Breakthrough Publications, 1993.

Harper F: Care of the older horse. In Horse Industry Handbook. Lexington, KY, American Youth Horse Council, 1993.

Harper F: The digestive system of the horse. Fact sheet: Horse Information. Knoxville, TN, University of Tennessee Horse Extension Program, 1997.

Henneke DR, Potter GD, Kreider JL, et al: Relationship between condition score, physical measurement, and body fat percentage in mares. Equine Vet J 15:371, 1983.

Holland RE: Understanding the Older Horse. Lexington, KY, BloodHorse Publications, 1999.

Kellon EM: The Older Horse, 2nd ed. Ossining, NY, Breakthrough Publications, 1993.

Koop KJ: Equine Nutrition and Feeding Management Southern States [pamphlet]. available from Southern States Cooperative, Richmond, VA.

Marcella K: Big breath of fresh air: Treatment and prevention of heaves. The Mane Points, Fall, 1998.

Steward LE: Fencing & Facilities for Horses. University of Maryland, Maryland Cooperative Extension Service.

National Research Council Subcommittee on Horse Nutrition: Nutrient Requirements of Horses, 5th rev ed. Washington, DC, National Academy Press, 1989.

Ralston SL, Squires EL, Nockels CF: Digestion in the aged horse. J Equine Vet Sci 9:203, 1989.

Ralston SL: Clinical nutrition of adult horses. Vet Clin North Am 6:339, 1990.

Schryver H, Hintz F, Lowe JE: Feeding Horses. Cornell [University] Cooperative Extension Publication Information Bulletin 94. Ithaca, NY, Cornell University Cooperative Extension Office, 1992.

Index

Note to Reader: The letter "b" is used with page references to indicate boxes, the letter "f" indicates figures, and the letter "t" indicates tables.

Radiography *(Continued)*
  of skull tumors, 154
Ragwort, liver toxicity and, 210
Ranitidine, gastric ulceration and, 124
Records, oldest horse, 2-3
Rectal biopsies, 118
Rectal prolapse, acupuncture and, 93
Recurrent airway obstruction
  albuterol and, 185f
  anesthesia and, 34-35
  bronchodilator therapy for, 184-185
  clinical signs of, 181, 181b
  complicating factors for, 185-186
  diagnosis of, 181-182, 182b
  environmental management of, 183
  inflammation and, 180, 183-184
  lavage results of, 182f
  management of, 186b
  overview of, 179-180, 247
  pathophysiology of, 180-181, 180b
  pharmaceutical management of, 186-187
  prognosis for, 187
  treatment of, 182-183
Reflexes, 223, 224f
Regurgitant jets, 42, 43f
Regurgitation, 34, 41-44, 43f, 45f, 46f
Rehmannia 6, 98-99, 98b, 99t
Relationships, 6-8, 8-9
Remission therapy, 99b
Renal disease. *See* Kidneys
Renin, aortic insufficiency and, 43, 44
Reproduction. *See* Breeding
Reproductive disorders
  anatomic changes of mares and, 193-194
  breeding and, 197-198
  cyclic characteristics and, 195-196
  embryo viability and, 196-197
  endocrine glands and, 195-196, 198-199
  infertility, 62, 93
  nutrition and, 199
  oocyte viability and, 197
  ovaries and, 195
  papillomas of genitalia, 148-149
  preovulatory follicles and, 196
  testes and, 198, 199
  tumors of genitalia, 162-163
  uterotubal junction and oviduct and, 194-195
  uterus and, 194
Respiratory function, 28-29, 28t, 70
Resting arterial oxygen partial pressure, 28-29, 180, 181
Restriction in lateral bending, 110
Retina, disorders of, 174-175
Retinopathy, 174-175, 174f, 175f
Rhabdomyosarcomas, 151
Rhinitis, chronic, 20f
Rhythmic gaits, 224
Rifampin, pulmonary disease and, 189
Ringbone, 17f, 220, 250
Risks, anesthesia and, 25
Roached back, 109, 110

S
Sacroiliac joint, 112-113, 140
Sacrum, 113, 140
Salmeterol xinafoate, 185
Sand colic, 13, 125, 132, 133-134
Sarcoid, 147, 149

Sarcomas. *See also* Hemangiosarcomas; Lymphosarcomas
  of bone or cartilage, 152, 153, 154, 190
  colic and, 159, 160
  intestinal, 128
  muscular, 159
Schwannomas, 151
Sclerosis, arthritis and, 136-137
Seedy toe, 219
Segmental acupuncture, 90
Selective breeding. *See* Breeding
Seminomas, 163, 191
Senecio jacobea, 210
Senile retinopathy, 174-175, 174f, 175f
Sensitization, pain and, 82
Sensory contact, 8
Septic arthritis, 250
Serotonin agonists, anesthesia and, 35-36
Sertoli cell tumors, 163
Serum hepatitis, 210
Shelter, importance of, 12
Shi points, 87-88
Shi quan Da Bu Tang, 97, 97t, 98b
Shoeing, 143-144, 219-220, 245, 250
Si jhun, 94-95
Si Jun Zi Tang, 96, 96t, 97
Si Wu Tang, 97
Silent aortic insufficiency, 42
Sinovitis, arthritis and, 136
Sinusitis, dental, 57
Skeletal muscle, anesthesia and, 28t
Skin blood flow, exercise and, 73, 75
Skin, tumors of, 147-151
Skull, tumors of, 154
Sleep disorders, 227-229, 228f, 229f
Sludge formation, 202
Small colon disorders, 127-128
Small intestine disorders, 124-125
Smooth mouth, 55-56, 56f, 57
Social support, attachments and, 9, 10
Somatic dysfunction, pain and, 82-83, 83b
Sorbitol dehydrogenase, 213
Soybean products, 12
Spavins, 250
Specialty feeds, 3, 12
Spermatogenesis, 198
Spinal cord, 165, 206
Spironolactone, 43
Spleen, tumors of, 160f, 161
Spondylosis deformans, 89, 139-140, 227f
Squamous cell carcinomas
  of bladder, 162, 203
  esophageal, 119
  exploratory celiotomy and, 133
  of eyes, 22f, 178
  gastrointestinal, 128, 128f, 159-160, 160f
  of head, 153-155
  of hoof, 153
  incidence of, 147
  of larynx and pharynx, 155
  microscopic view of, 149f
  of oral cavity, 154
  overview of, 20
  pulmonary, 191
  of vulva, 23f
Squamous papillomas, 148-149
Squamous ulceration, 122
Stallions, reproductive disorders of, 198-199